SO-BJL-506

Black Jack

Volume 3

Osamu Tezuka

 VERTICAL.

Delafield Public Library
Delafield, WI 53018
262-646-6230
www.delafieldlibrary.org

Translation—Camellia Nieh
Production—Glen Isip
Akane Ishida
Lawrence Leung

Copyright © 2009 by Tezuka Productions
Translation Copyright © 2009 by Camellia Nieh and Vertical, Inc.

This is a work of fiction.

All rights reserved.

Published by Vertical, Inc., New York.

Originally published in Japanese as *Burakku Jakku 3*
by Akita Shoten, Tokyo, 1987.
Burakku Jakku first serialized in *Shukan Shonen Champion*,
Akita Shoten, 1973–83.

ISBN: 978-1-934287-41-5

Manufactured in the United States of America

First Edition

Third Printing

Vertical, Inc.
451 Park Avenue South 7th Floor
New York, NY 10016
www.vertical-inc.com

CONTENTS

DISOWNED SON

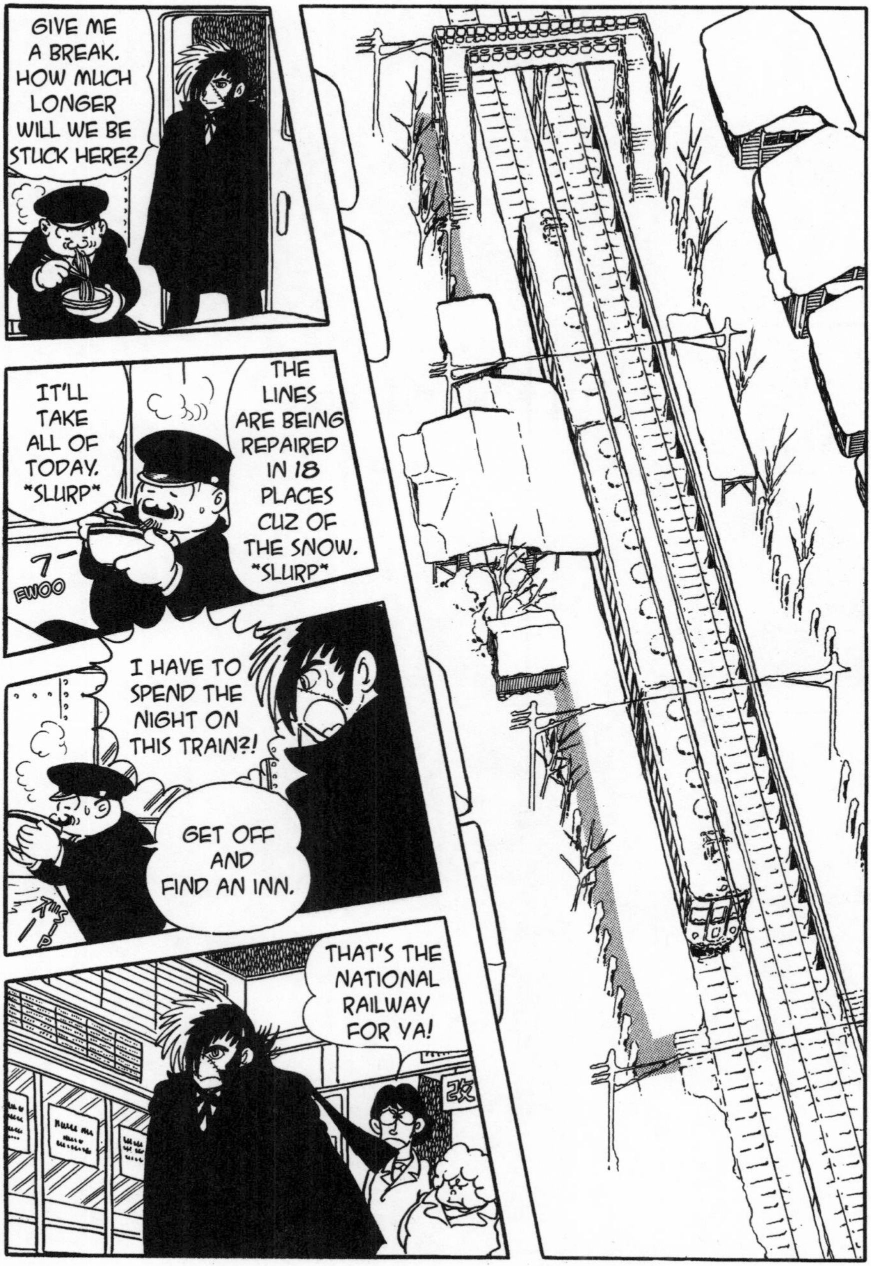
GIVE ME A BREAK. HOW MUCH LONGER WILL WE BE STUCK HERE?
THE LINES ARE BEING REPAIRED IN 18 PLACES CUZ OF THE SNOW. *SLURP*
IT'LL TAKE ALL OF TODAY. *SLURP*
FWOO
I HAVE TO SPEND THE NIGHT ON THIS TRAIN?!
GET OFF AND FIND AN INN.
THAT'S THE NATIONAL RAILWAY FOR YA!

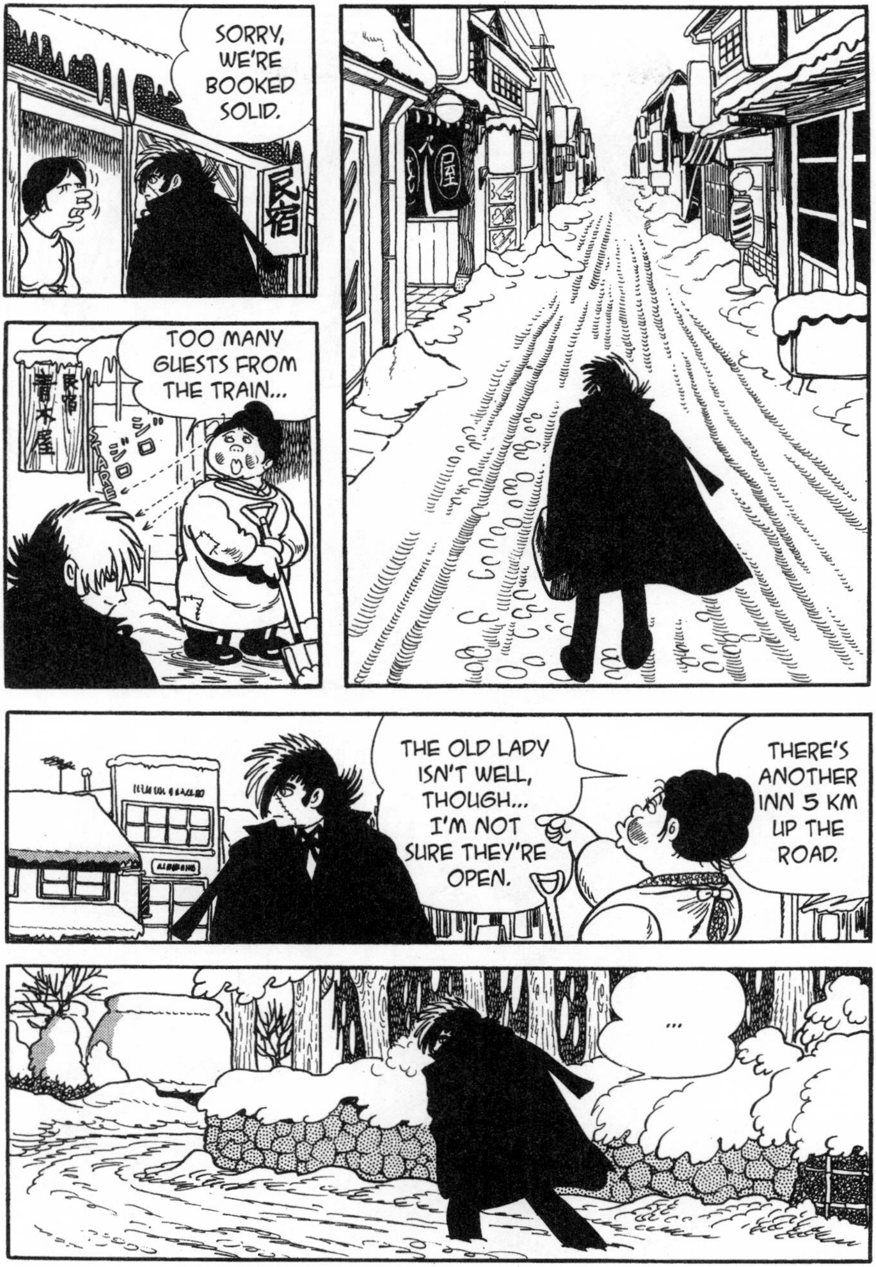

SORRY, WE'RE BOOKED SOLID.
民宿
TOO MANY GUESTS FROM THE TRAIN...
民宿 青木屋
ジロ ジロ
STARE
THERE'S ANOTHER INN 5 KM UP THE ROAD.
THE OLD LADY ISN'T WELL, THOUGH... I'M NOT SURE THEY'RE OPEN.
...

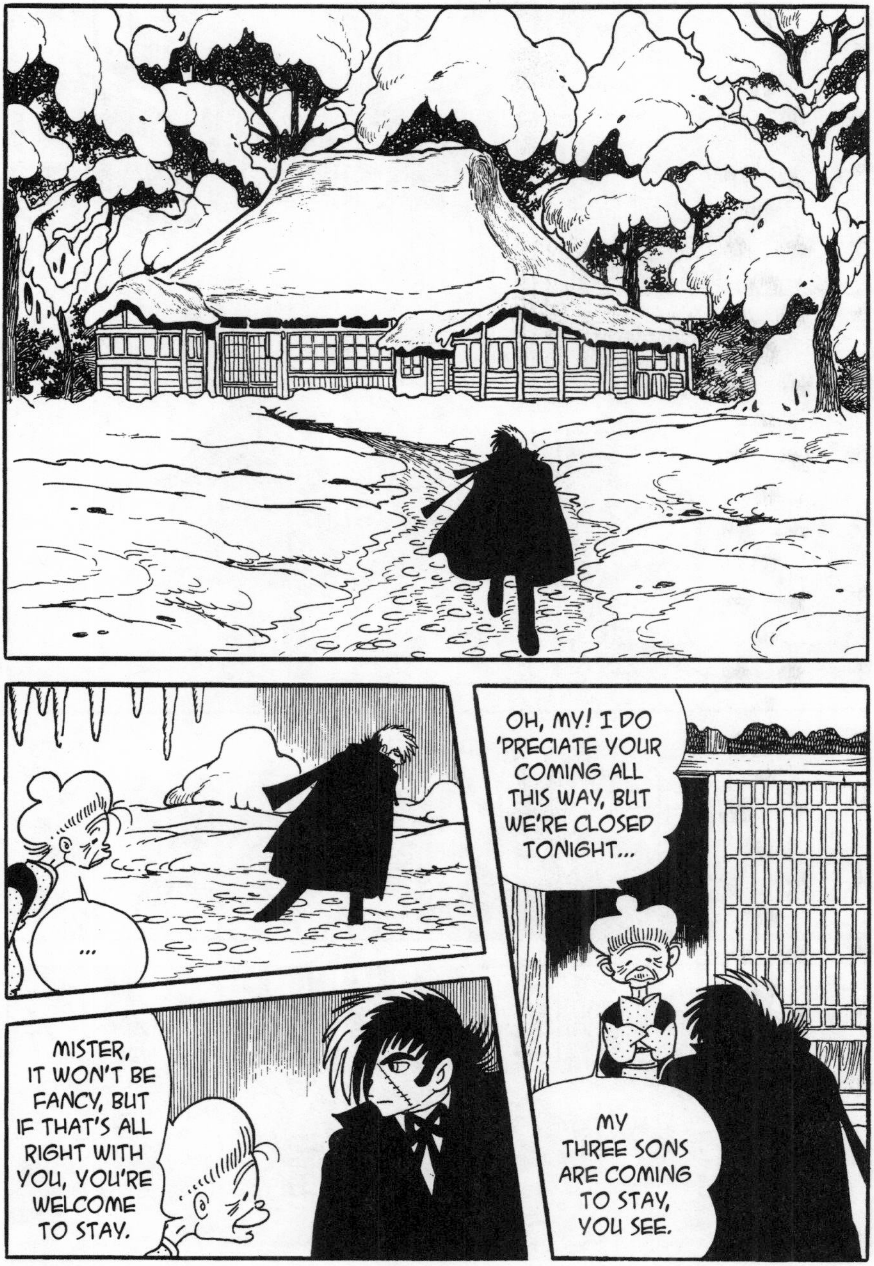
OH, MY! I DO 'PRECIATE YOUR COMING ALL THIS WAY, BUT WE'RE CLOSED TONIGHT...
MY THREE SONS ARE COMING TO STAY, YOU SEE.
...
MISTER, IT WON'T BE FANCY, BUT IF THAT'S ALL RIGHT WITH YOU, YOU'RE WELCOME TO STAY.

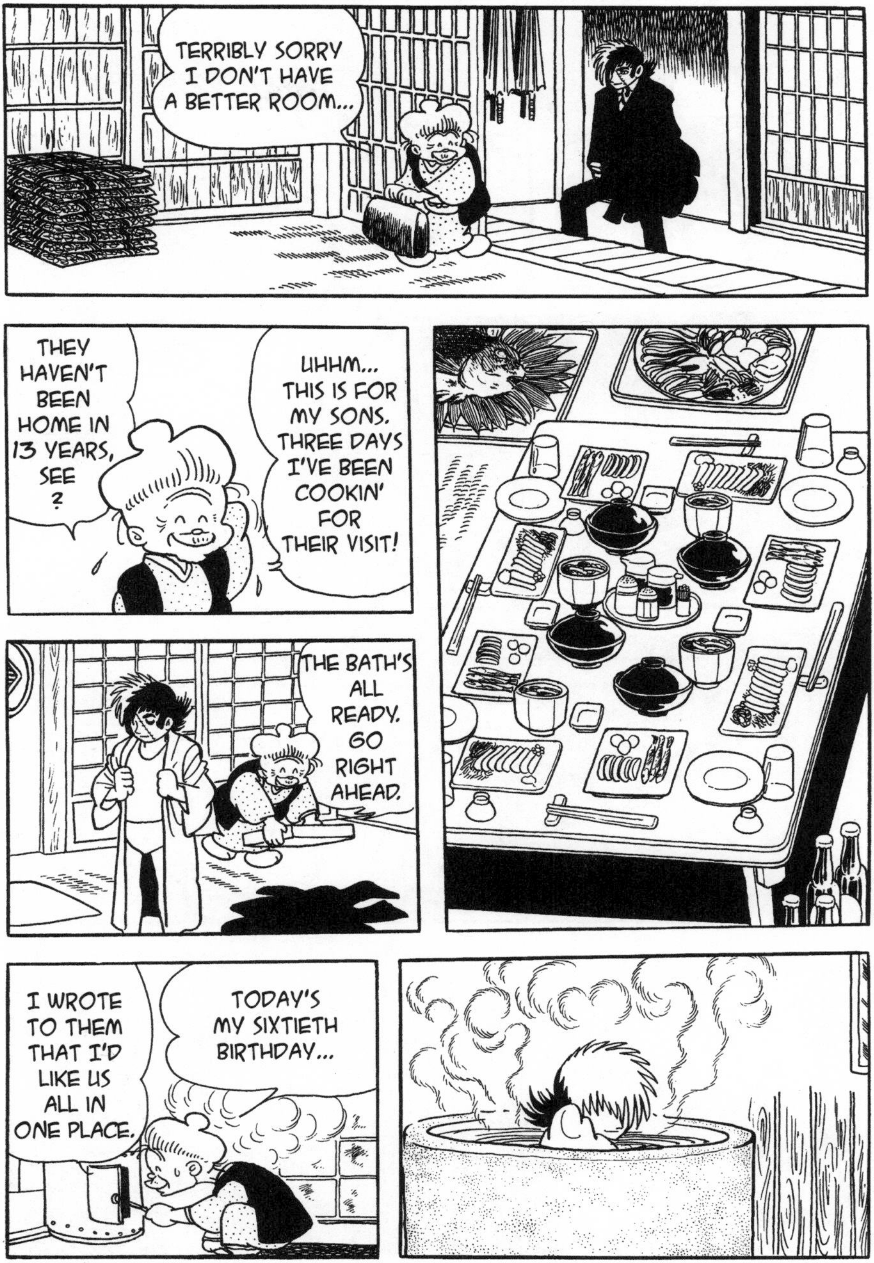
TERRIBLY SORRY I DON'T HAVE A BETTER ROOM...
UHHM... THIS IS FOR MY SONS. THREE DAYS I'VE BEEN COOKIN' FOR THEIR VISIT!
THEY HAVEN'T BEEN HOME IN 13 YEARS, SEE?
THE BATH'S ALL READY. GO RIGHT AHEAD.
TODAY'S MY SIXTIETH BIRTHDAY...
I WROTE TO THEM THAT I'D LIKE US ALL IN ONE PLACE.

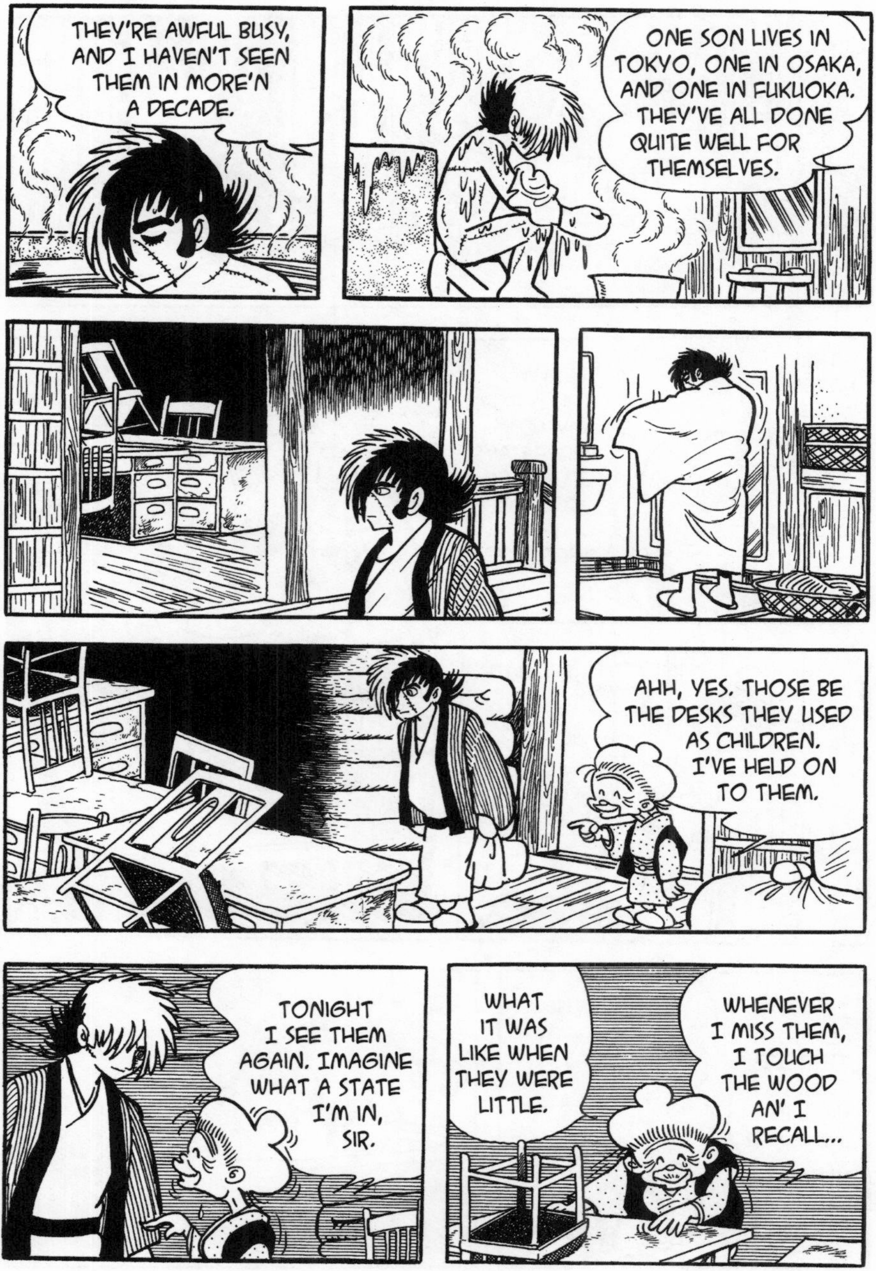
ONE SON LIVES IN TOKYO, ONE IN OSAKA, AND ONE IN FUKUOKA. THEY'VE ALL DONE QUITE WELL FOR THEMSELVES.
THEY'RE AWFUL BUSY, AND I HAVEN'T SEEN THEM IN MORE'N A DECADE.
AHH, YES. THOSE BE THE DESKS THEY USED AS CHILDREN. I'VE HELD ON TO THEM.
WHENEVER I MISS THEM, I TOUCH THE WOOD AN' I RECALL...
WHAT IT WAS LIKE WHEN THEY WERE LITTLE.
TONIGHT I SEE THEM AGAIN. IMAGINE WHAT A STATE I'M IN, SIR.

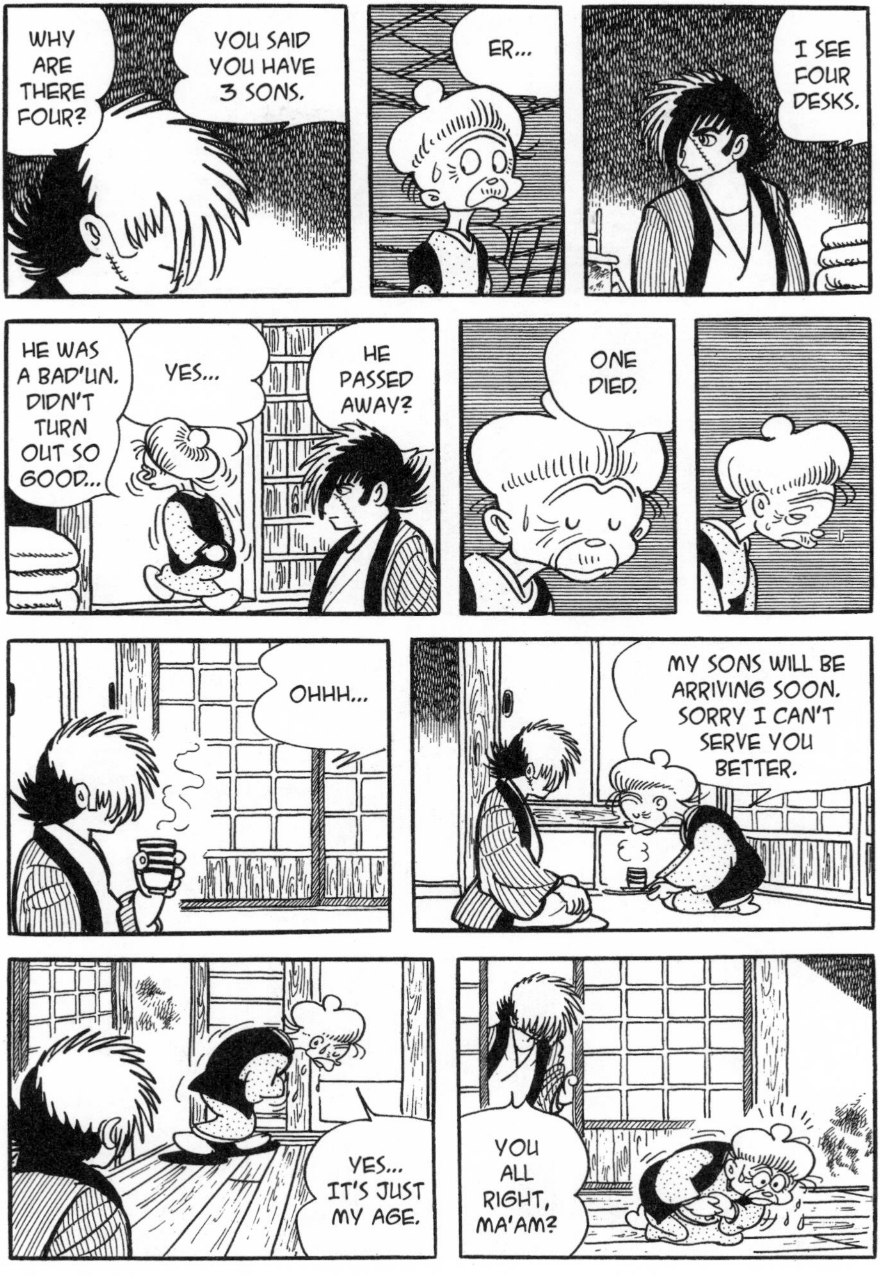
I SEE FOUR DESKS.
ER...
YOU SAID YOU HAVE 3 SONS.
WHY ARE THERE FOUR?
ONE DIED.
HE PASSED AWAY?
YES...
HE WAS A BAD'UN. DIDN'T TURN OUT SO GOOD...
MY SONS WILL BE ARRIVING SOON. SORRY I CAN'T SERVE YOU BETTER.
OHHH...
YOU ALL RIGHT, MA'AM?
YES... IT'S JUST MY AGE.

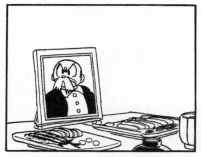

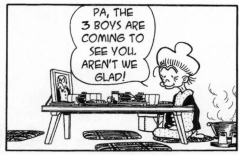

PA, THE 3 BOYS ARE COMING TO SEE YOU. AREN'T WE GLAD!
SUCH GOOD BOYS...
YOU DIDN'T LIVE TO SEE THEM MAKE IT IN THE WORLD.
ALL THREE HAVE WIVES AND EVEN THEIR OWN KIDS!
OH...! ONE OF THEM'S HERE!
WHICH COULD IT BE?
TAP
TAP
TWO TELE-GRAMS FOR YOU.
MY, MY! AND IN THIS WEATHER, TOO.
BIRTHDAY WISHES?

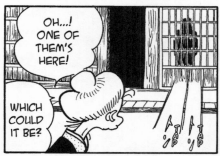

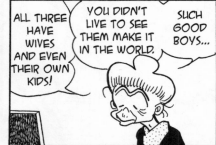

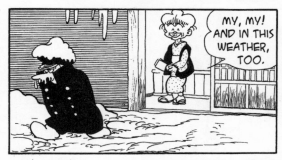

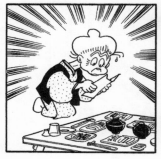

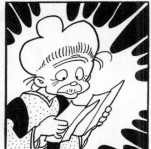

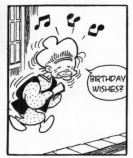

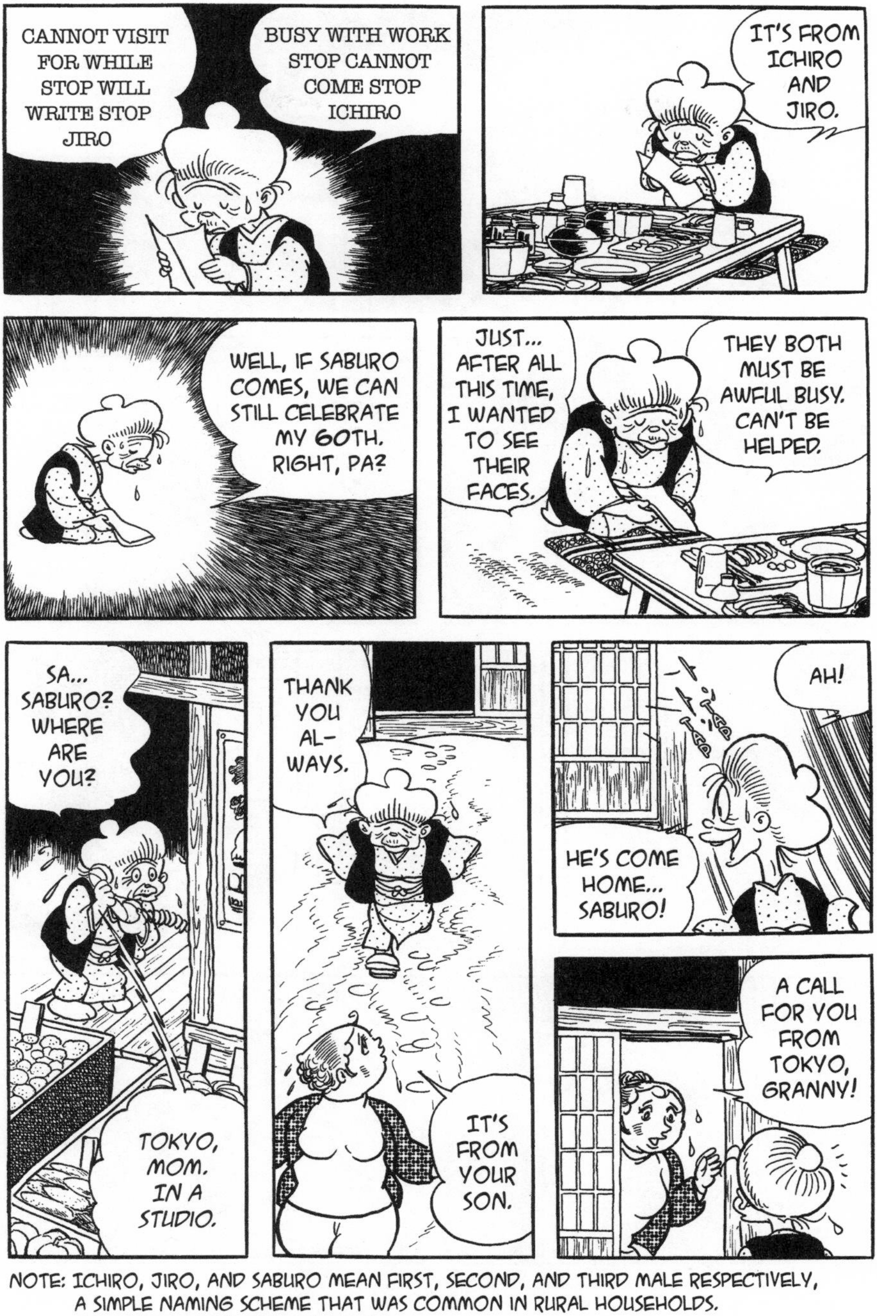
IT'S FROM ICHIRO AND JIRO.
BUSY WITH WORK STOP CANNOT COME STOP ICHIRO
CANNOT VISIT FOR WHILE STOP WILL WRITE STOP JIRO
THEY BOTH MUST BE AWFUL BUSY. CAN'T BE HELPED.
JUST... AFTER ALL THIS TIME, I WANTED TO SEE THEIR FACES.
WELL, IF SABURO COMES, WE CAN STILL CELEBRATE MY 60TH. RIGHT, PA?
AH!
HE'S COME HOME... SABURO!
A CALL FOR YOU FROM TOKYO, GRANNY!
THANK YOU AL-WAYS.
IT'S FROM YOUR SON.
SA... SABURO? WHERE ARE YOU?
TOKYO, MOM. IN A STUDIO.

NOTE: ICHIRO, JIRO, AND SABURO MEAN FIRST, SECOND, AND THIRD MALE RESPECTIVELY, A SIMPLE NAMING SCHEME THAT WAS COMMON IN RURAL HOUSEHOLDS. THE FOURTH SON WOULD BE SHIRO.

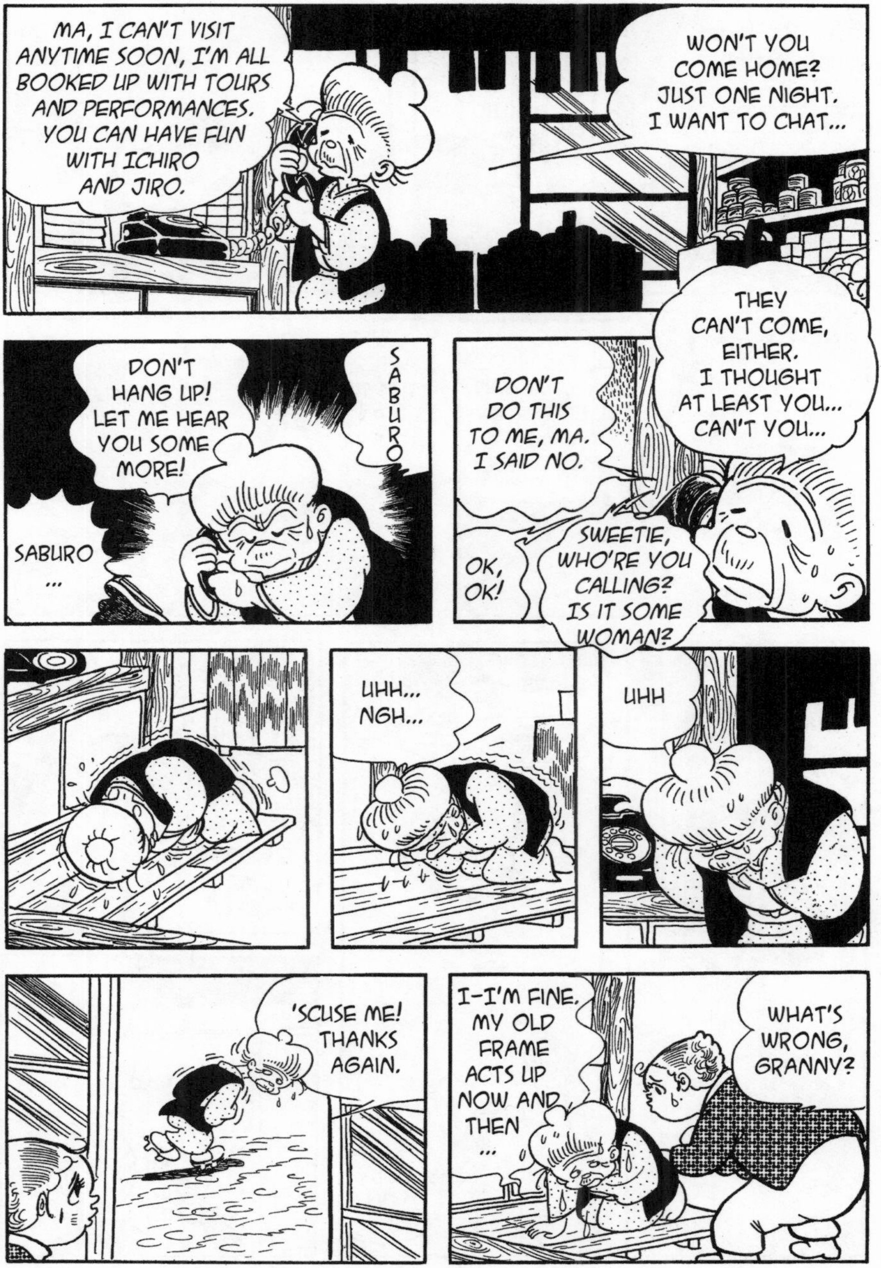
WON'T YOU COME HOME? JUST ONE NIGHT. I WANT TO CHAT...
MA, I CAN'T VISIT ANYTIME SOON, I'M ALL BOOKED UP WITH TOURS AND PERFORMANCES. YOU CAN HAVE FUN WITH ICHIRO AND JIRO.
THEY CAN'T COME, EITHER. I THOUGHT AT LEAST YOU... CAN'T YOU...
DON'T DO THIS TO ME, MA. I SAID NO.
SWEETIE, WHO'RE YOU CALLING? IS IT SOME WOMAN?
OK, OK!
SABURO
DON'T HANG UP! LET ME HEAR YOU SOME MORE!
SABURO ...
UHH
UHH... NGH...
WHAT'S WRONG, GRANNY?
I-I'M FINE. MY OLD FRAME ACTS UP NOW AND THEN ...
'SCUSE ME! THANKS AGAIN.

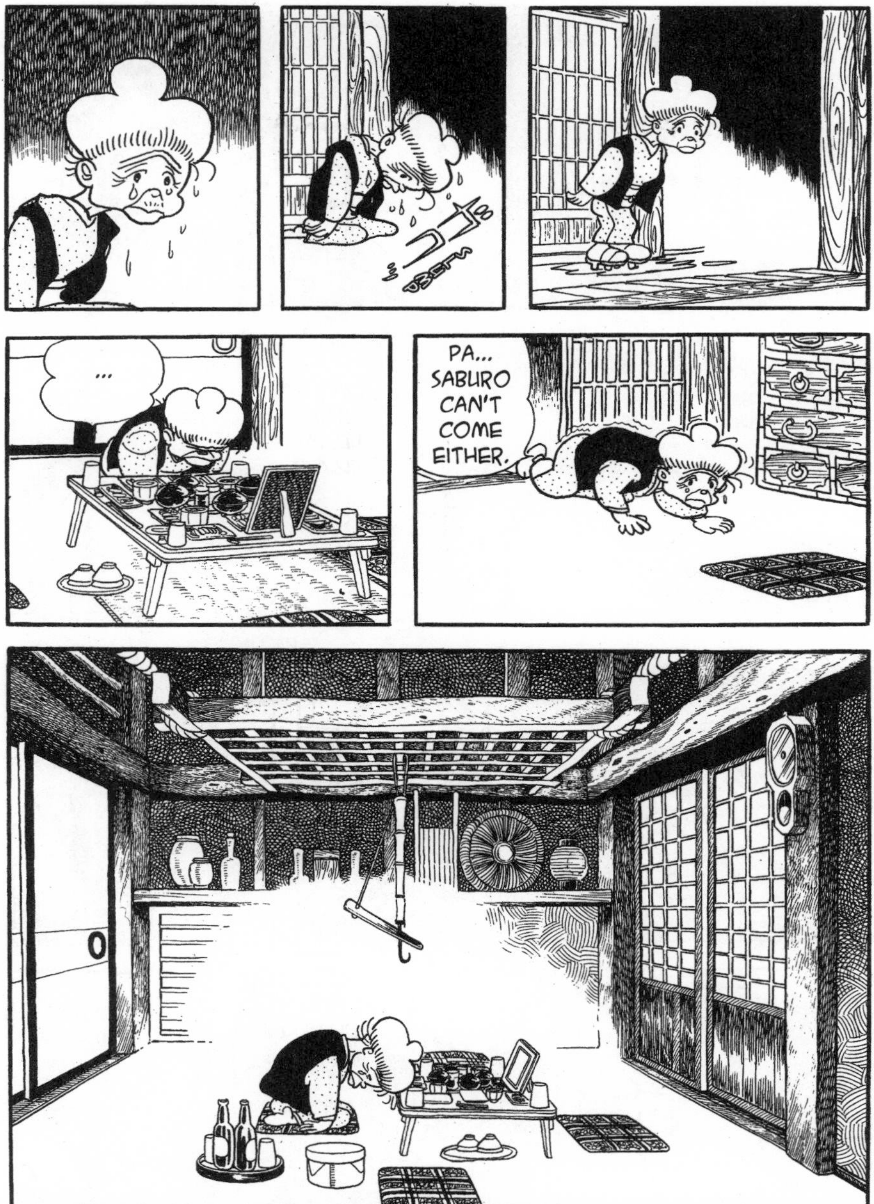
PA... SABURO CAN'T COME EITHER.
...

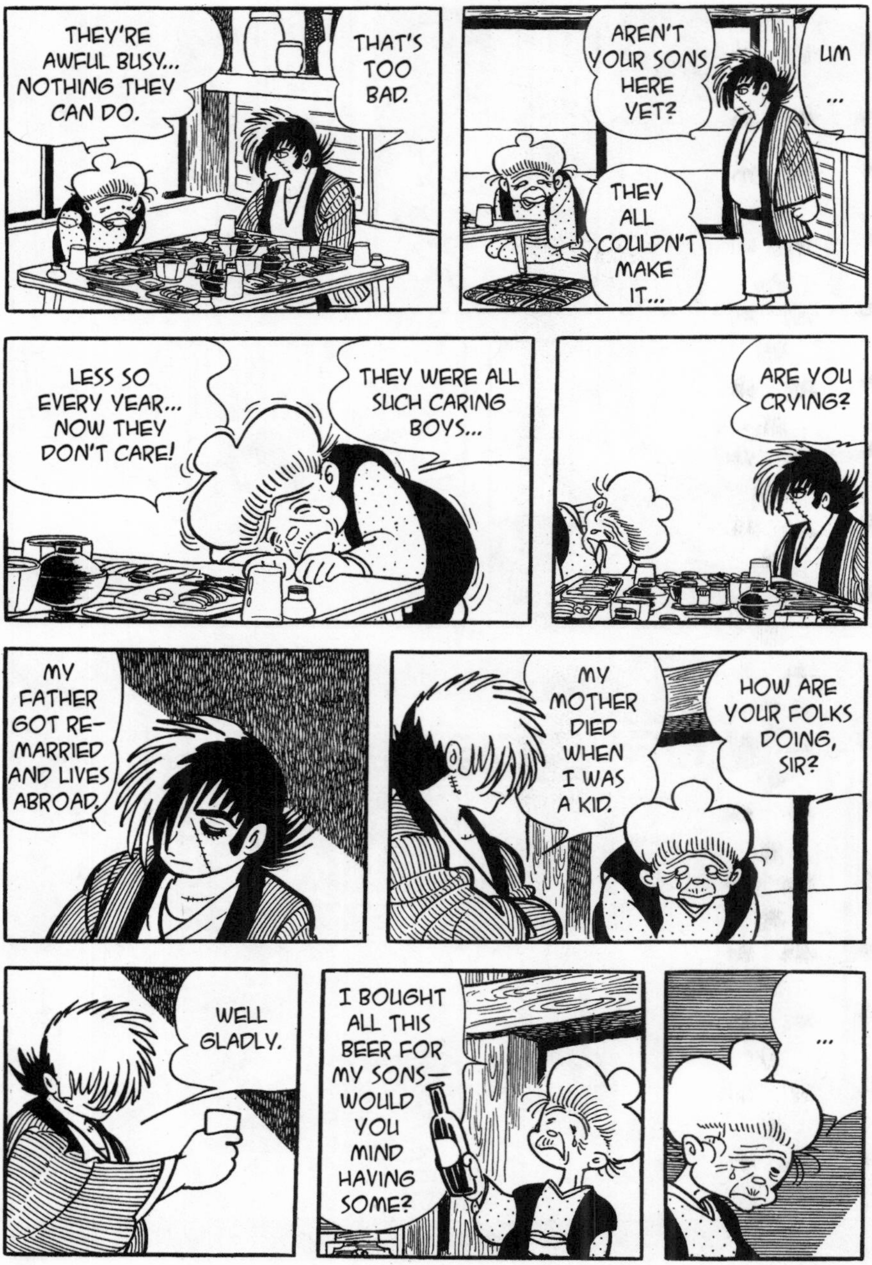
UM ...
AREN'T YOUR SONS HERE YET?
THEY ALL COULDN'T MAKE IT...
THAT'S TOO BAD.
THEY'RE AWFUL BUSY... NOTHING THEY CAN DO.
ARE YOU CRYING?
THEY WERE ALL SUCH CARING BOYS...
LESS SO EVERY YEAR... NOW THEY DON'T CARE!
HOW ARE YOUR FOLKS DOING, SIR?
MY MOTHER DIED WHEN I WAS A KID.
MY FATHER GOT RE-MARRIED AND LIVES ABROAD.
...
I BOUGHT ALL THIS BEER FOR MY SONS—WOULD YOU MIND HAVING SOME?
WELL GLADLY.

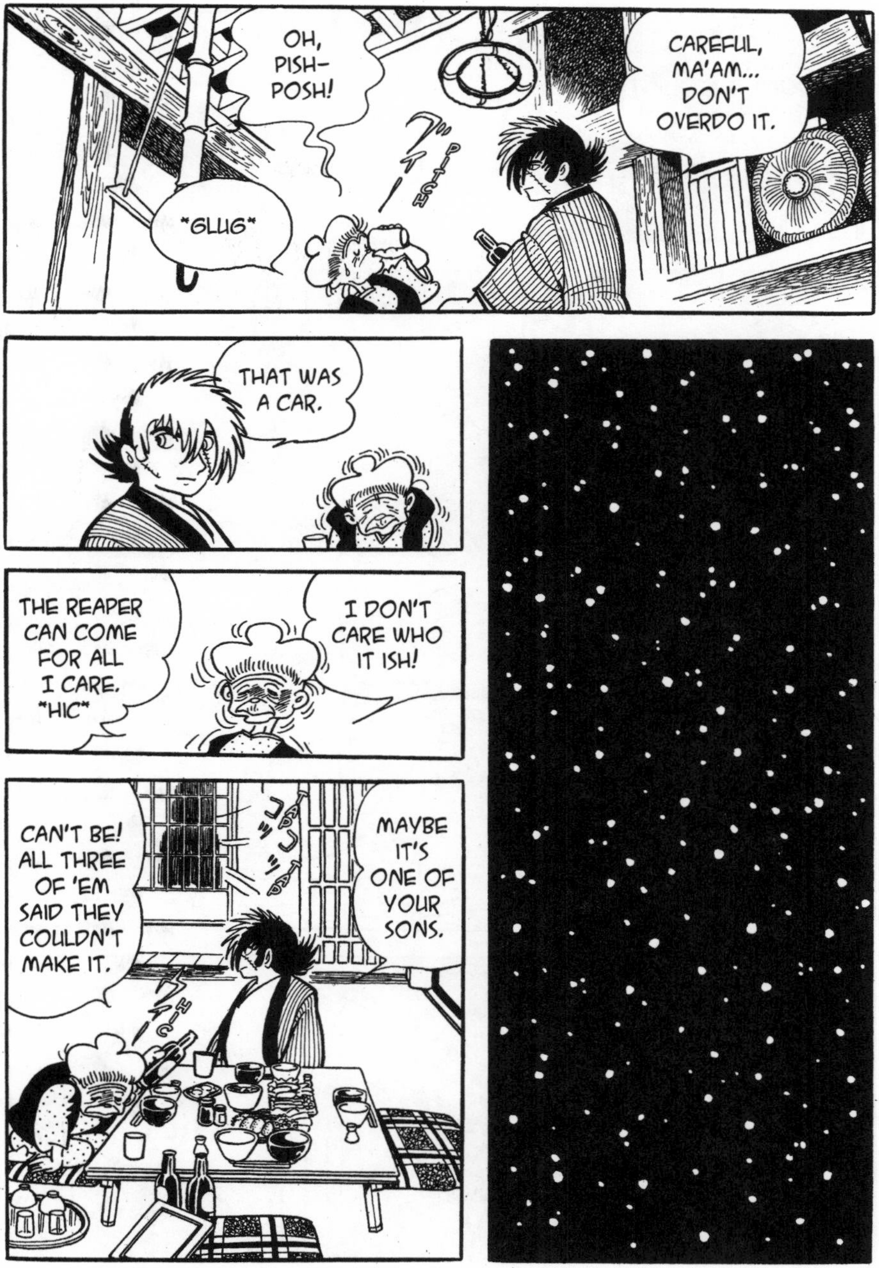
CAREFUL, MA'AM... DON'T OVERDO IT.
PITCH
OH, PISH-POSH!
GLUG
THAT WAS A CAR.
I DON'T CARE WHO IT ISH!
THE REAPER CAN COME FOR ALL I CARE. *HIC*
MAYBE IT'S ONE OF YOUR SONS.
TAP TAP
HIC
CAN'T BE! ALL THREE OF 'EM SAID THEY COULDN'T MAKE IT.

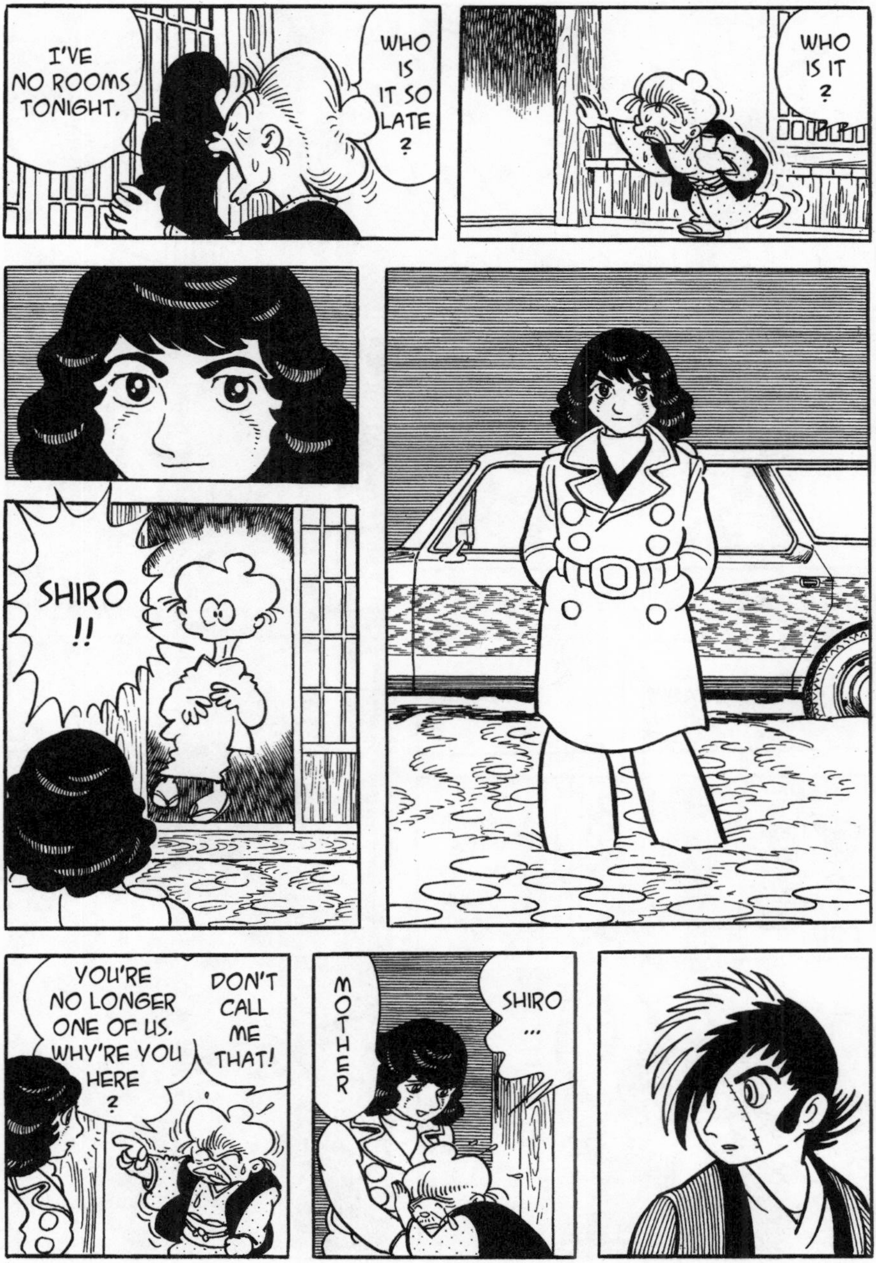
WHO IS IT ?
WHO IS IT SO LATE ?
I'VE NO ROOMS TONIGHT.
SHIRO !!
SHIRO ...
MOTHER
DON'T CALL ME THAT!
YOU'RE NO LONGER ONE OF US. WHY'RE YOU HERE ?

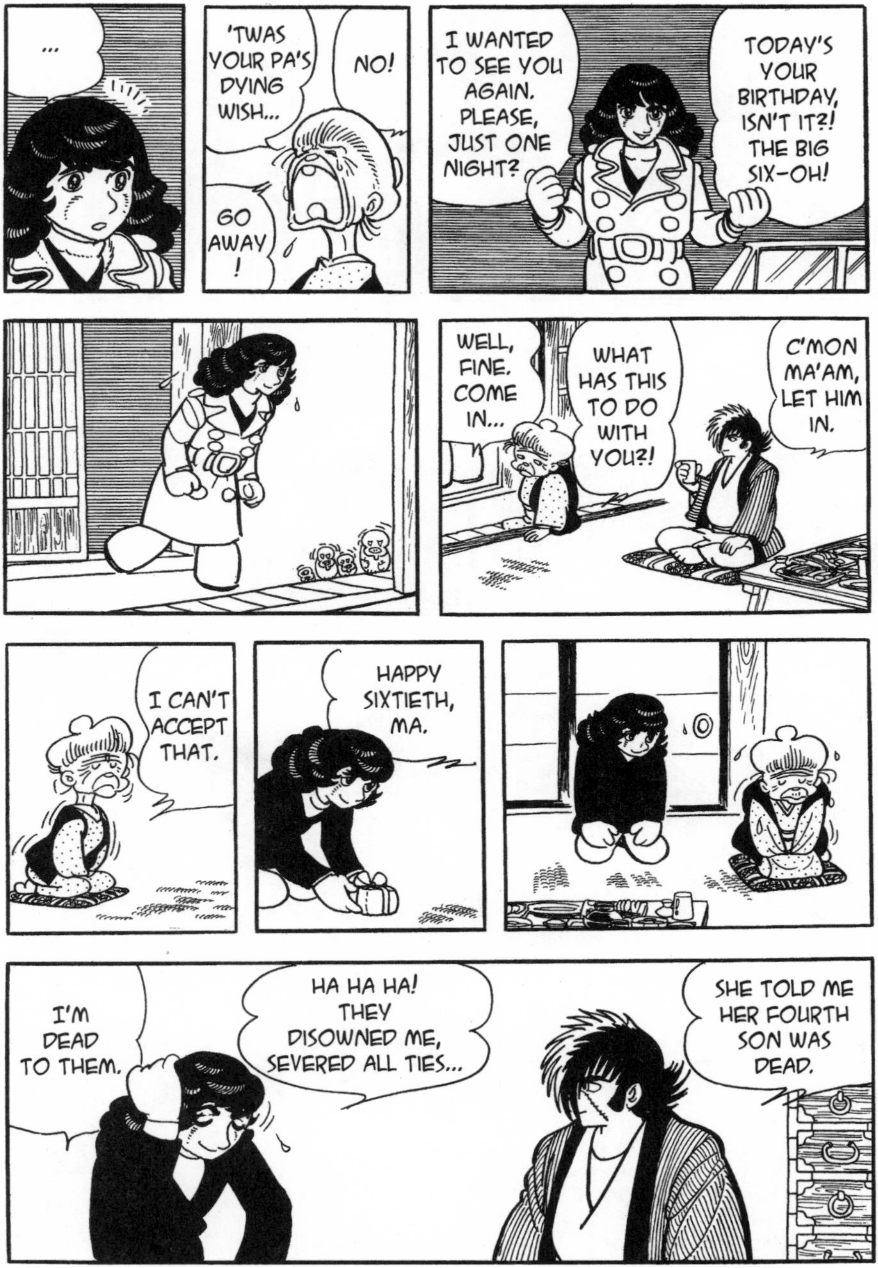
TODAY'S YOUR BIRTHDAY, ISN'T IT?! THE BIG SIX-OH!
I WANTED TO SEE YOU AGAIN. PLEASE, JUST ONE NIGHT?
NO!
'TWAS YOUR PA'S DYING WISH...
GO AWAY!
...
C'MON MA'AM, LET HIM IN.
WHAT HAS THIS TO DO WITH YOU?!
WELL, FINE. COME IN...
HAPPY SIXTIETH, MA.
I CAN'T ACCEPT THAT.
SHE TOLD ME HER FOURTH SON WAS DEAD.
HA HA HA! THEY DISOWNED ME, SEVERED ALL TIES...
I'M DEAD TO THEM.

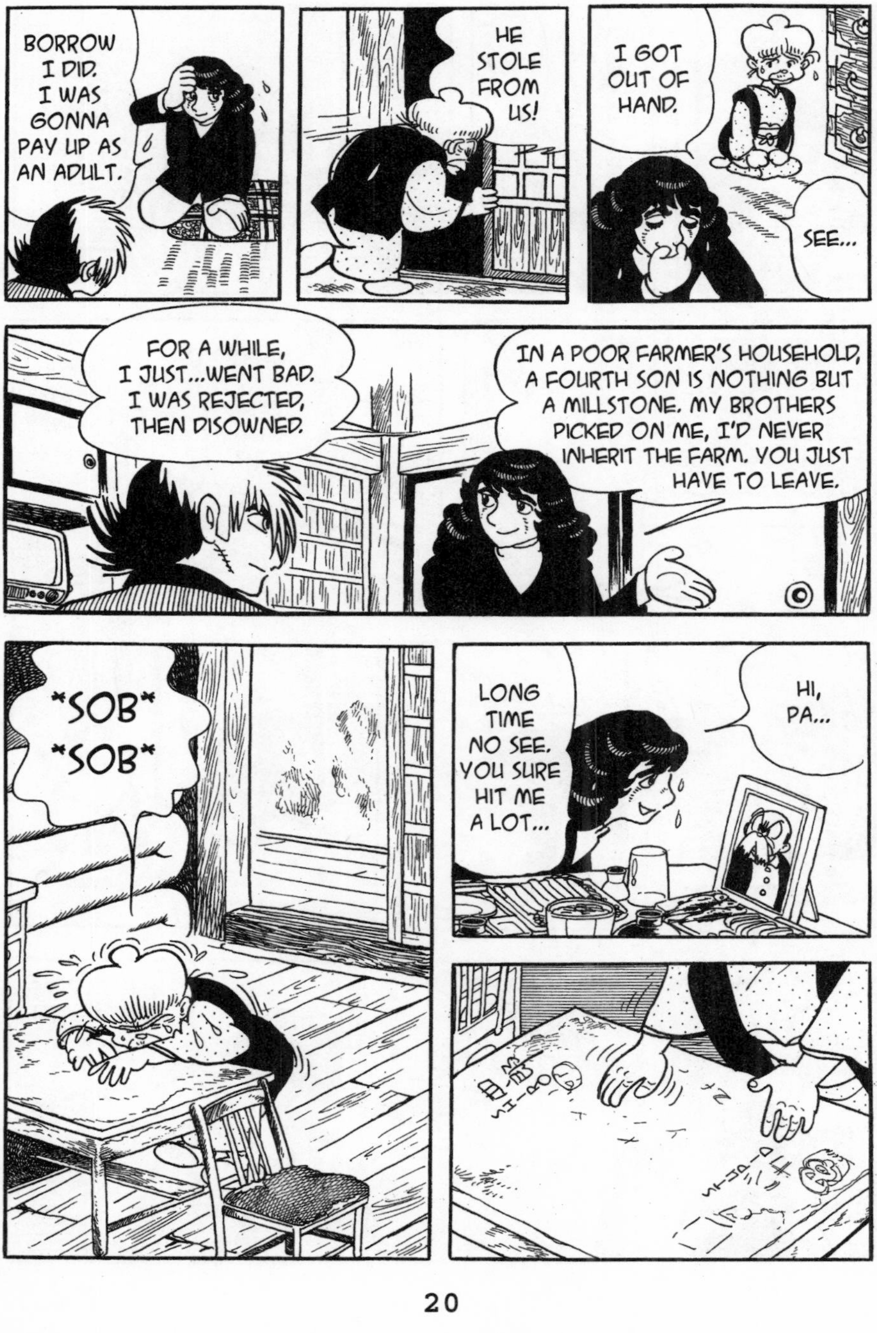
I GOT OUT OF HAND.
SEE...
HE STOLE FROM US!
BORROW I DID. I WAS GONNA PAY UP AS AN ADULT.
IN A POOR FARMER'S HOUSEHOLD, A FOURTH SON IS NOTHING BUT A MILLSTONE. MY BROTHERS PICKED ON ME, I'D NEVER INHERIT THE FARM. YOU JUST HAVE TO LEAVE.
FOR A WHILE, I JUST...WENT BAD. I WAS REJECTED, THEN DISOWNED.
HI, PA...
LONG TIME NO SEE. YOU SURE HIT ME A LOT...
SOB *SOB*

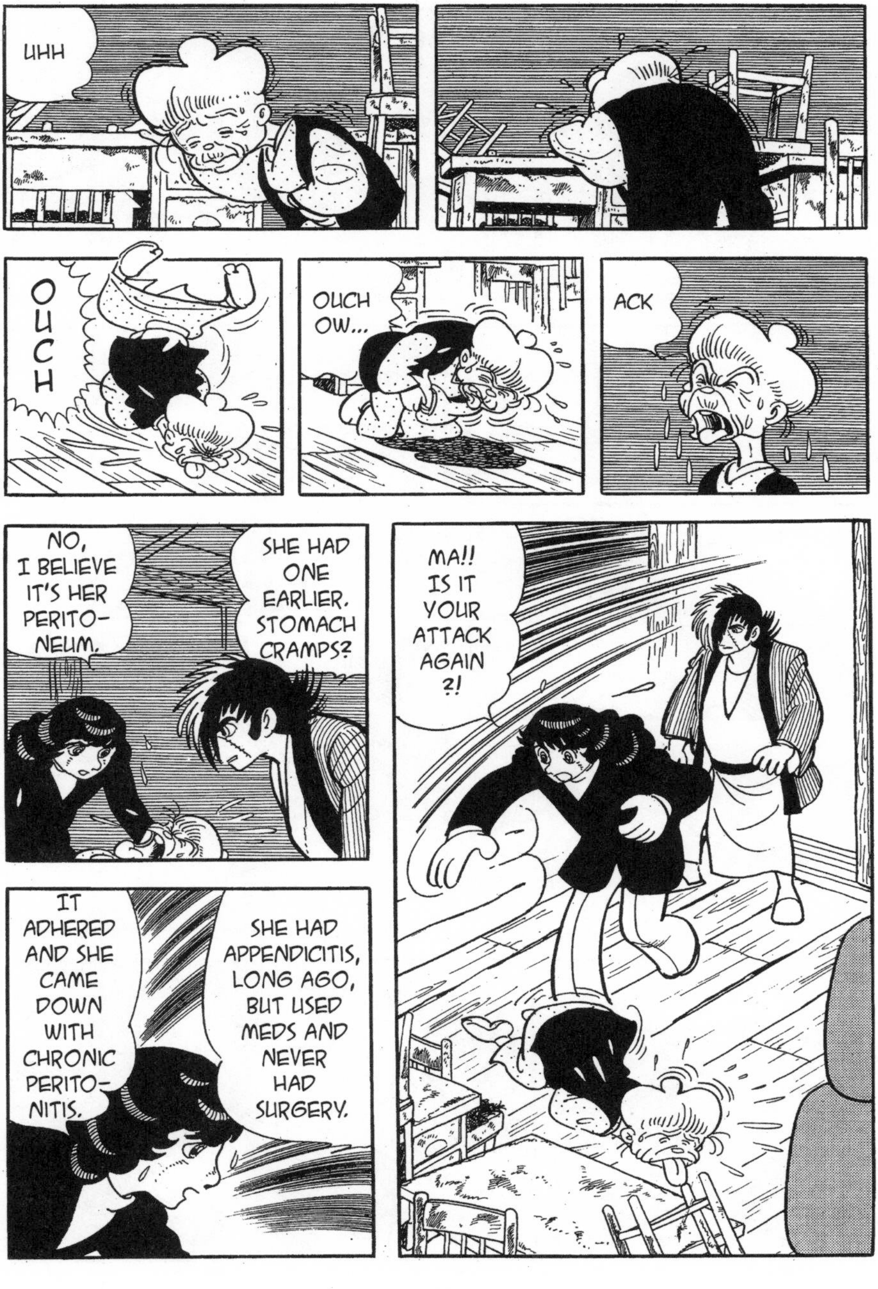
UHH
ACK
OUCH OW...
OUCH
MA!! IS IT YOUR ATTACK AGAIN ?!
SHE HAD ONE EARLIER. STOMACH CRAMPS?
NO, I BELIEVE IT'S HER PERITO- NEUM.
SHE HAD APPENDICITIS, LONG AGO, BUT USED MEDS AND NEVER HAD SURGERY.
IT ADHERED AND SHE CAME DOWN WITH CHRONIC PERITO- NITIS.

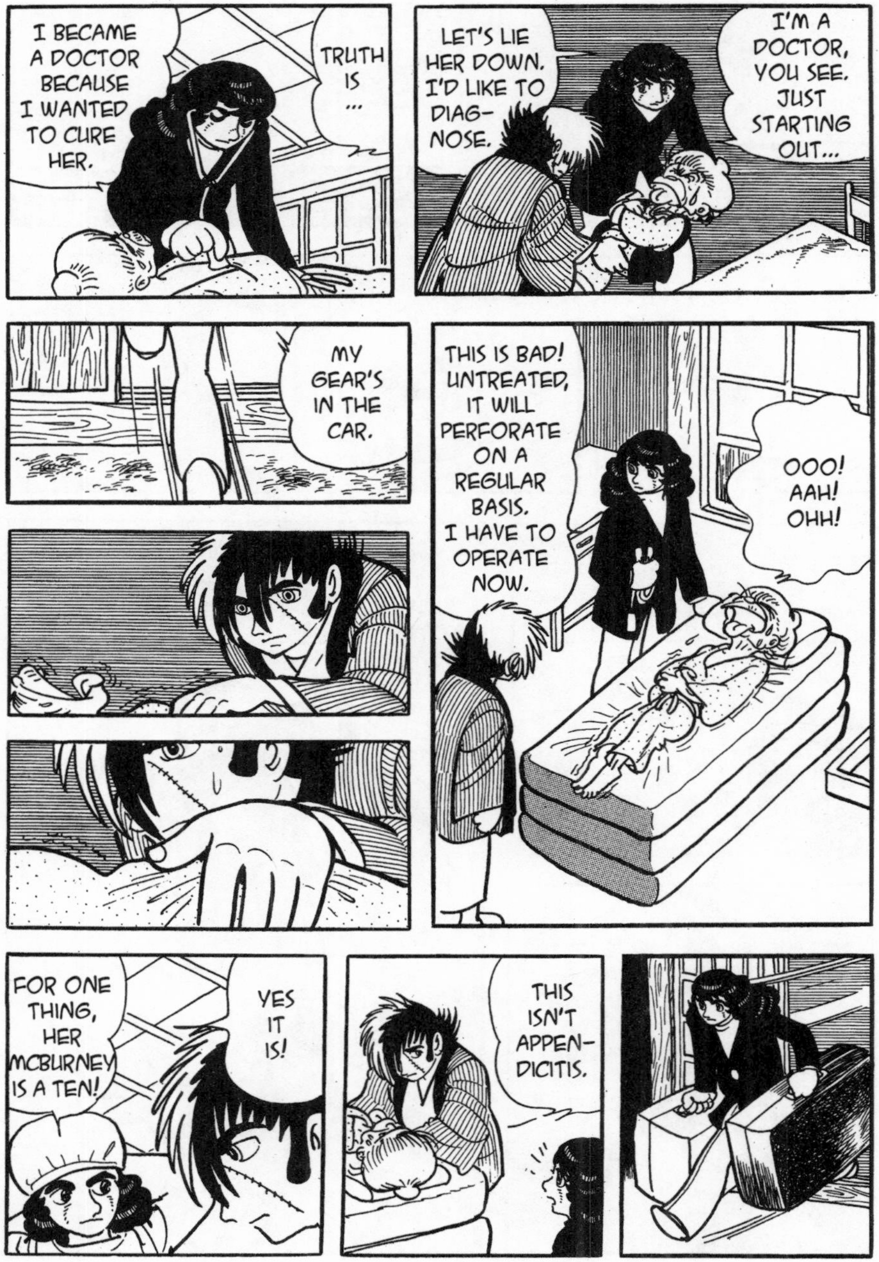
I'M A DOCTOR, YOU SEE. JUST STARTING OUT...
LET'S LIE HER DOWN. I'D LIKE TO DIAG-NOSE.
TRUTH IS ...
I BECAME A DOCTOR BECAUSE I WANTED TO CURE HER.
OOO! AAH! OHH!
THIS IS BAD! UNTREATED, IT WILL PERFORATE ON A REGULAR BASIS. I HAVE TO OPERATE NOW.
MY GEAR'S IN THE CAR.
THIS ISN'T APPEN-DICITIS.
YES IT IS!
FOR ONE THING, HER MCBURNEY IS A TEN!

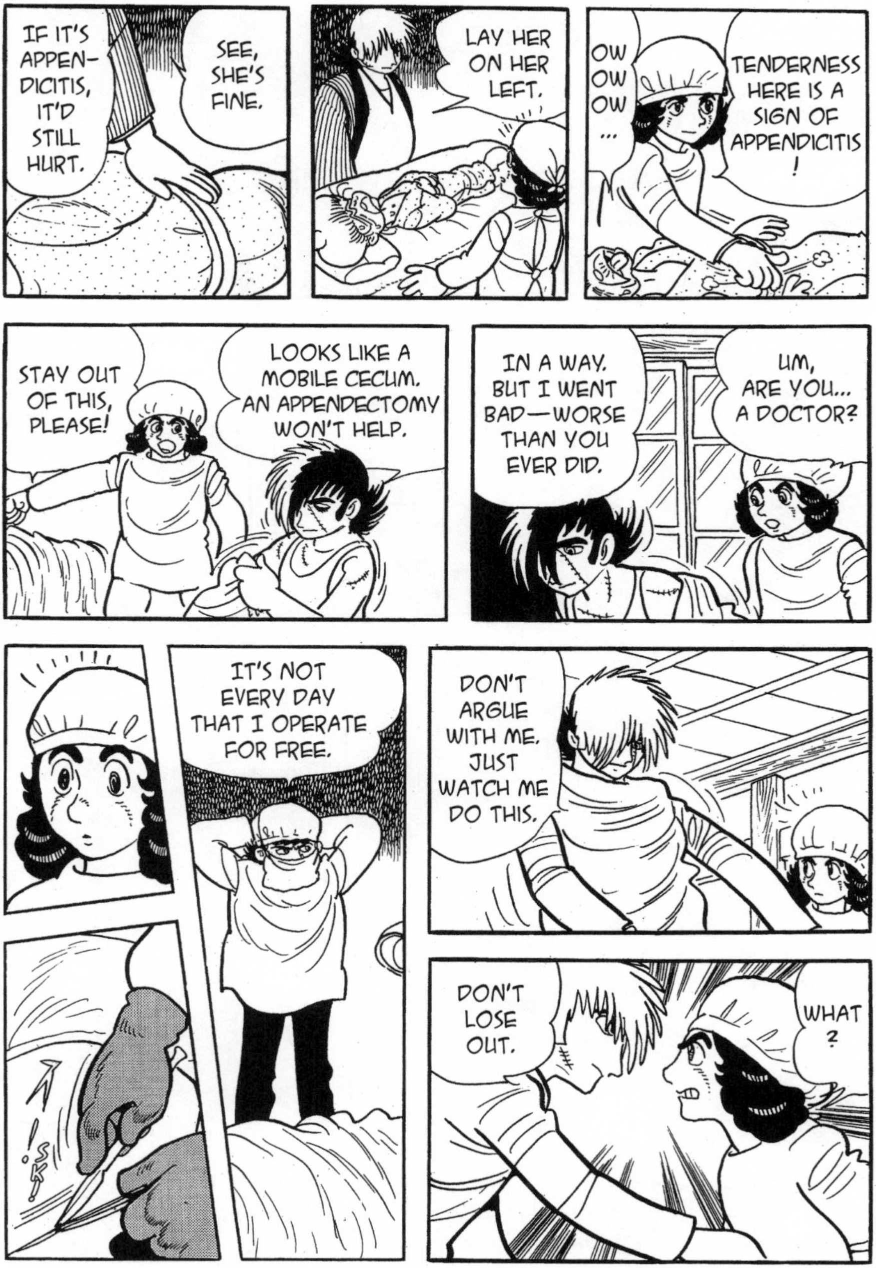
TENDERNESS HERE IS A SIGN OF APPENDICITIS!
OW OW OW ...
LAY HER ON HER LEFT.
SEE, SHE'S FINE.
IF IT'S APPENDICITIS, IT'D STILL HURT.
UM, ARE YOU... A DOCTOR?
IN A WAY. BUT I WENT BAD—WORSE THAN YOU EVER DID.
LOOKS LIKE A MOBILE CECUM. AN APPENDECTOMY WON'T HELP.
STAY OUT OF THIS, PLEASE!
DON'T ARGUE WITH ME. JUST WATCH ME DO THIS.
WHAT?
DON'T LOSE OUT.
IT'S NOT EVERY DAY THAT I OPERATE FOR FREE.
SK!

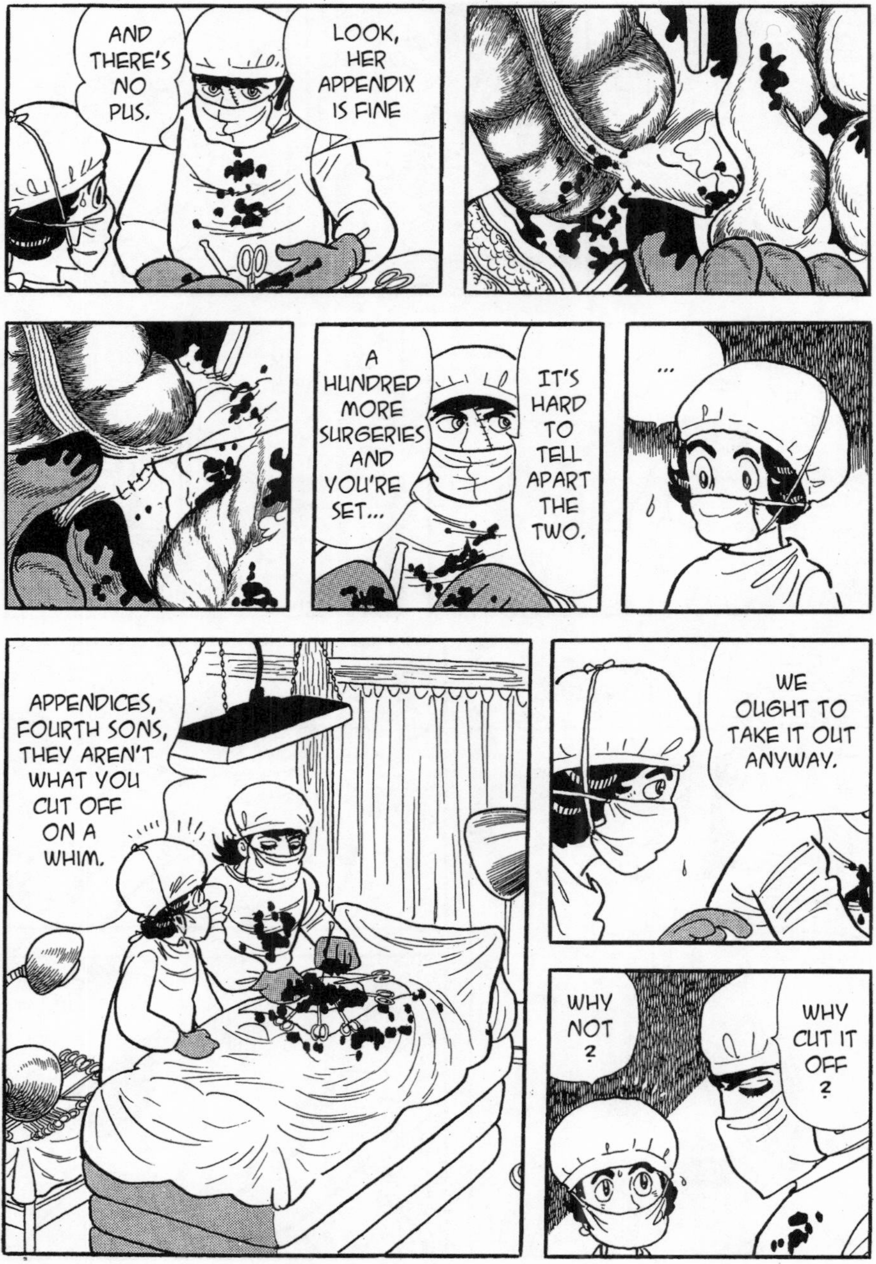
LOOK, HER APPENDIX IS FINE
AND THERE'S NO PUS.
...
IT'S HARD TO TELL APART THE TWO.
A HUNDRED MORE SURGERIES AND YOU'RE SET...
WE OUGHT TO TAKE IT OUT ANYWAY.
WHY CUT IT OFF?
WHY NOT?
APPENDICES, FOURTH SONS, THEY AREN'T WHAT YOU CUT OFF ON A WHIM.

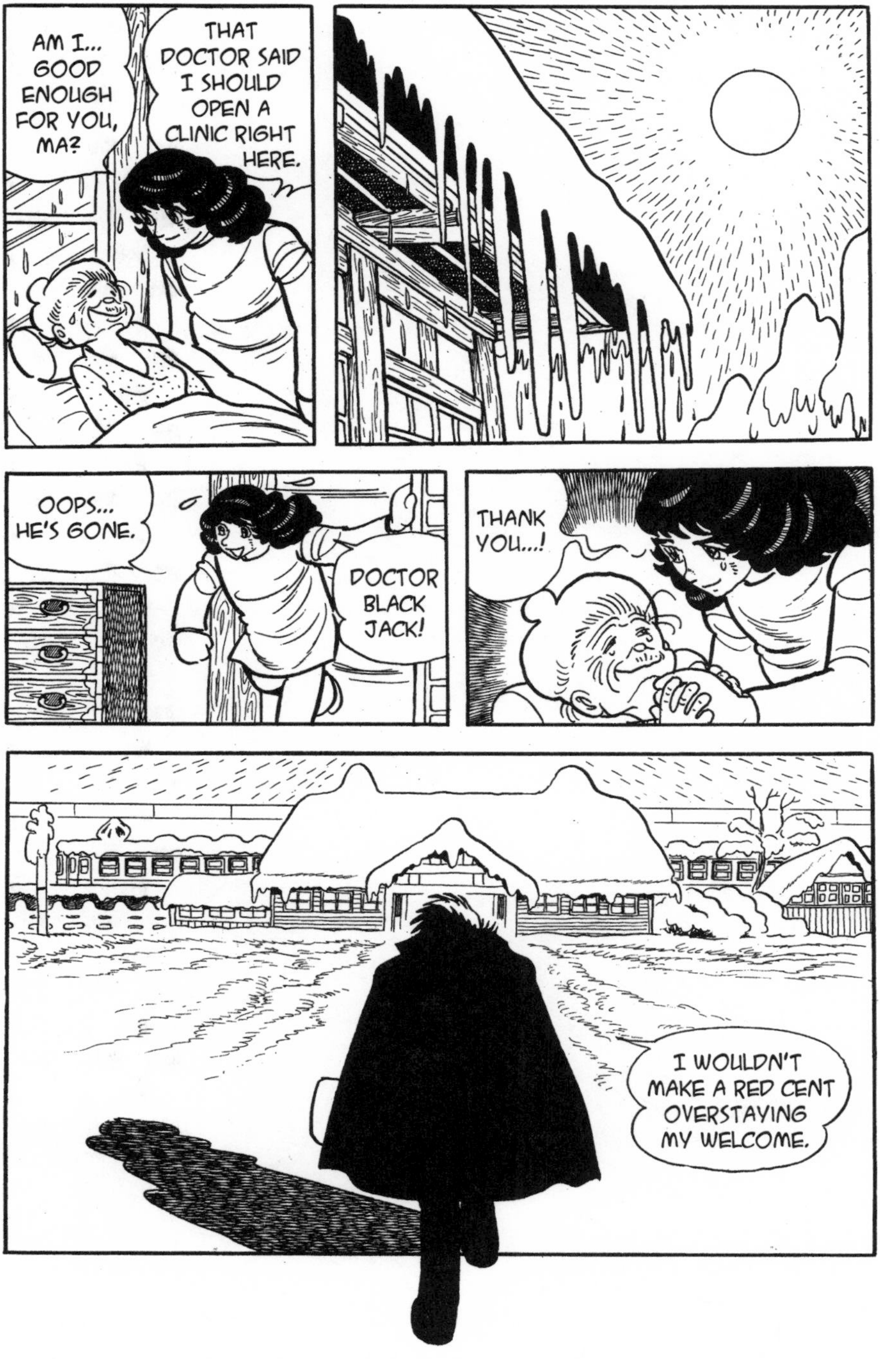
THAT DOCTOR SAID I SHOULD OPEN A CLINIC RIGHT HERE.
AM I... GOOD ENOUGH FOR YOU, MA?
THANK YOU...!
DOCTOR BLACK JACK!
OOPS... HE'S GONE.
I WOULDN'T MAKE A RED CENT OVERSTAYING MY WELCOME.

SHRINKING

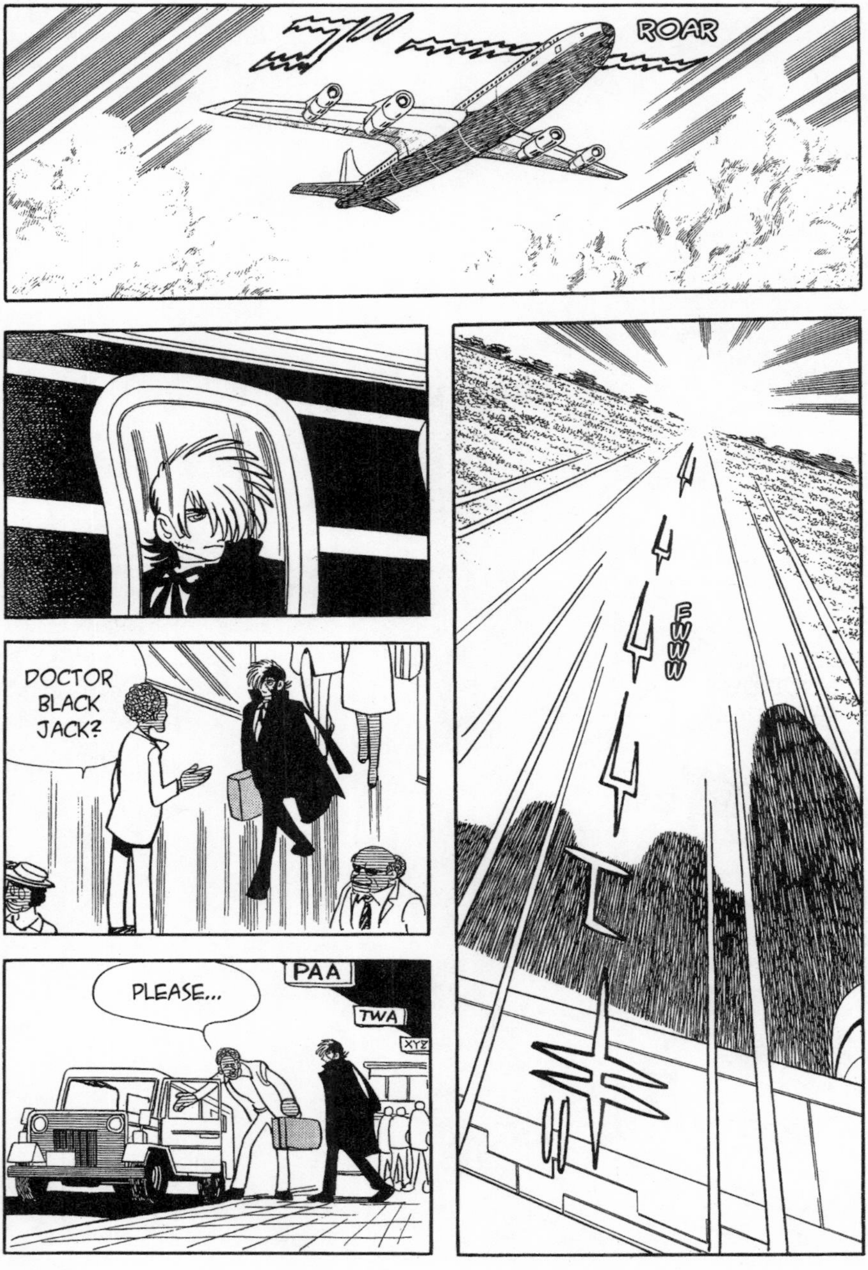
ROAR
FWWW
DOCTOR BLACK JACK?
PLEASE...
PAA
TWA

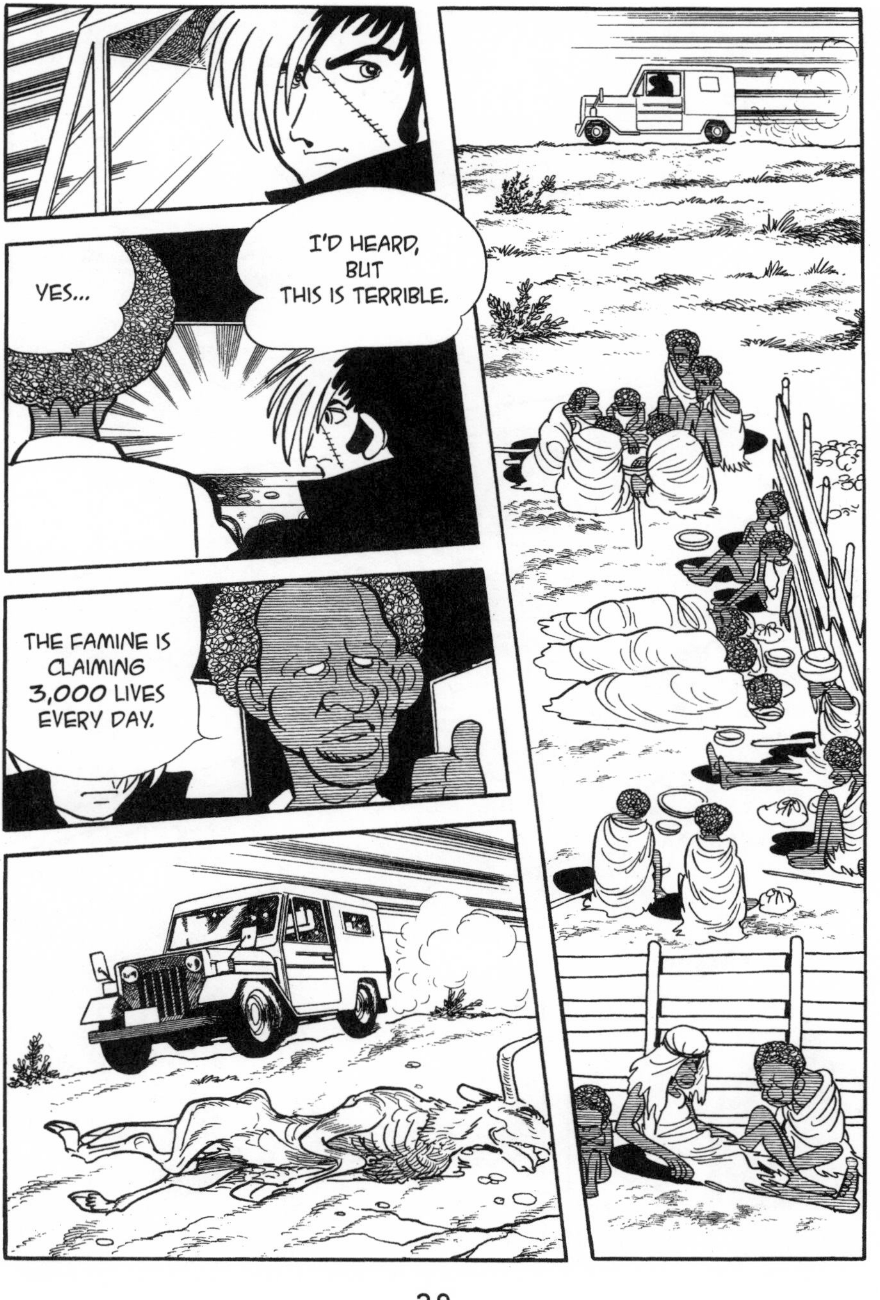
I'D HEARD, BUT THIS IS TERRIBLE.
YES...
THE FAMINE IS CLAIMING 3,000 LIVES EVERY DAY.

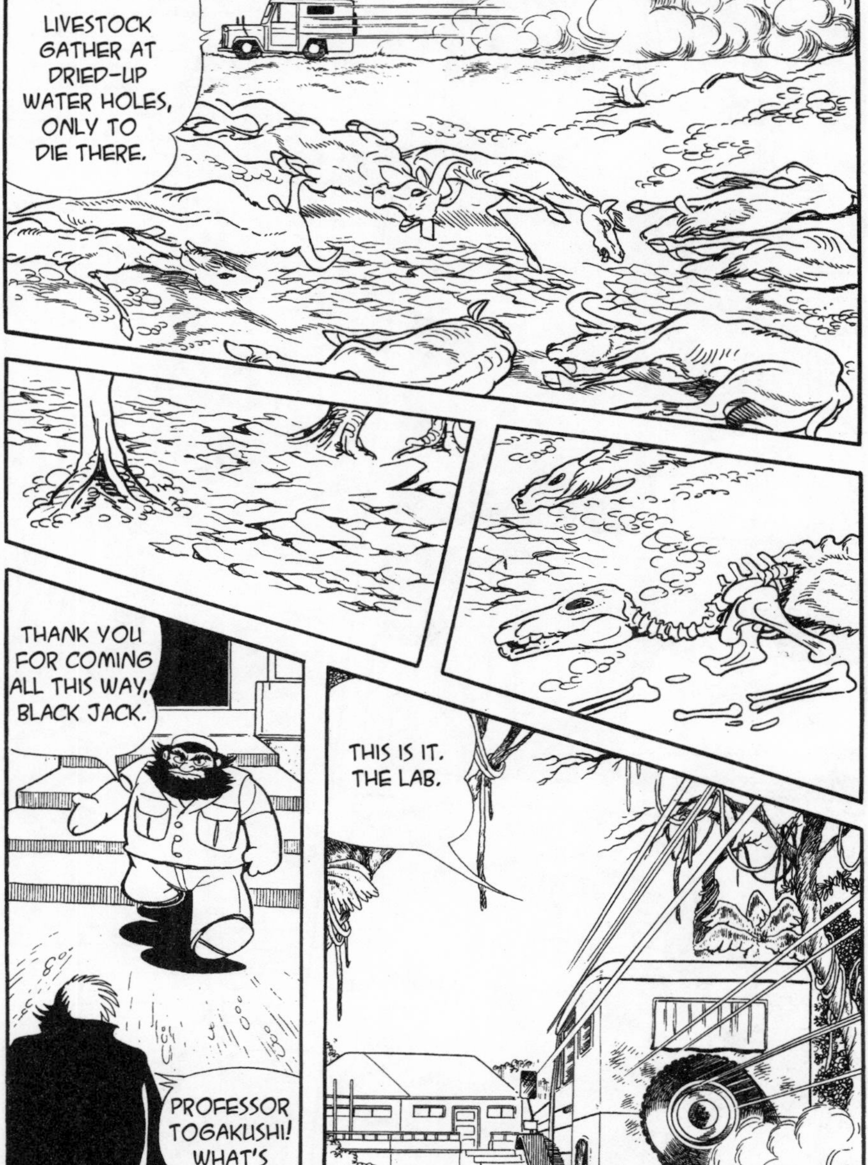
LIVESTOCK GATHER AT DRIED-UP WATER HOLES, ONLY TO DIE THERE.
THIS IS IT. THE LAB.
THANK YOU FOR COMING ALL THIS WAY, BLACK JACK.
PROFESSOR TOGAKUSHI! WHAT'S THE DEAL HERE?

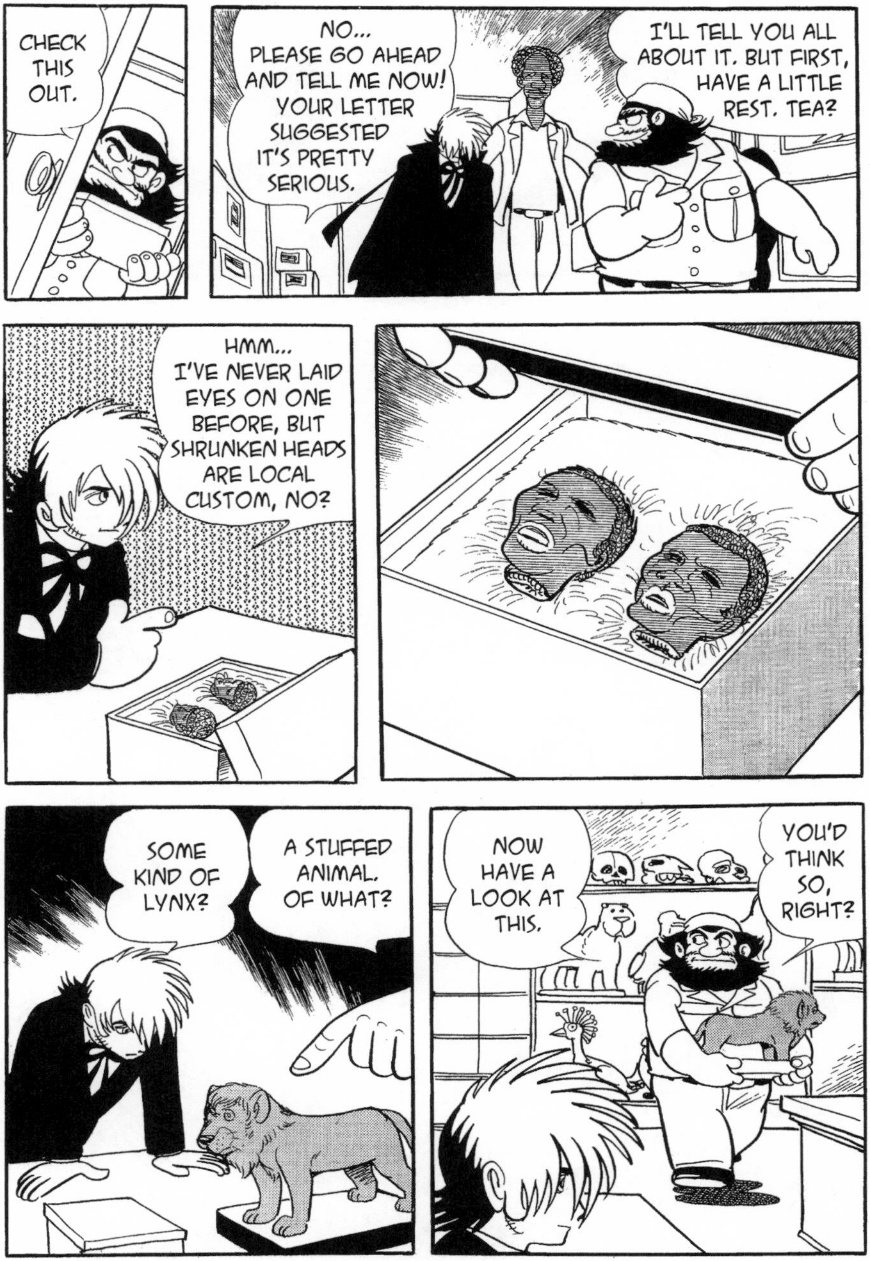
I'LL TELL YOU ALL ABOUT IT. BUT FIRST, HAVE A LITTLE REST. TEA?
NO... PLEASE GO AHEAD AND TELL ME NOW! YOUR LETTER SUGGESTED IT'S PRETTY SERIOUS.
CHECK THIS OUT.
HMM... I'VE NEVER LAID EYES ON ONE BEFORE, BUT SHRUNKEN HEADS ARE LOCAL CUSTOM, NO?
YOU'D THINK SO, RIGHT?
NOW HAVE A LOOK AT THIS.
A STUFFED ANIMAL, OF WHAT?
SOME KIND OF LYNX?

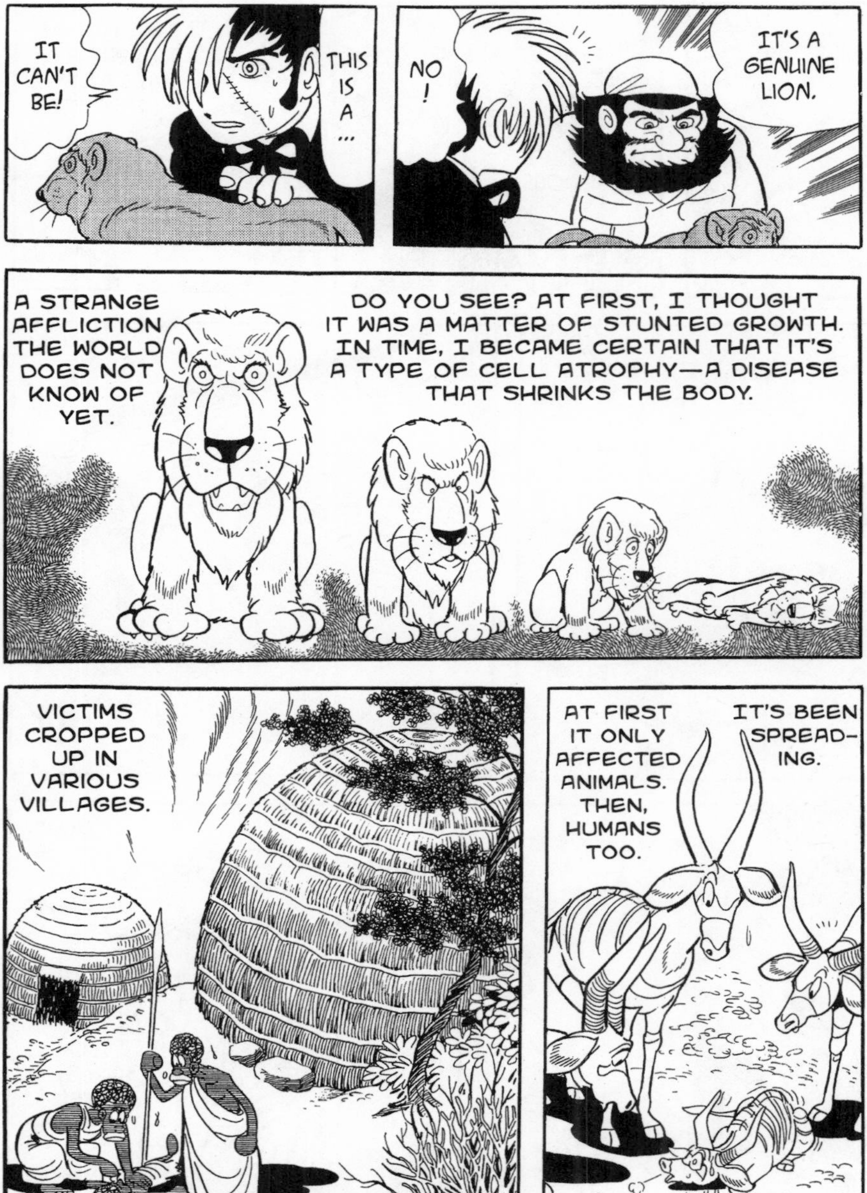
IT CAN'T BE!
THIS IS A ...
NO!
IT'S A GENUINE LION.
A STRANGE AFFLICTION THE WORLD DOES NOT KNOW OF YET.
DO YOU SEE? AT FIRST, I THOUGHT IT WAS A MATTER OF STUNTED GROWTH. IN TIME, I BECAME CERTAIN THAT IT'S A TYPE OF CELL ATROPHY—A DISEASE THAT SHRINKS THE BODY.
VICTIMS CROPPED UP IN VARIOUS VILLAGES.
AT FIRST IT ONLY AFFECTED ANIMALS. THEN, HUMANS TOO.
IT'S BEEN SPREAD-ING.

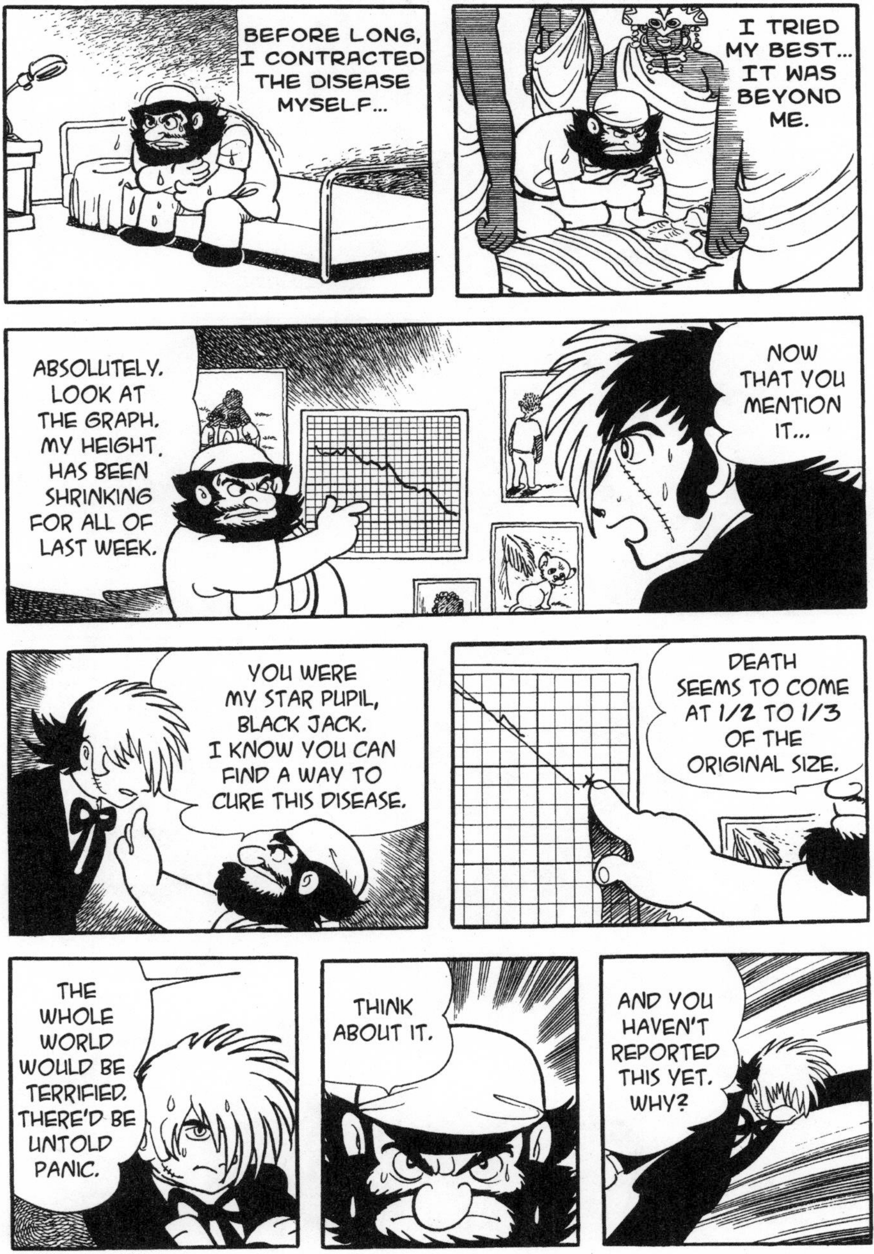
I TRIED MY BEST... IT WAS BEYOND ME.
BEFORE LONG, I CONTRACTED THE DISEASE MYSELF...
NOW THAT YOU MENTION IT...
ABSOLUTELY. LOOK AT THE GRAPH. MY HEIGHT HAS BEEN SHRINKING FOR ALL OF LAST WEEK.
DEATH SEEMS TO COME AT 1/2 TO 1/3 OF THE ORIGINAL SIZE.
YOU WERE MY STAR PUPIL, BLACK JACK. I KNOW YOU CAN FIND A WAY TO CURE THIS DISEASE.
AND YOU HAVEN'T REPORTED THIS YET. WHY?
THINK ABOUT IT.
THE WHOLE WORLD WOULD BE TERRIFIED. THERE'D BE UNTOLD PANIC.

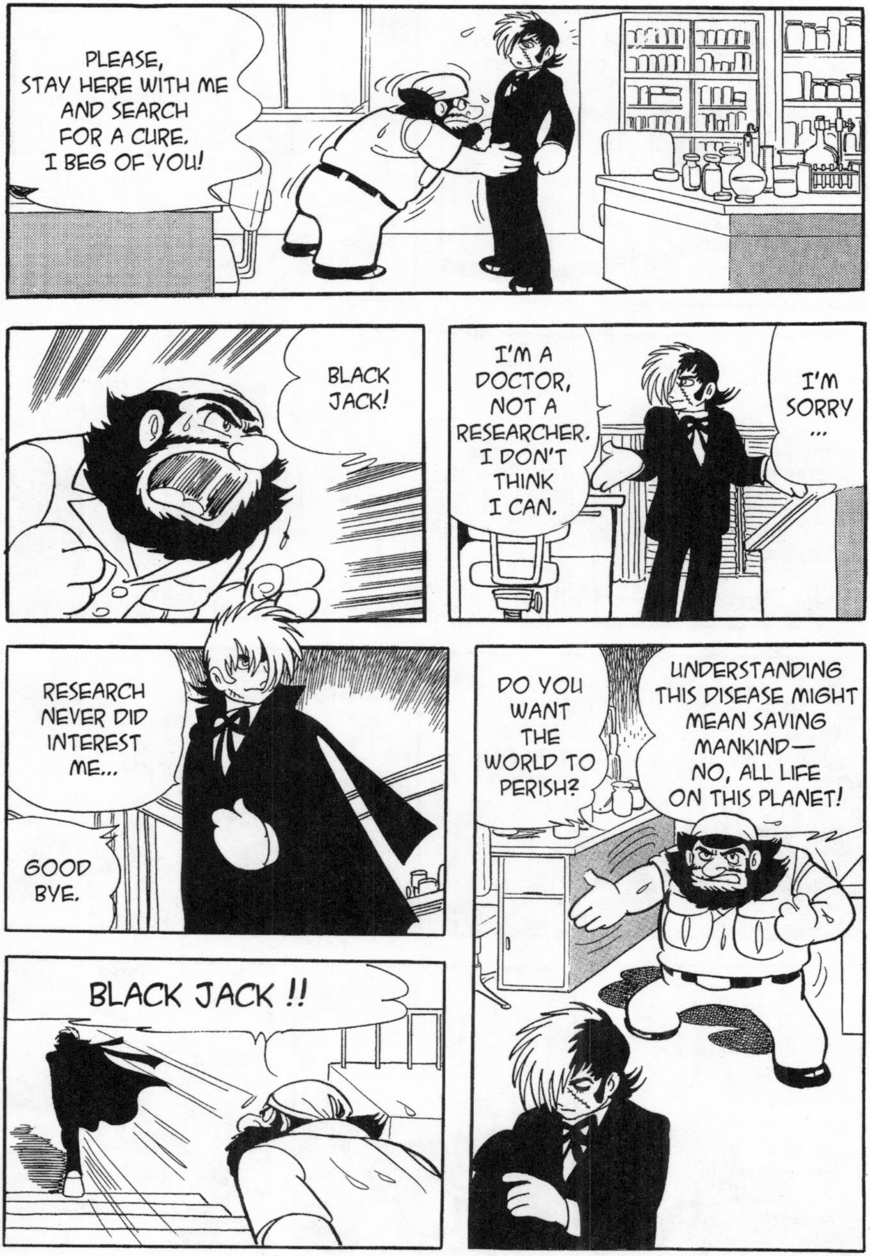
PLEASE, STAY HERE WITH ME AND SEARCH FOR A CURE. I BEG OF YOU!
I'M SORRY ...
I'M A DOCTOR, NOT A RESEARCHER. I DON'T THINK I CAN.
BLACK JACK!
UNDERSTANDING THIS DISEASE MIGHT MEAN SAVING MANKIND— NO, ALL LIFE ON THIS PLANET!
DO YOU WANT THE WORLD TO PERISH?
RESEARCH NEVER DID INTEREST ME...
GOOD BYE.
BLACK JACK !!

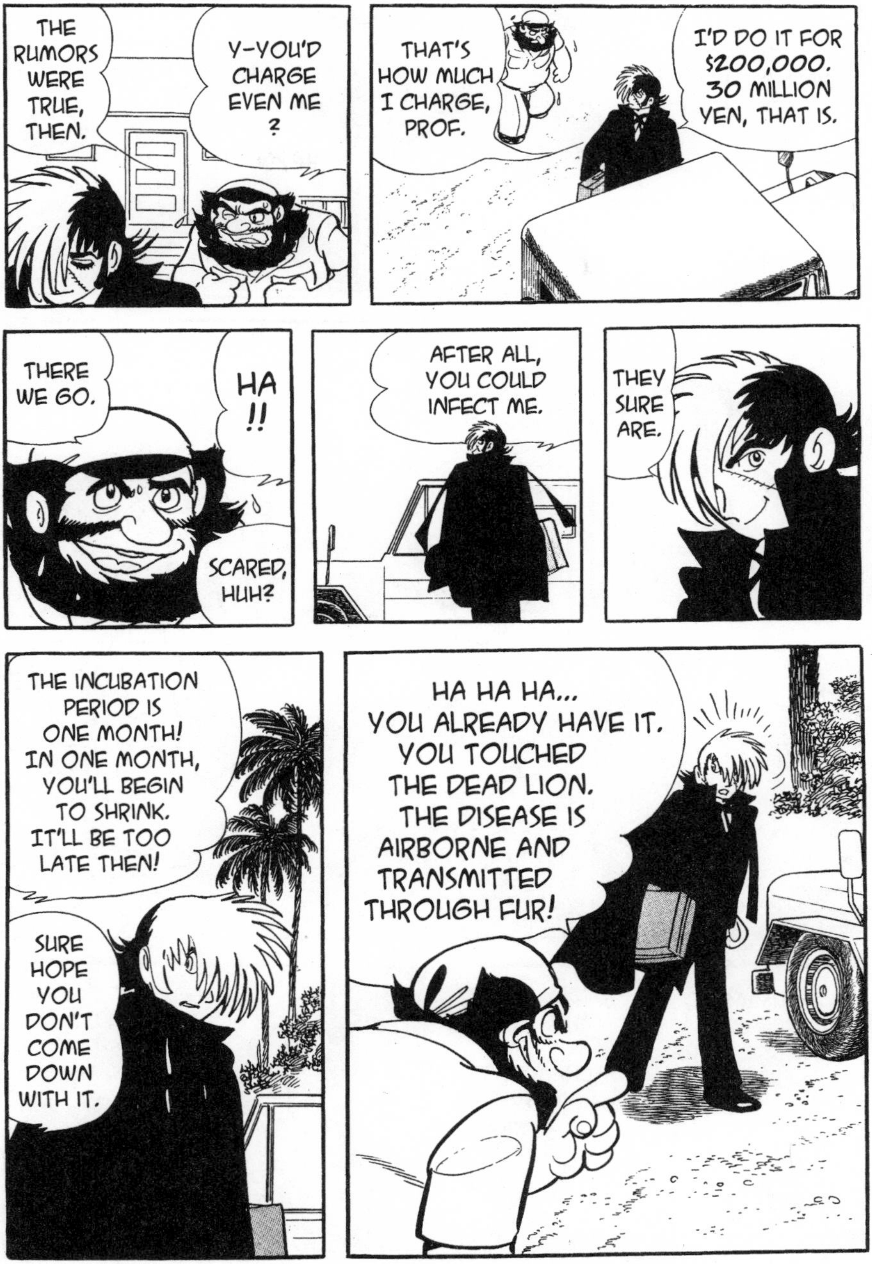
I'D DO IT FOR $200,000. 30 MILLION YEN, THAT IS.
THAT'S HOW MUCH I CHARGE, PROF.
Y-YOU'D CHARGE EVEN ME ?
THE RUMORS WERE TRUE, THEN.
THEY SURE ARE.
AFTER ALL, YOU COULD INFECT ME.
HA !!
THERE WE GO.
SCARED, HUH?
HA HA HA... YOU ALREADY HAVE IT. YOU TOUCHED THE DEAD LION. THE DISEASE IS AIRBORNE AND TRANSMITTED THROUGH FUR!
THE INCUBATION PERIOD IS ONE MONTH! IN ONE MONTH, YOU'LL BEGIN TO SHRINK. IT'LL BE TOO LATE THEN!
SURE HOPE YOU DON'T COME DOWN WITH IT.

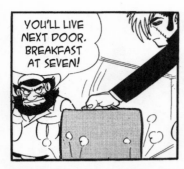

...
YOU'LL LIVE NEXT DOOR. BREAKFAST AT SEVEN!
DAY 5. SURE ENOUGH, THE PROF'S BODY IS SHRINKING...
HE'S LOST 30 CM SINCE I BEGAN MY DIAGNOSIS!
TISSUE EXAMS, X-RAYS... I'VE TRIED THEM ALL. NO LUCK.
THIS ISN'T A DISEASE. THERE MUST BE SOME OTHER EXPLANATION.
EVERY CELL IS SHRINKING WITHOUT CHANGING STRUCTURE!
WHAT'S MORE, OLDER CELLS CONTINUE TO BE REPLACED...

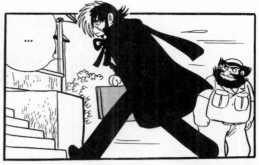

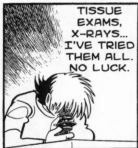

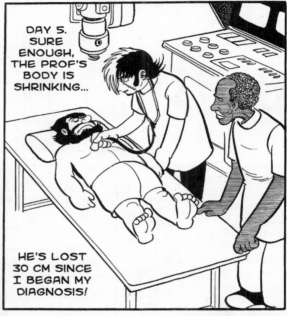

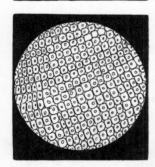

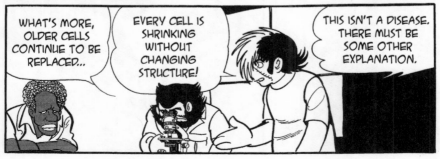

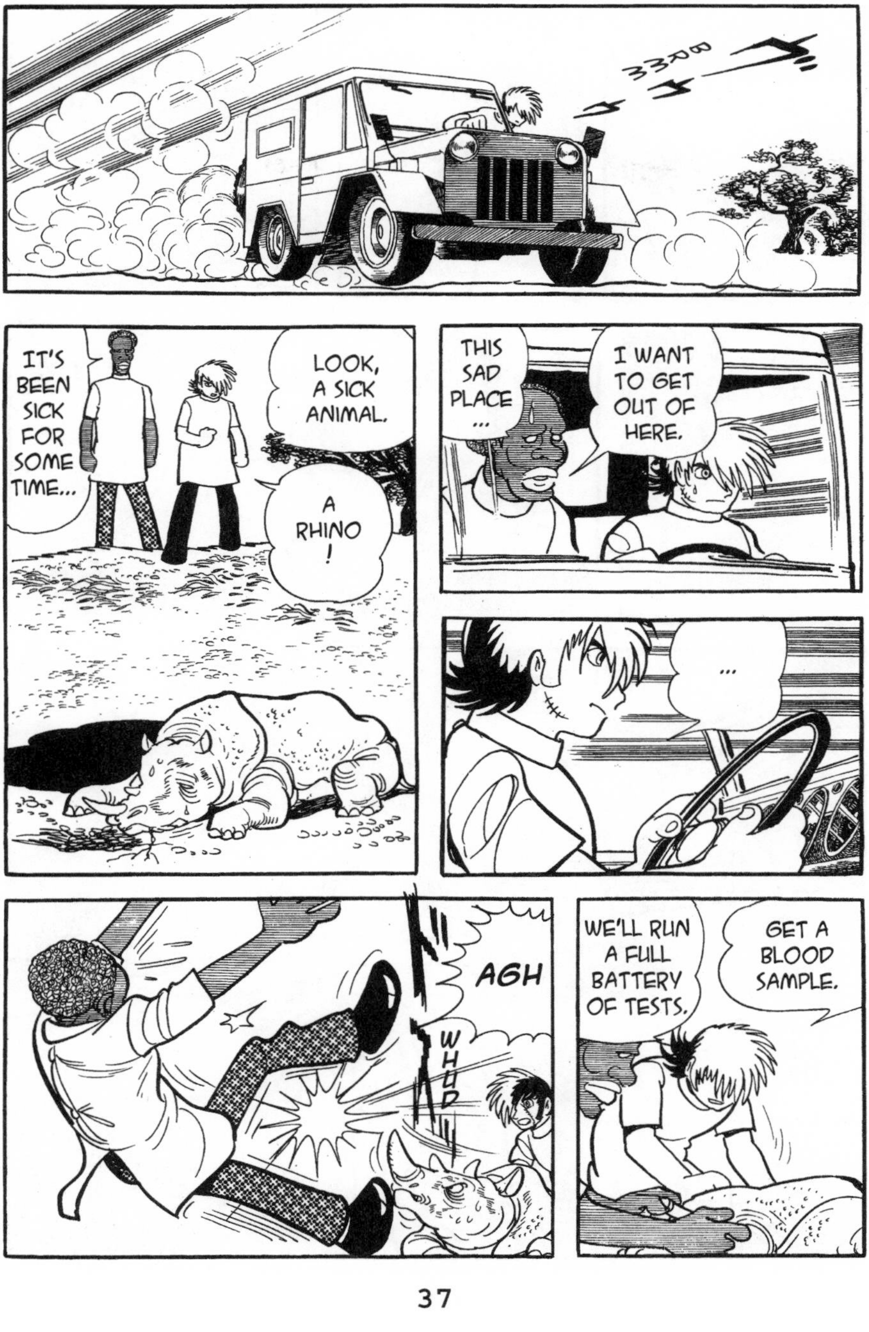
I WANT TO GET OUT OF HERE.
THIS SAD PLACE ...
...
LOOK, A SICK ANIMAL.
A RHINO!
IT'S BEEN SICK FOR SOME TIME...
GET A BLOOD SAMPLE.
WE'LL RUN A FULL BATTERY OF TESTS.
AGH
WHUD

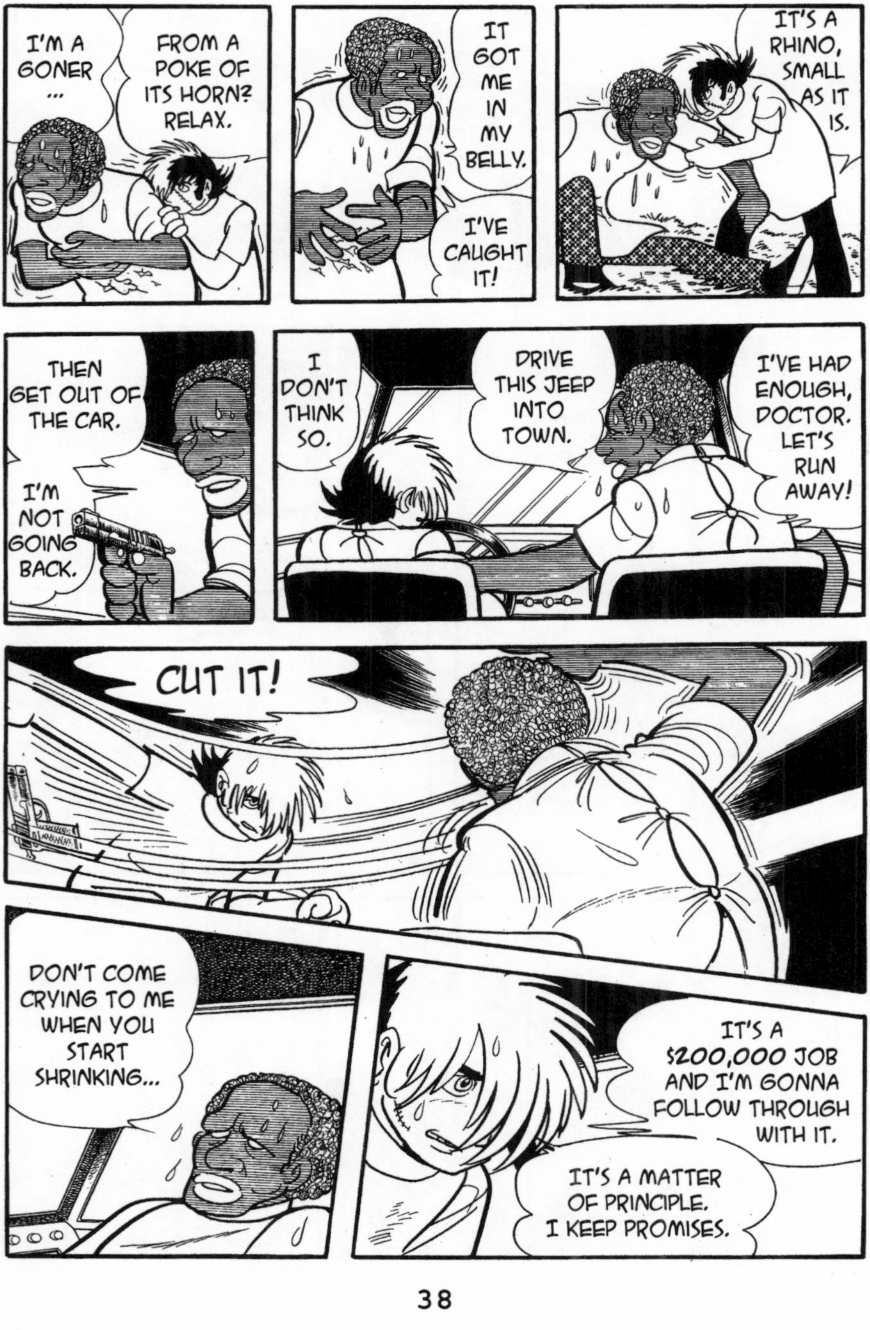
IT'S A RHINO, SMALL AS IT IS.
IT GOT ME IN MY BELLY.
I'VE CAUGHT IT!
I'M A GONER ...
FROM A POKE OF ITS HORN? RELAX.
I'VE HAD ENOUGH, DOCTOR. LET'S RUN AWAY!
DRIVE THIS JEEP INTO TOWN.
I DON'T THINK SO.
THEN GET OUT OF THE CAR.
I'M NOT GOING BACK.
CUT IT!
IT'S A $200,000 JOB AND I'M GONNA FOLLOW THROUGH WITH IT.
IT'S A MATTER OF PRINCIPLE. I KEEP PROMISES.
DON'T COME CRYING TO ME WHEN YOU START SHRINKING...

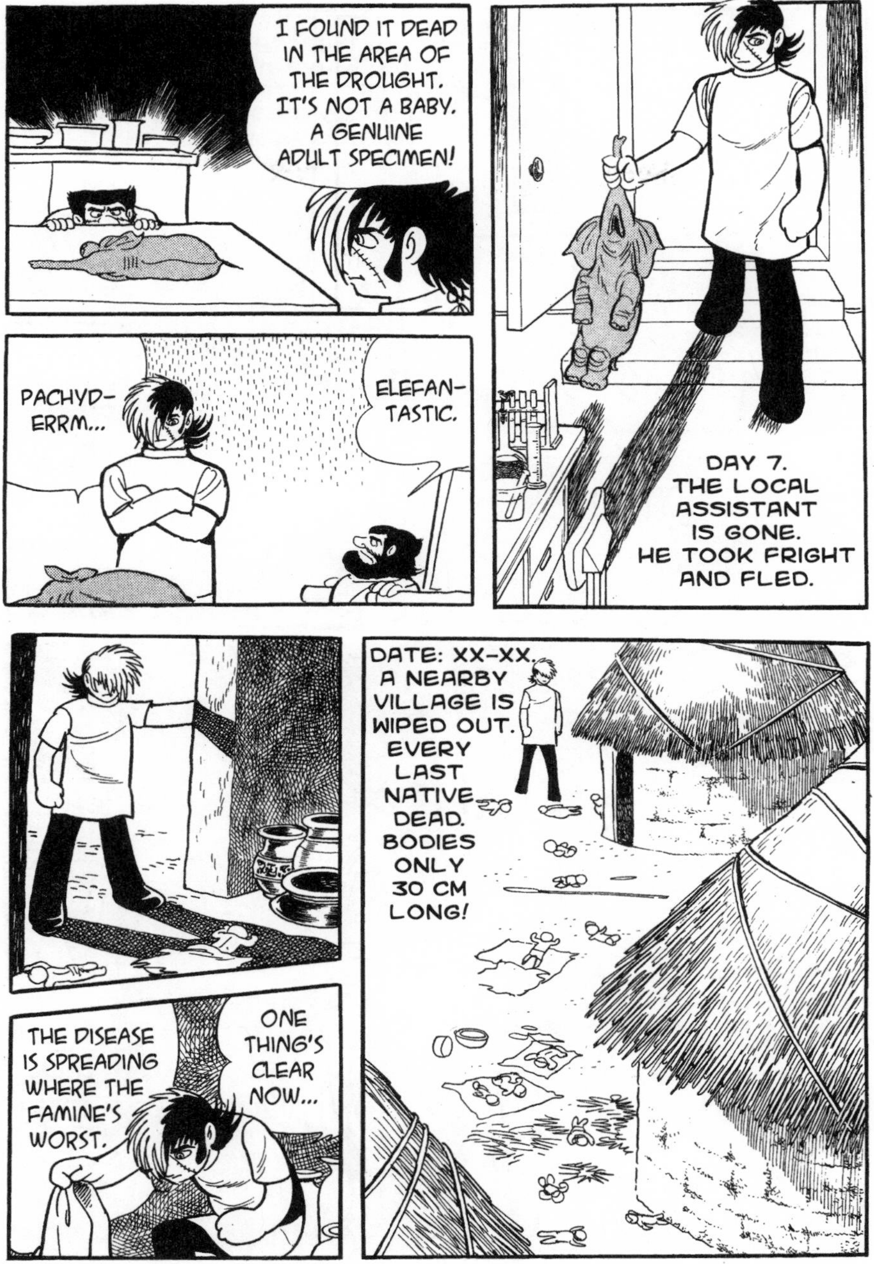
DAY 7. THE LOCAL ASSISTANT IS GONE. HE TOOK FRIGHT AND FLED.
I FOUND IT DEAD IN THE AREA OF THE DROUGHT. IT'S NOT A BABY. A GENUINE ADULT SPECIMEN!
ELEFAN-TASTIC.
PACHYD-ERRM...
DATE: XX-XX. A NEARBY VILLAGE IS WIPED OUT. EVERY LAST NATIVE DEAD. BODIES ONLY 30 CM LONG!
ONE THING'S CLEAR NOW...
THE DISEASE IS SPREADING WHERE THE FAMINE'S WORST.

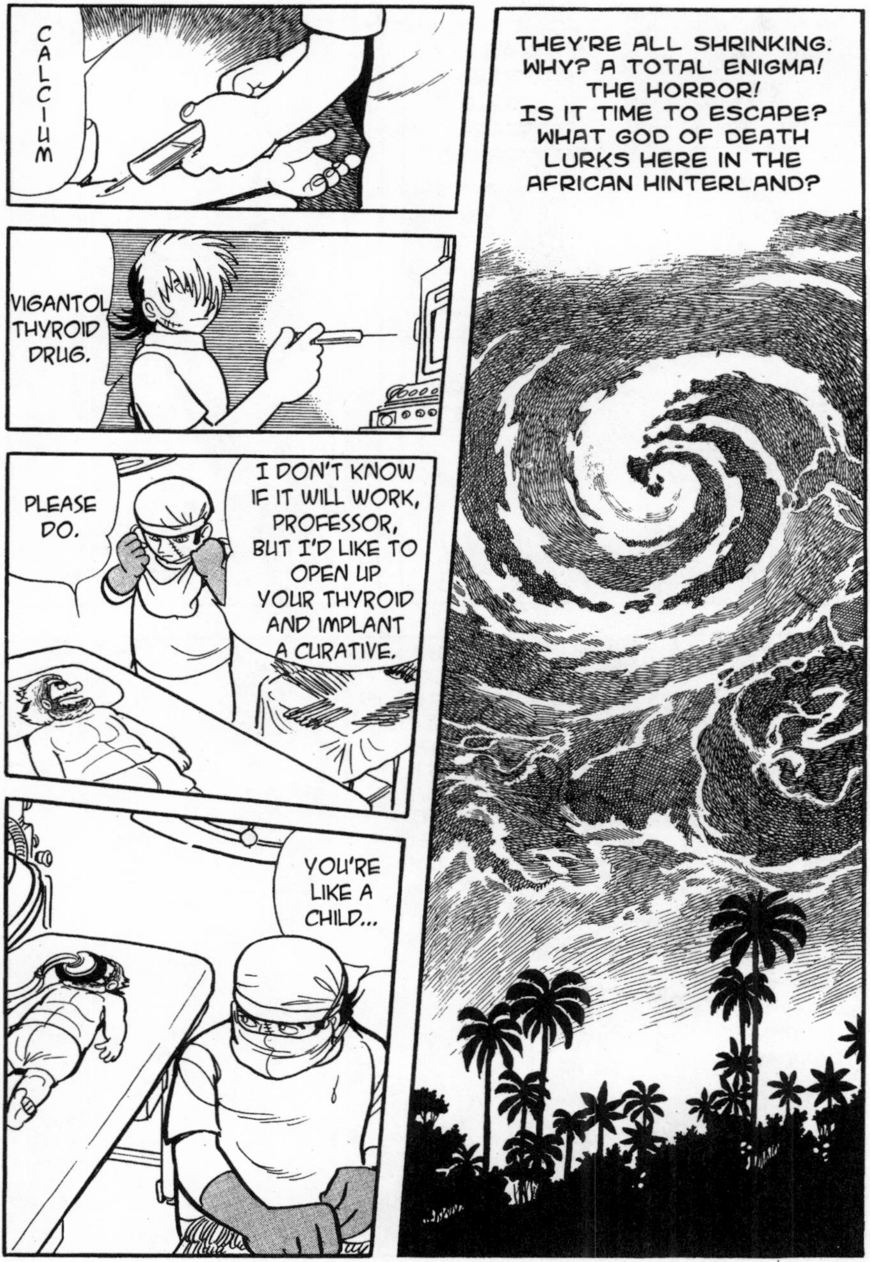
THEY'RE ALL SHRINKING. WHY? A TOTAL ENIGMA! THE HORROR! IS IT TIME TO ESCAPE? WHAT GOD OF DEATH LURKS HERE IN THE AFRICAN HINTERLAND?
CALCIUM
VIGANTOL THYROID DRUG.
I DON'T KNOW IF IT WILL WORK, PROFESSOR, BUT I'D LIKE TO OPEN UP YOUR THYROID AND IMPLANT A CURATIVE.
PLEASE DO.
YOU'RE LIKE A CHILD...

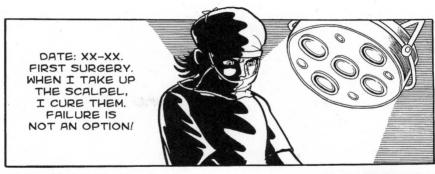

DATE: XX–XX.
FIRST SURGERY.
WHEN I TAKE UP
THE SCALPEL,
I CURE THEM.
FAILURE IS
NOT AN OPTION!

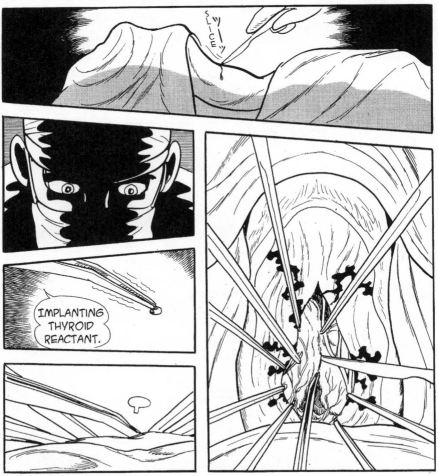

IMPLANTING
THYROID
REACTANT.

41

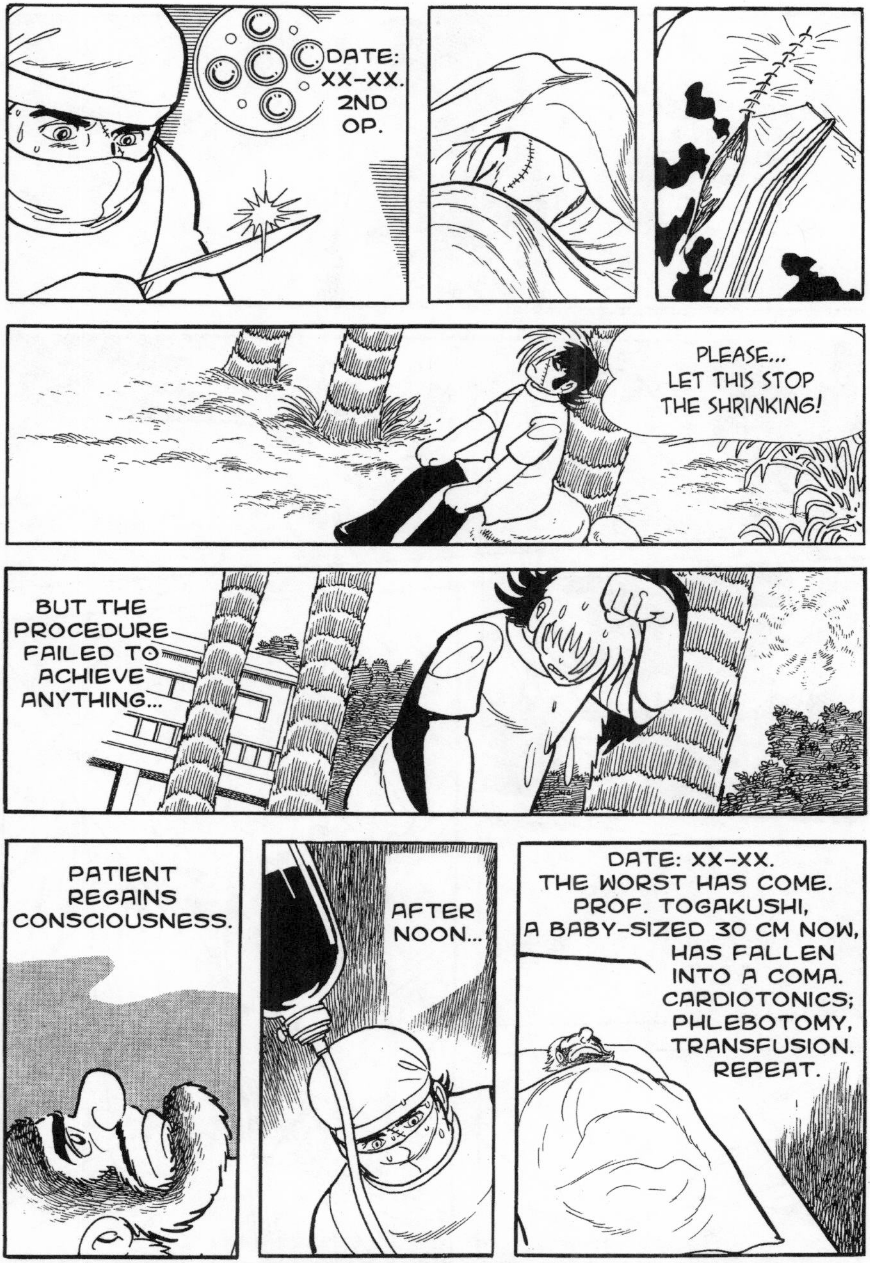
DATE: XX-XX. 2ND OP.
PLEASE... LET THIS STOP THE SHRINKING!
BUT THE PROCEDURE FAILED TO ACHIEVE ANYTHING...
DATE: XX-XX. THE WORST HAS COME. PROF. TOGAKUSHI, A BABY-SIZED 30 CM NOW, HAS FALLEN INTO A COMA. CARDIOTONICS; PHLEBOTOMY, TRANSFUSION. REPEAT.
AFTER NOON...
PATIENT REGAINS CONSCIOUSNESS.

NOTE: A "PHLEBOTOMY" LETS A PORTION OF BLOOD FROM THE PATIENT'S VEIN AND IS USED TO TREAT HIGH BLOOD PRESSURE AND CEREBRAL HEMORRHAGING.

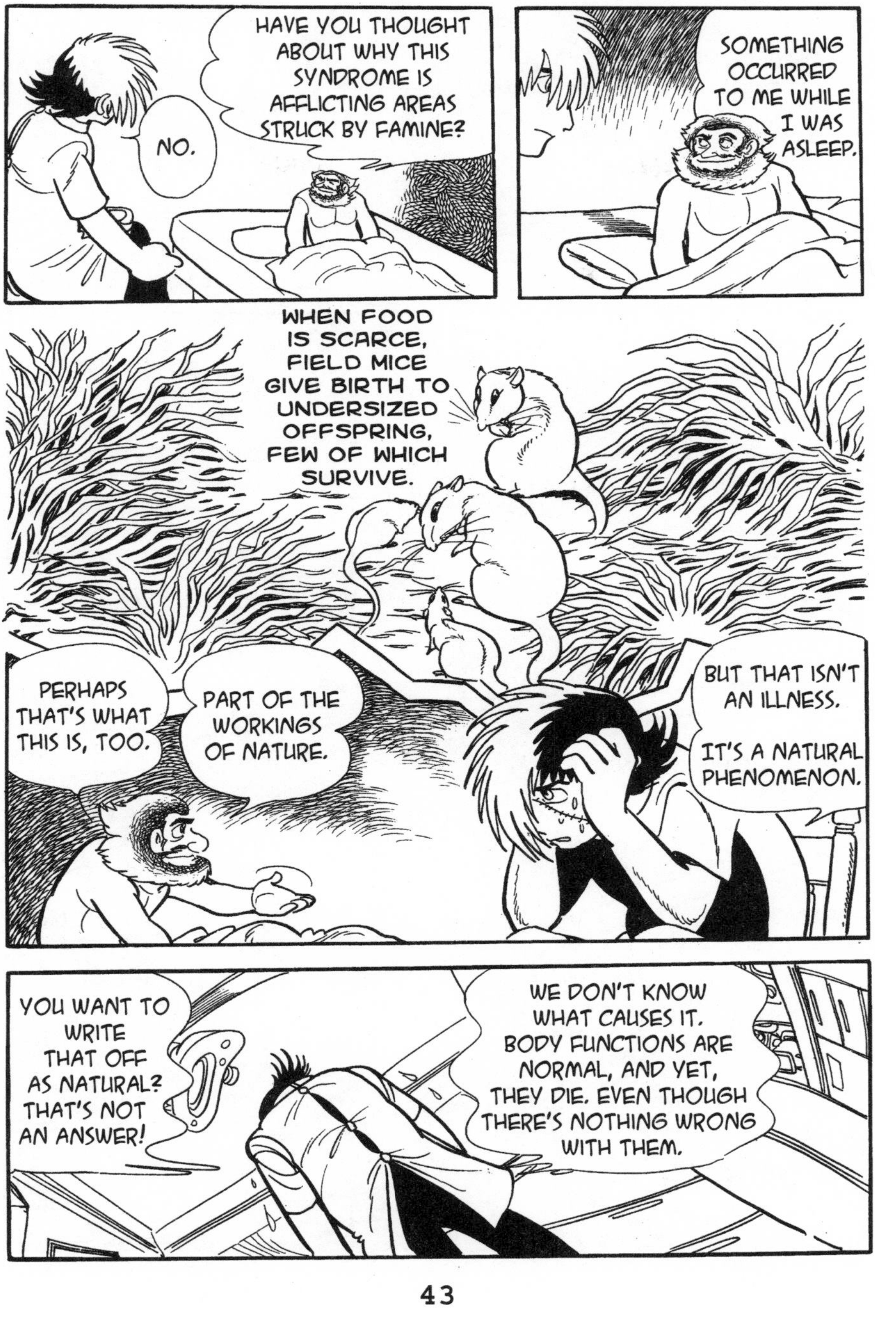
SOMETHING OCCURRED TO ME WHILE I WAS ASLEEP.
HAVE YOU THOUGHT ABOUT WHY THIS SYNDROME IS AFFLICTING AREAS STRUCK BY FAMINE?
NO.
WHEN FOOD IS SCARCE, FIELD MICE GIVE BIRTH TO UNDERSIZED OFFSPRING, FEW OF WHICH SURVIVE.
BUT THAT ISN'T AN ILLNESS.
IT'S A NATURAL PHENOMENON.
PERHAPS THAT'S WHAT THIS IS, TOO.
PART OF THE WORKINGS OF NATURE.
WE DON'T KNOW WHAT CAUSES IT. BODY FUNCTIONS ARE NORMAL, AND YET, THEY DIE. EVEN THOUGH THERE'S NOTHING WRONG WITH THEM.
YOU WANT TO WRITE THAT OFF AS NATURAL? THAT'S NOT AN ANSWER!

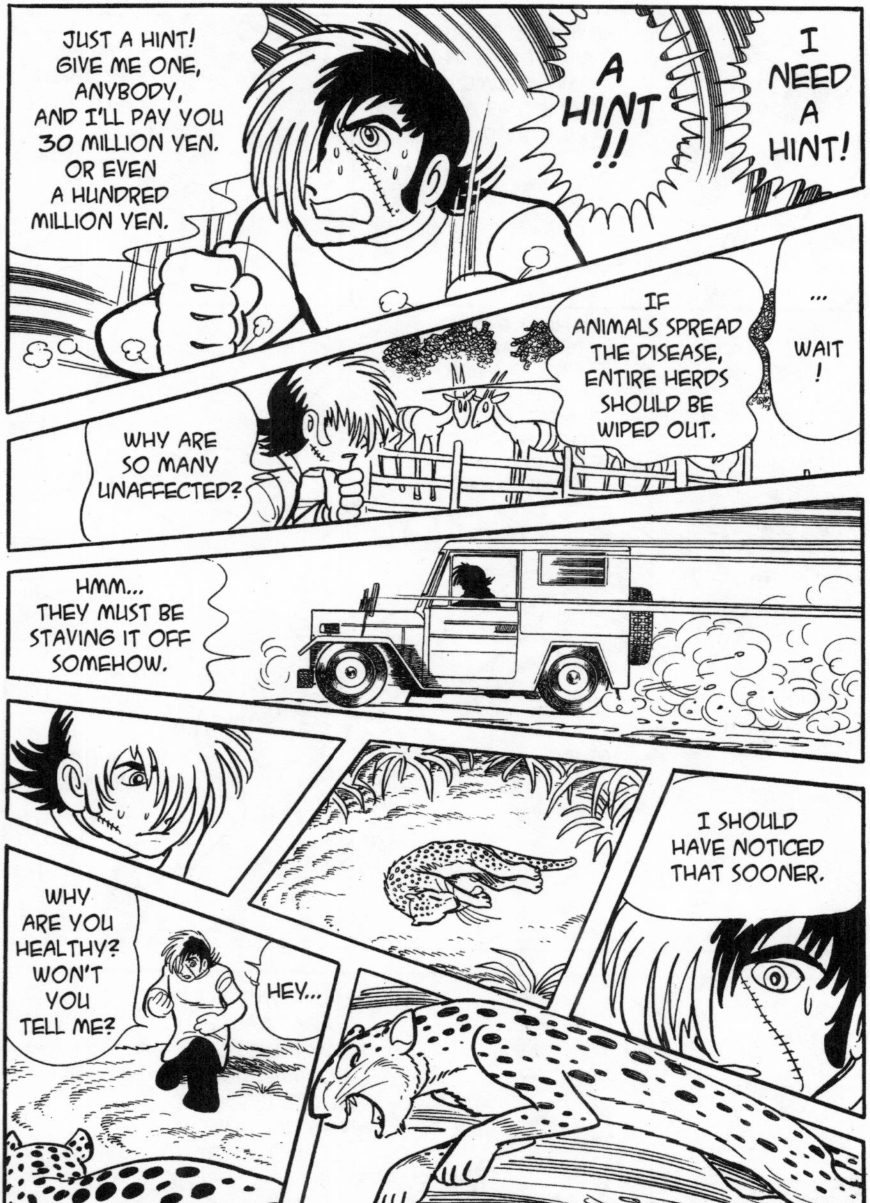
I NEED A HINT!
A HINT!!
JUST A HINT! GIVE ME ONE, ANYBODY, AND I'LL PAY YOU 30 MILLION YEN. OR EVEN A HUNDRED MILLION YEN.
... WAIT!
IF ANIMALS SPREAD THE DISEASE, ENTIRE HERDS SHOULD BE WIPED OUT.
WHY ARE SO MANY UNAFFECTED?
HMM... THEY MUST BE STAVING IT OFF SOMEHOW.
I SHOULD HAVE NOTICED THAT SOONER.
HEY...
WHY ARE YOU HEALTHY? WON'T YOU TELL ME?

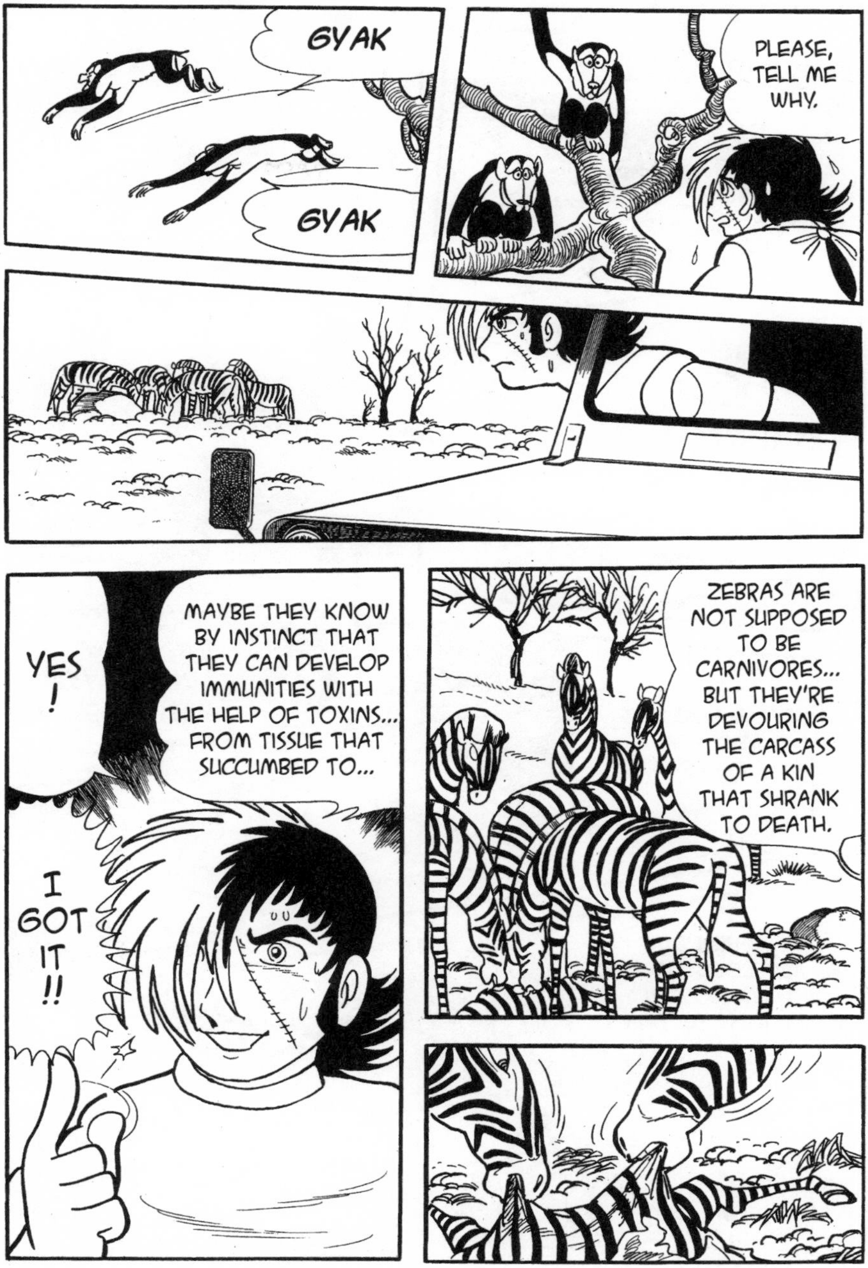
PLEASE, TELL ME WHY.
GYAK
GYAK
ZEBRAS ARE NOT SUPPOSED TO BE CARNIVORES... BUT THEY'RE DEVOURING THE CARCASS OF A KIN THAT SHRANK TO DEATH.
MAYBE THEY KNOW BY INSTINCT THAT THEY CAN DEVELOP IMMUNITIES WITH THE HELP OF TOXINS... FROM TISSUE THAT SUCCUMBED TO...
YES!
I GOT IT!!

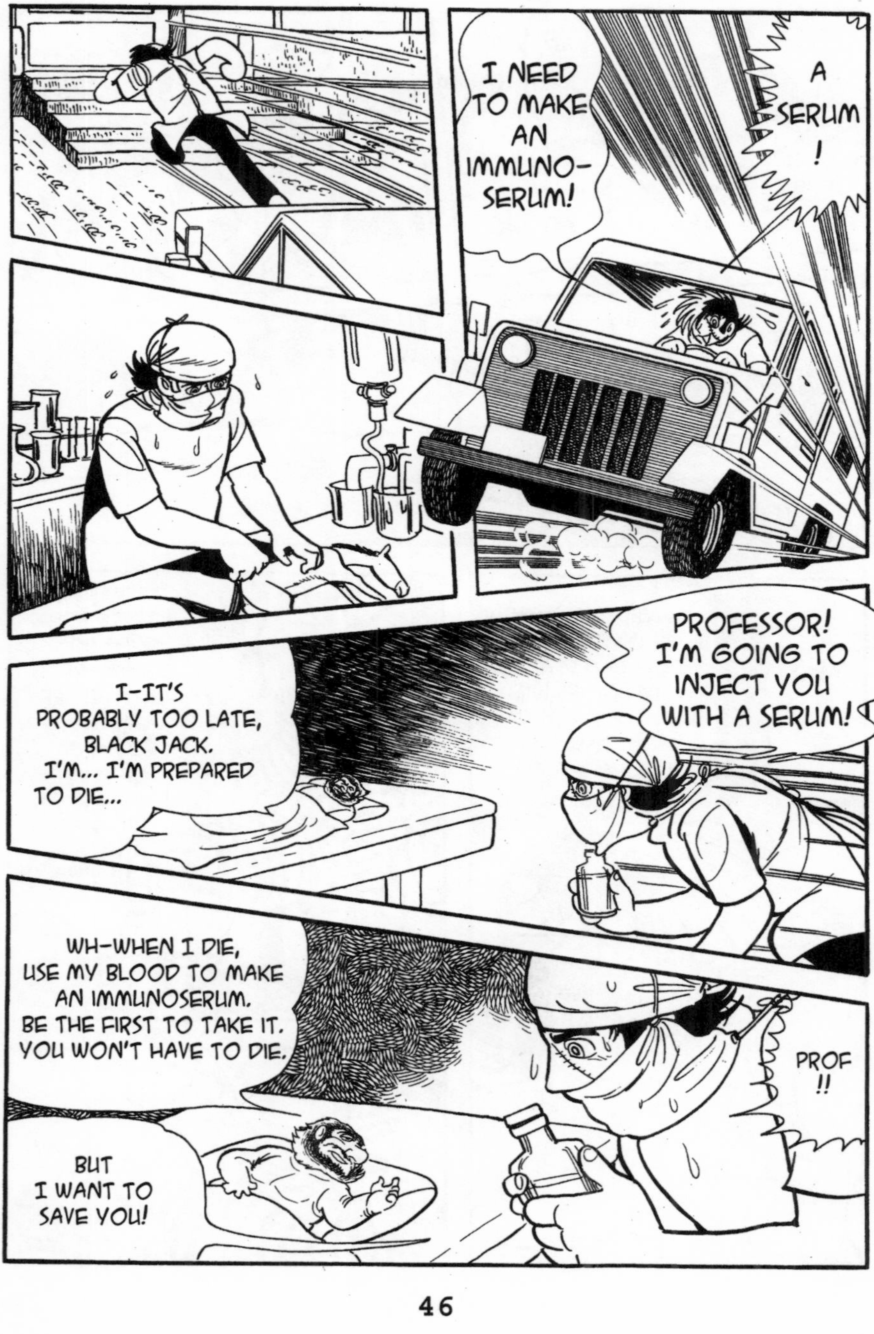
A SERUM!
I NEED TO MAKE AN IMMUNO-SERUM!
PROFESSOR! I'M GOING TO INJECT YOU WITH A SERUM!
I-IT'S PROBABLY TOO LATE, BLACK JACK. I'M... I'M PREPARED TO DIE...
PROF!!
WH-WHEN I DIE, USE MY BLOOD TO MAKE AN IMMUNOSERUM. BE THE FIRST TO TAKE IT. YOU WON'T HAVE TO DIE.
BUT I WANT TO SAVE YOU!

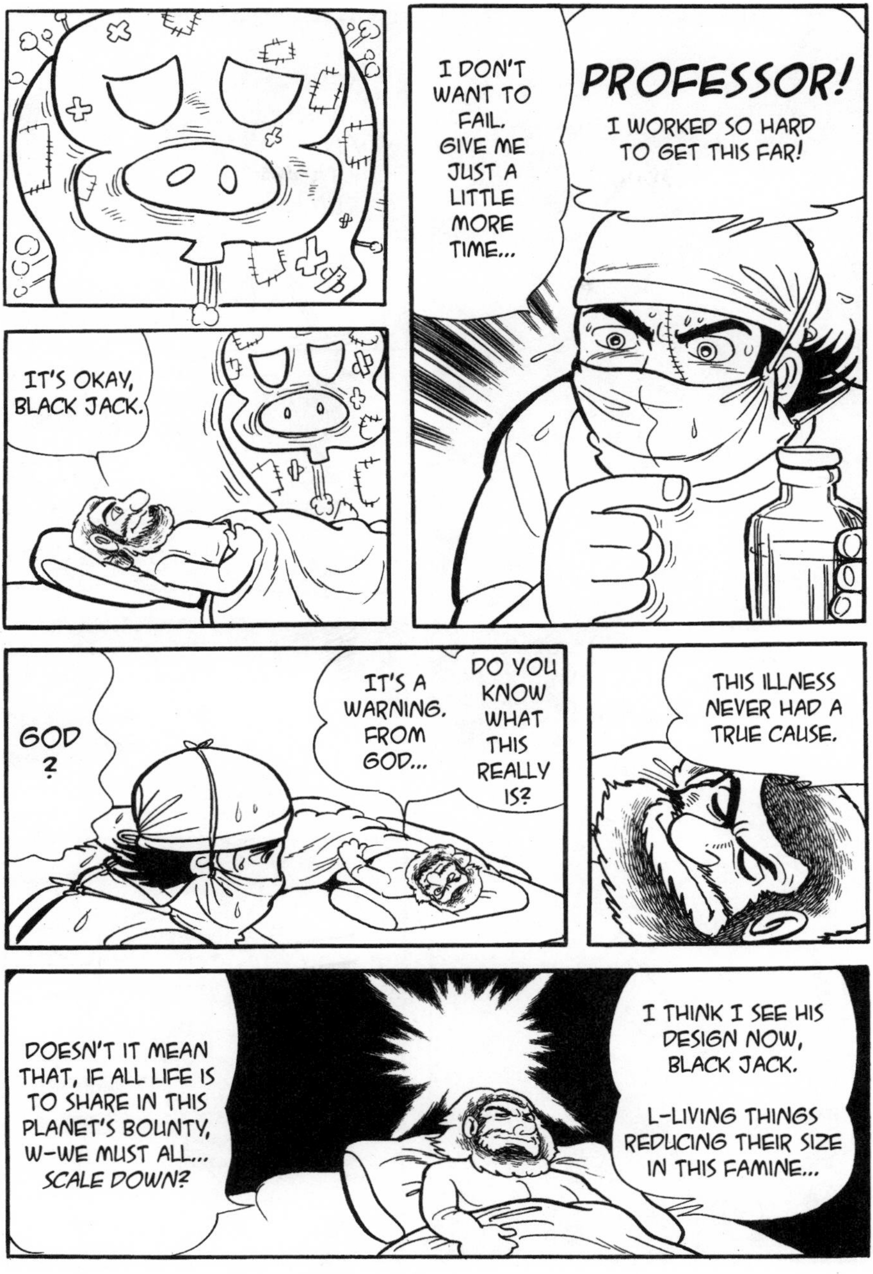
PROFESSOR! I WORKED SO HARD TO GET THIS FAR!
I DON'T WANT TO FAIL. GIVE ME JUST A LITTLE MORE TIME...
IT'S OKAY, BLACK JACK.
THIS ILLNESS NEVER HAD A TRUE CAUSE.
DO YOU KNOW WHAT THIS REALLY IS?
IT'S A WARNING. FROM GOD...
GOD?
I THINK I SEE HIS DESIGN NOW, BLACK JACK.
L-LIVING THINGS REDUCING THEIR SIZE IN THIS FAMINE...
DOESN'T IT MEAN THAT, IF ALL LIFE IS TO SHARE IN THIS PLANET'S BOUNTY, W-WE MUST ALL... *SCALE DOWN?*

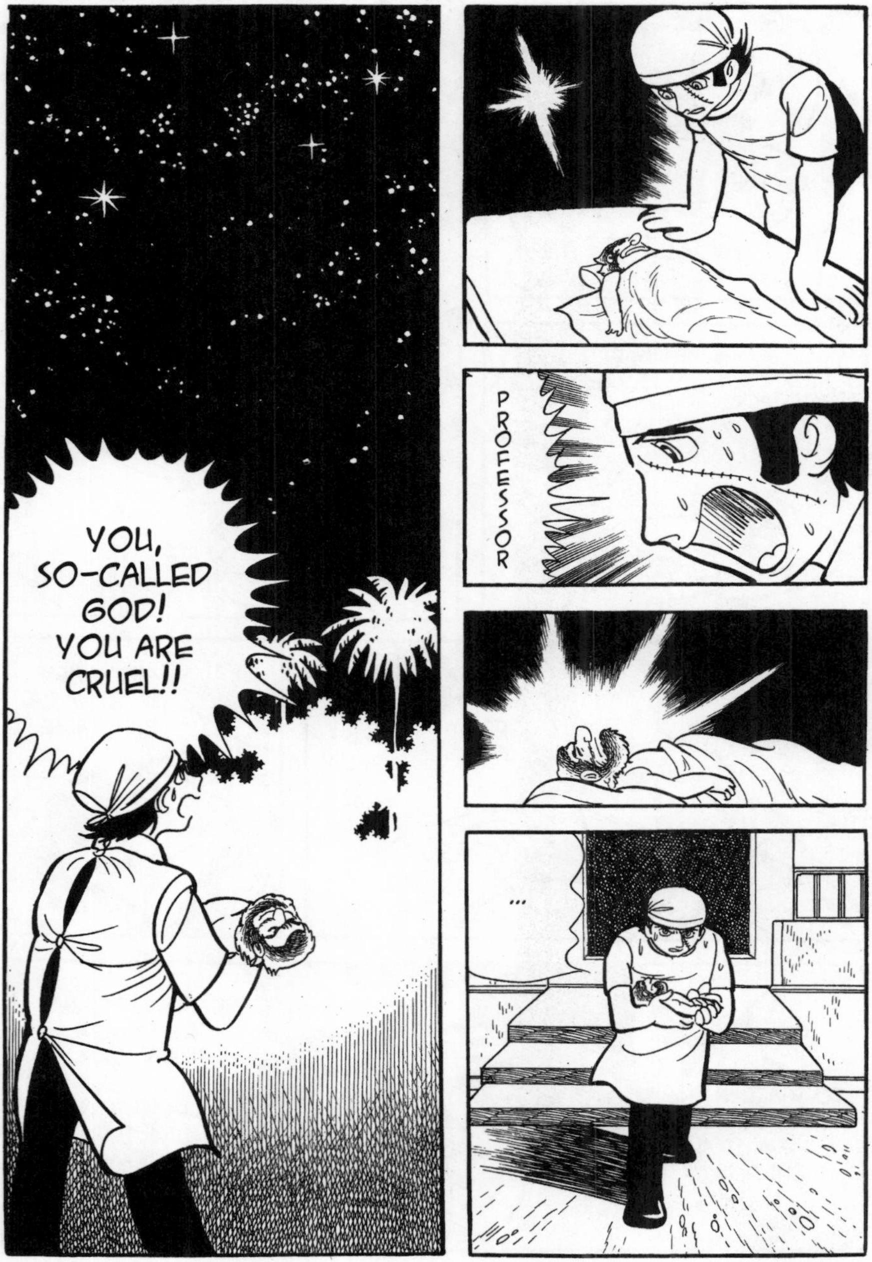
PROFESSOR
...
YOU, SO-CALLED GOD! YOU ARE CRUEL!!

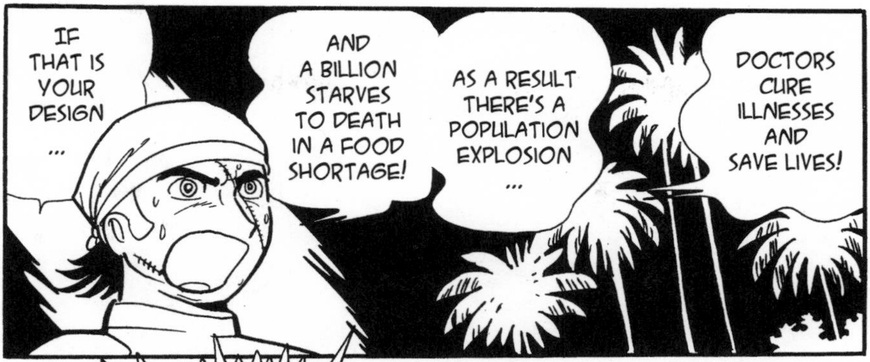
DOCTORS CURE ILLNESSES AND SAVE LIVES!
AS A RESULT THERE'S A POPULATION EXPLOSION ...
AND A BILLION STARVES TO DEATH IN A FOOD SHORTAGE!
IF THAT IS YOUR DESIGN ...

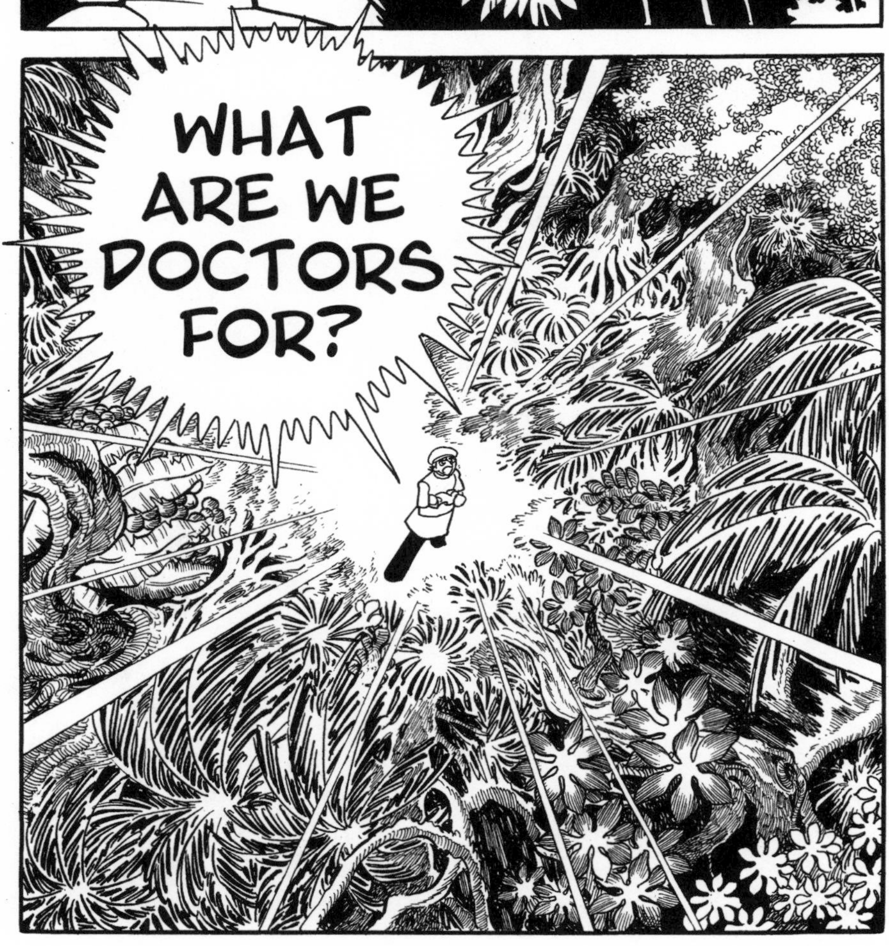
WHAT ARE WE DOCTORS FOR?

DINGOES

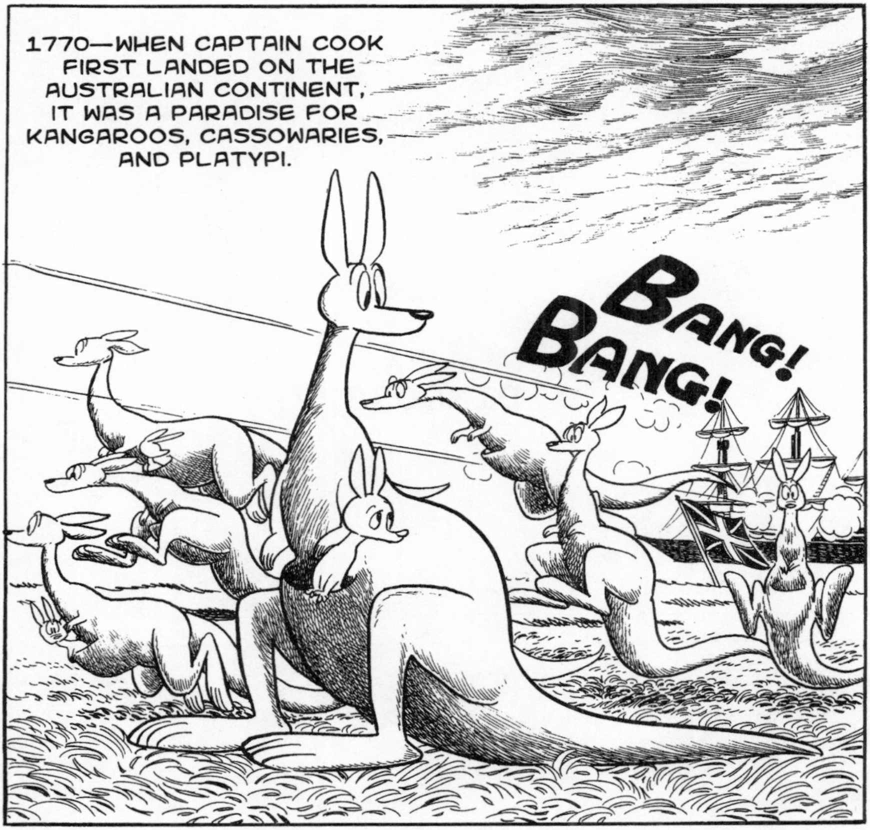
1770—WHEN CAPTAIN COOK FIRST LANDED ON THE AUSTRALIAN CONTINENT, IT WAS A PARADISE FOR KANGAROOS, CASSOWARIES, AND PLATYPI.
BANG!
BANG!

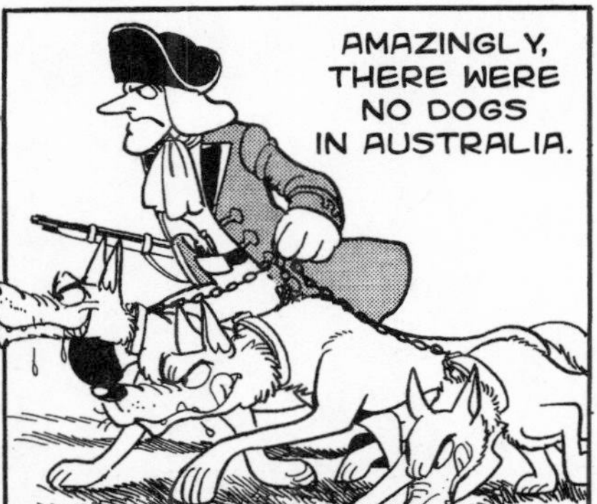
AMAZINGLY, THERE WERE NO DOGS IN AUSTRALIA.

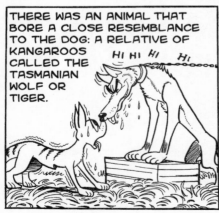

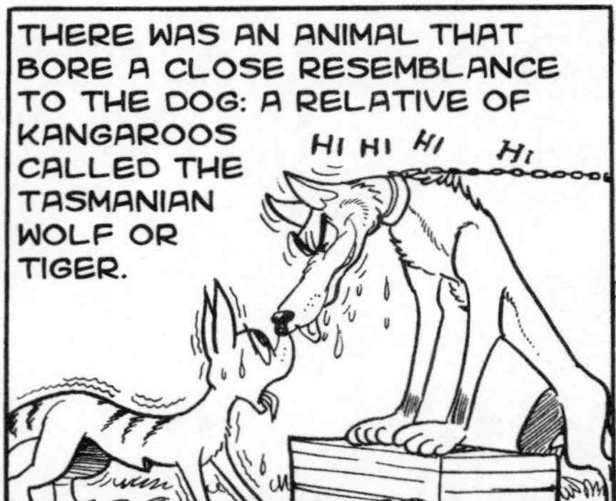
THERE WAS AN ANIMAL THAT BORE A CLOSE RESEMBLANCE TO THE DOG: A RELATIVE OF KANGAROOS CALLED THE TASMANIAN WOLF OR TIGER.
HI HI HI HI

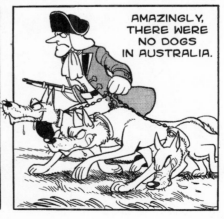

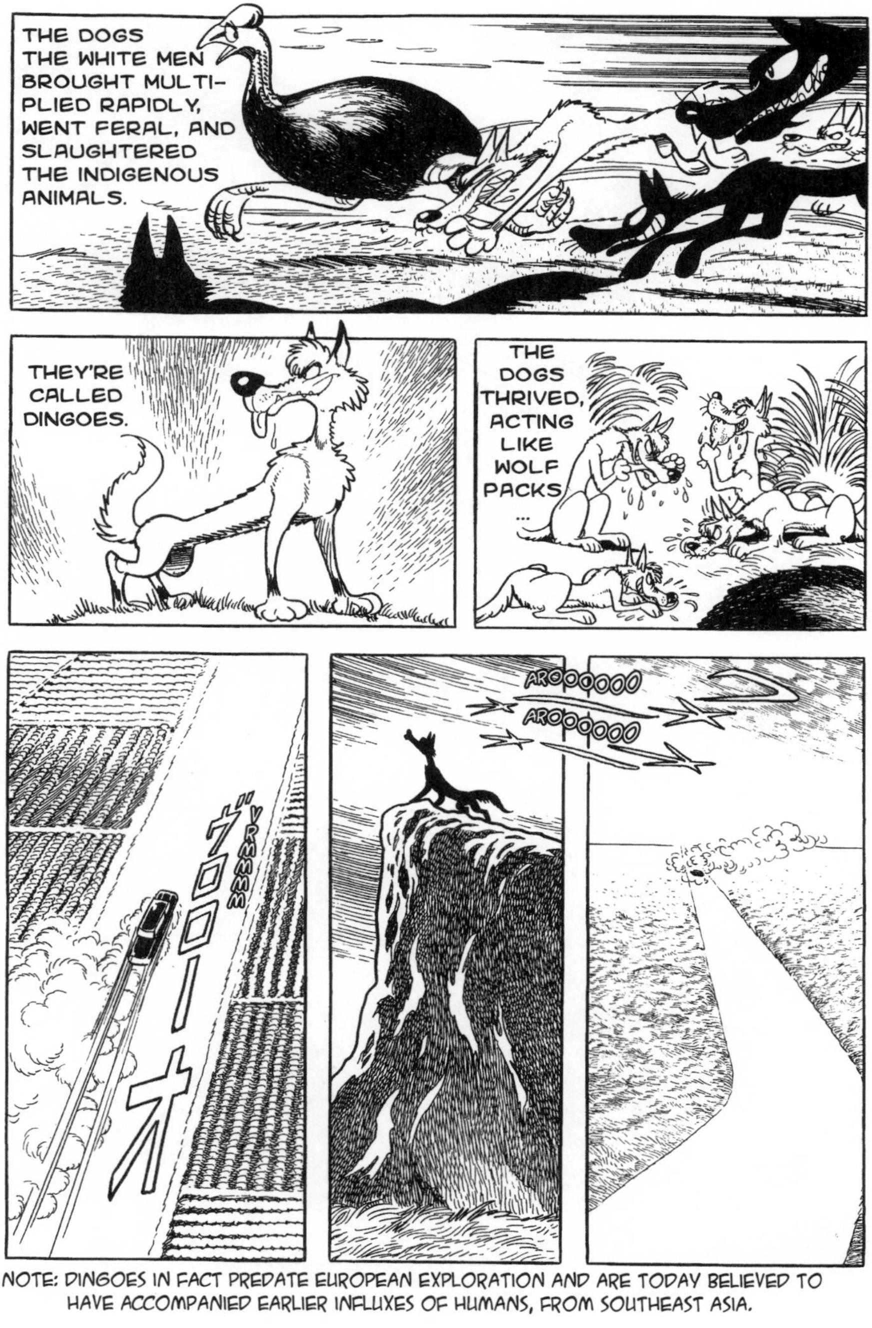
THE DOGS THE WHITE MEN BROUGHT MULTI-PLIED RAPIDLY, WENT FERAL, AND SLAUGHTERED THE INDIGENOUS ANIMALS.
THE DOGS THRIVED, ACTING LIKE WOLF PACKS ...
THEY'RE CALLED DINGOES.
AROOOOOO
AROOOOOO
ヴロローーオ
VRMMMM

NOTE: DINGOES IN FACT PREDATE EUROPEAN EXPLORATION AND ARE TODAY BELIEVED TO HAVE ACCOMPANIED EARLIER INFLUXES OF HUMANS, FROM SOUTHEAST ASIA.

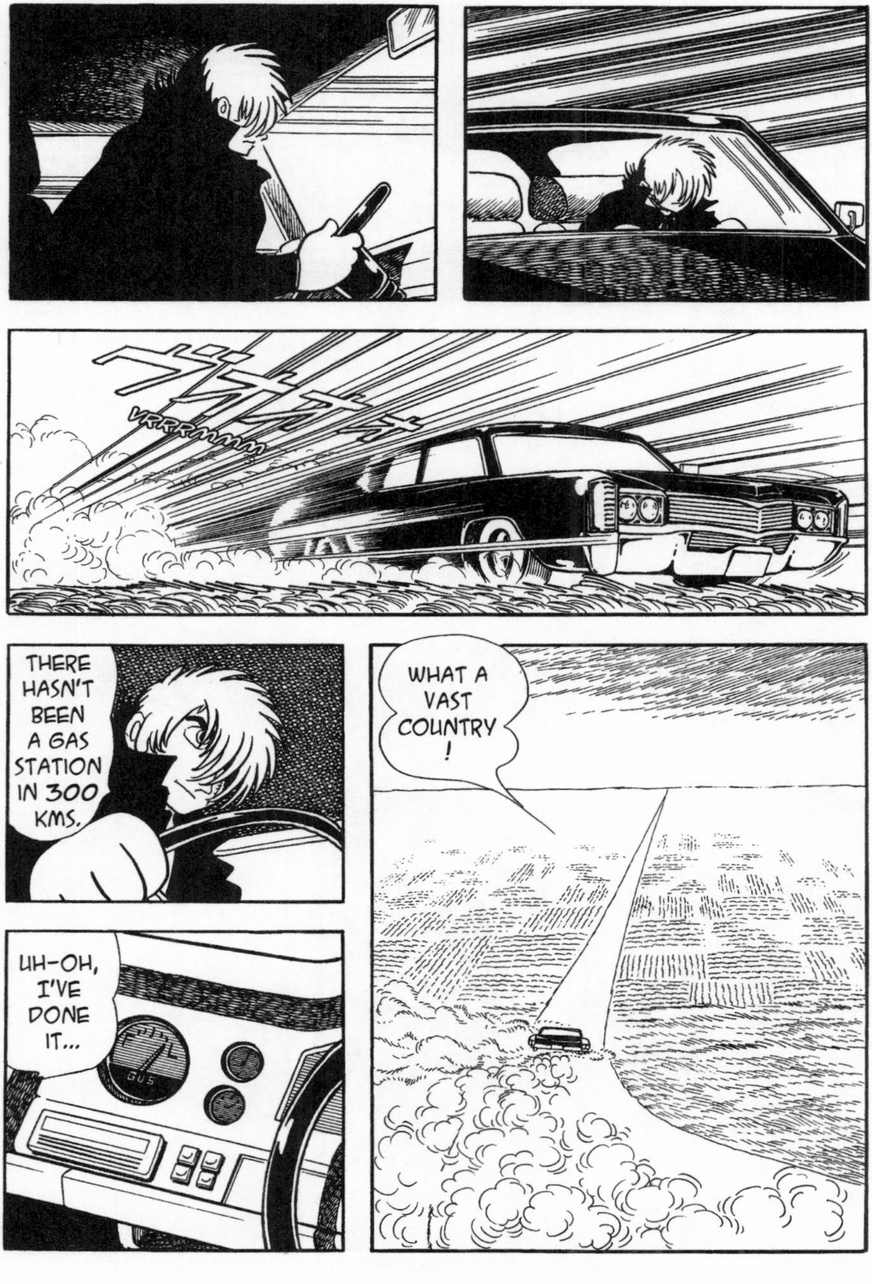
ヴオオオオ
VRRRMMMM
WHAT A VAST COUNTRY !
THERE HASN'T BEEN A GAS STATION IN 300 KMS.
UH-OH, I'VE DONE IT...

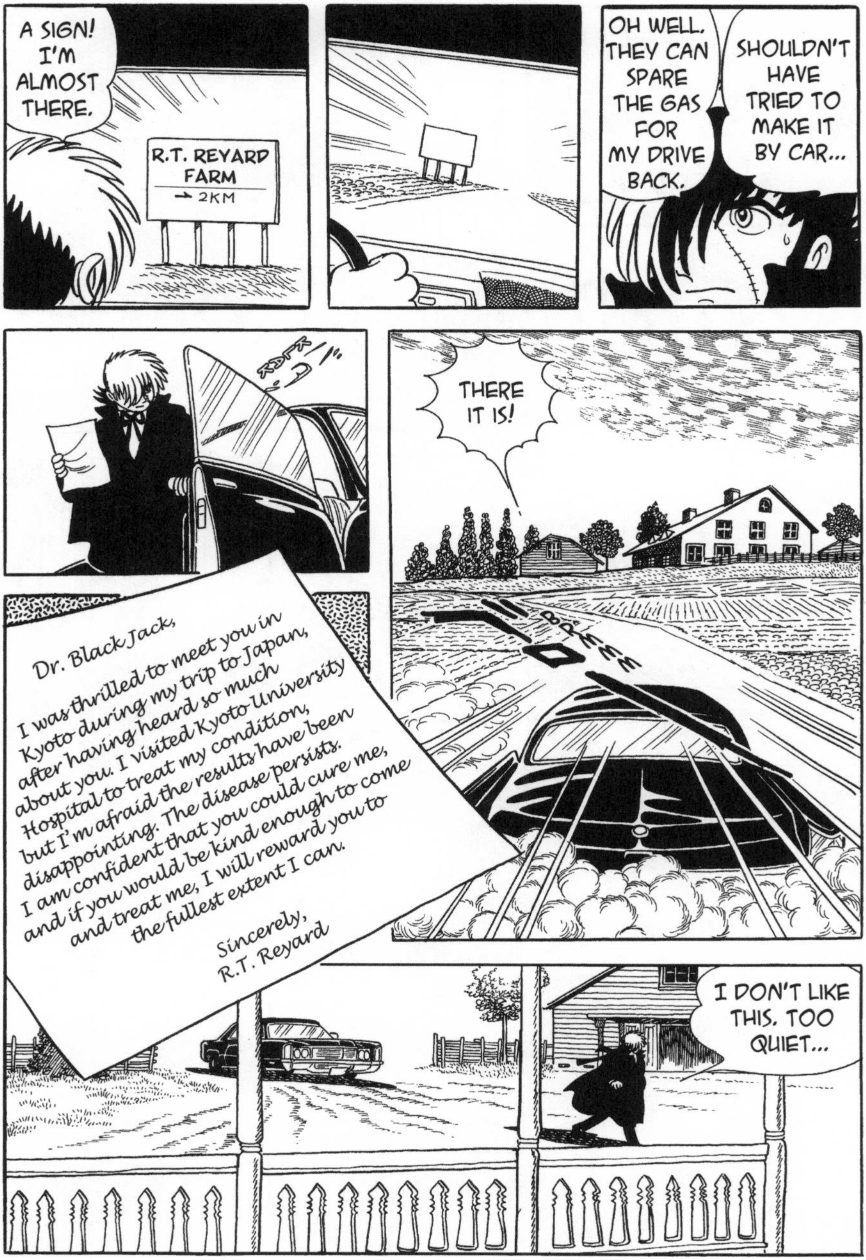
SHOULDN'T HAVE TRIED TO MAKE IT BY CAR...
OH WELL. THEY CAN SPARE THE GAS FOR MY DRIVE BACK.
R.T. REYARD FARM → 2KM
A SIGN! I'M ALMOST THERE.
THERE IT IS!
Dr. Black Jack,
I was thrilled to meet you in Kyoto during my trip to Japan, after having heard so much about you. I visited Kyoto University Hospital to treat my condition, but I'm afraid the results have been disappointing. The disease persists. I am confident that you could cure me, and if you would be kind enough to come and treat me, I will reward you to the fullest extent I can.
Sincerely,
R.T. Reyard
I DON'T LIKE THIS. TOO QUIET...

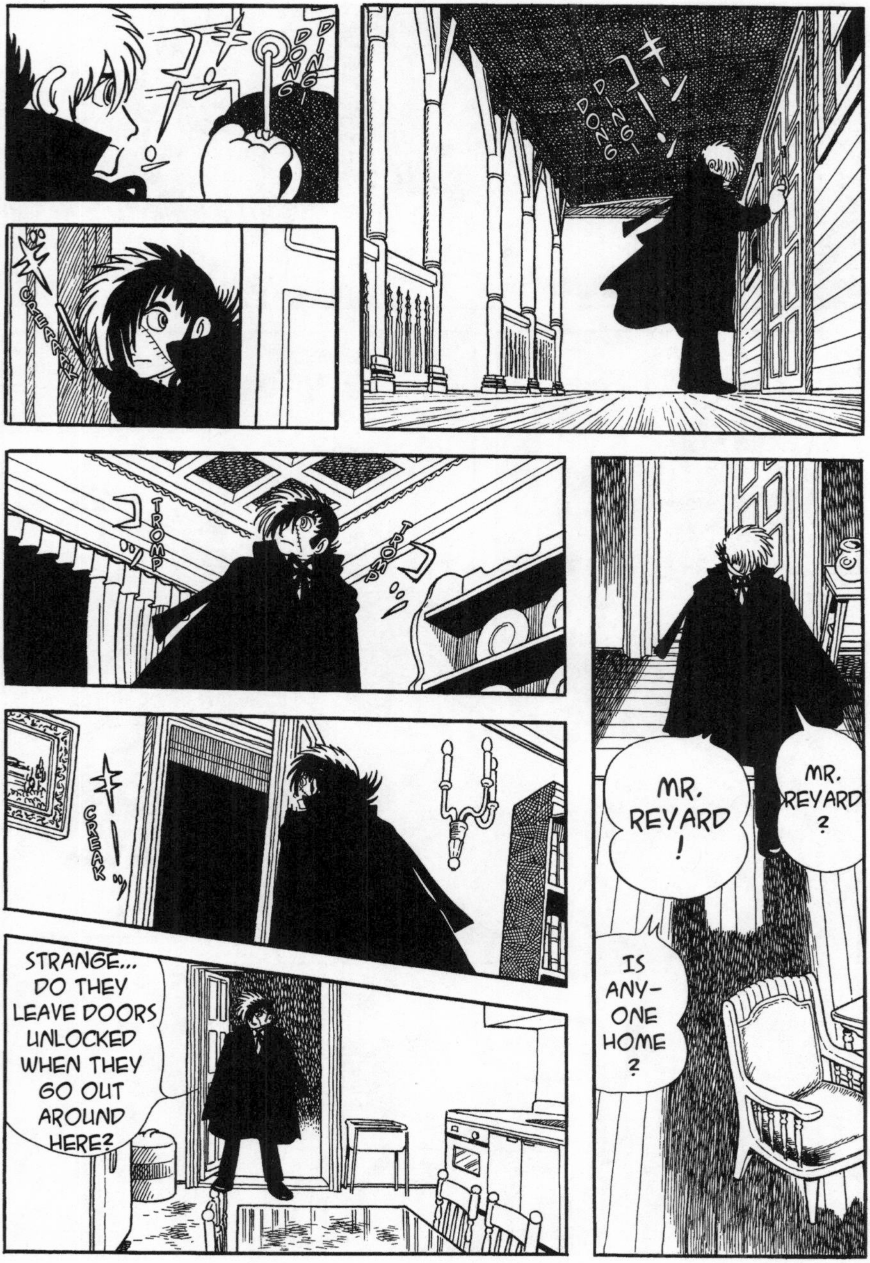
DING DONG
DING DONG
CREAAAK
MR. REYARD!
MR. REYARD?
IS ANYONE HOME?
TROMP
TROMP
CREAK
STRANGE... DO THEY LEAVE DOORS UNLOCKED WHEN THEY GO OUT AROUND HERE?

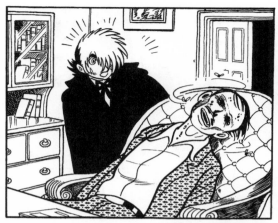

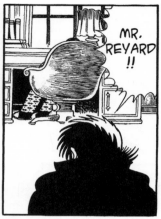

MR. REYARD!!
DEAD... AND HAVE BEEN FOR DAYS...
THE WHOLE FAMILY!
NO WOUNDS... SO IT WASN'T A ROBBERY, OR WILD BEASTS...

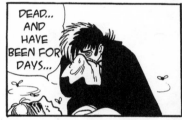

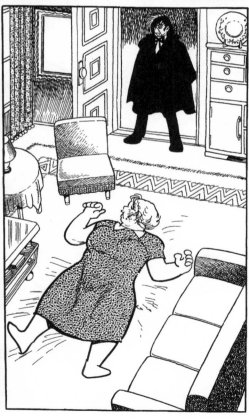

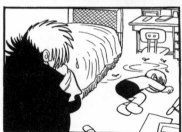

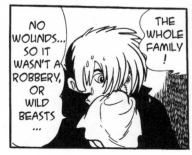

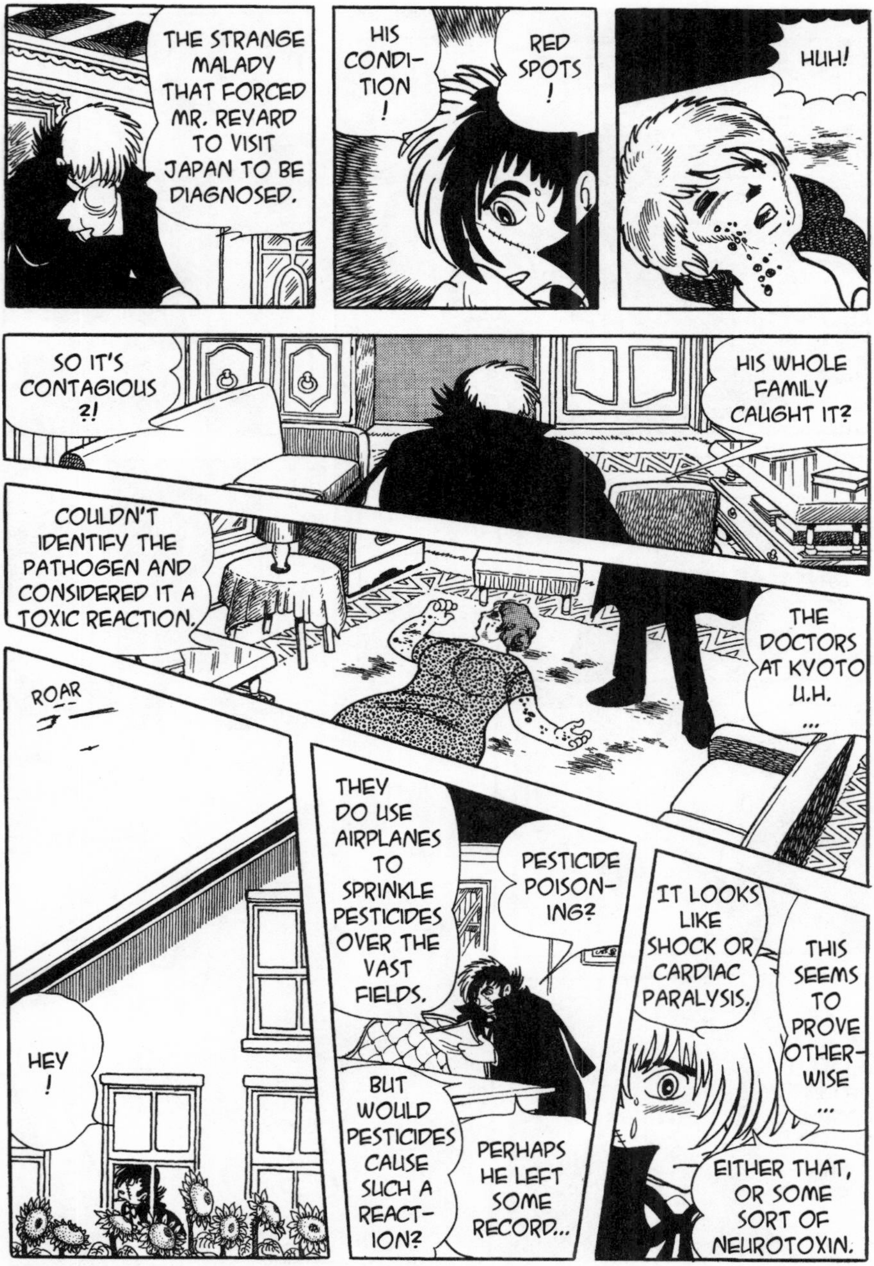
HUH!
RED SPOTS !
HIS CONDITION !
THE STRANGE MALADY THAT FORCED MR. REYARD TO VISIT JAPAN TO BE DIAGNOSED.
HIS WHOLE FAMILY CAUGHT IT?
SO IT'S CONTAGIOUS ?!
THE DOCTORS AT KYOTO U.H. ...
COULDN'T IDENTIFY THE PATHOGEN AND CONSIDERED IT A TOXIC REACTION.
IT LOOKS LIKE SHOCK OR CARDIAC PARALYSIS.
THIS SEEMS TO PROVE OTHERWISE ...
EITHER THAT, OR SOME SORT OF NEUROTOXIN.
PESTICIDE POISONING?
THEY DO USE AIRPLANES TO SPRINKLE PESTICIDES OVER THE VAST FIELDS.
BUT WOULD PESTICIDES CAUSE SUCH A REACTION?
PERHAPS HE LEFT SOME RECORD...
ROAR
HEY !

BRRMMMM
WHAT LUCK! A PRIVATE AIRCRAFT.
おーい
HULLOO!
おーい
おーい
HULLOO!
WHRRRRRR
WHOA!!
BOOM

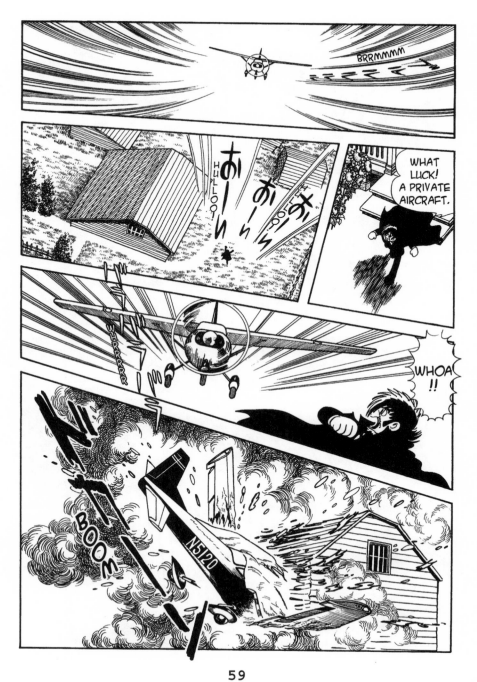

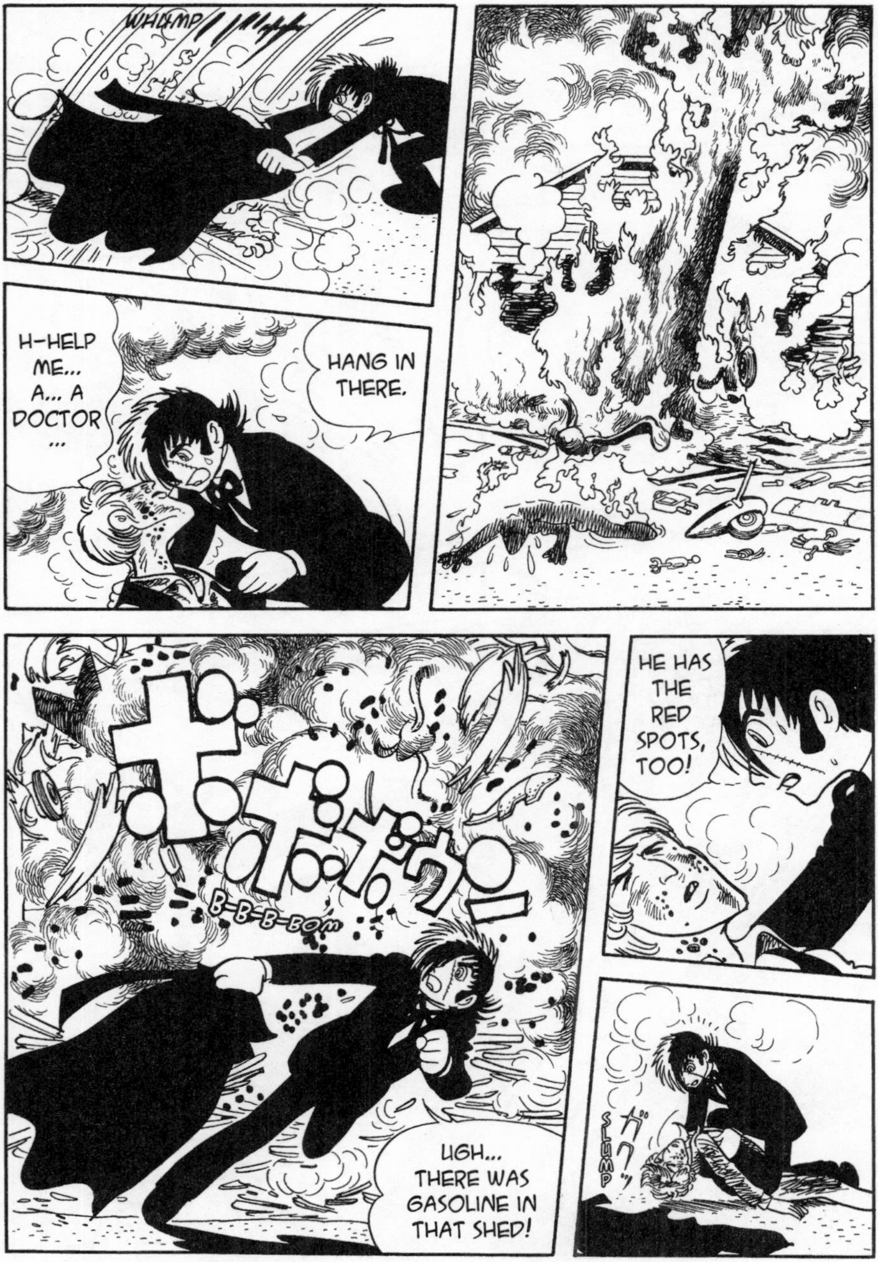
WHUMP
H-HELP ME... A... A DOCTOR ...
HANG IN THERE.
HE HAS THE RED SPOTS, TOO!
SLUMP
B-B-B-BOM
UGH... THERE WAS GASOLINE IN THAT SHED!

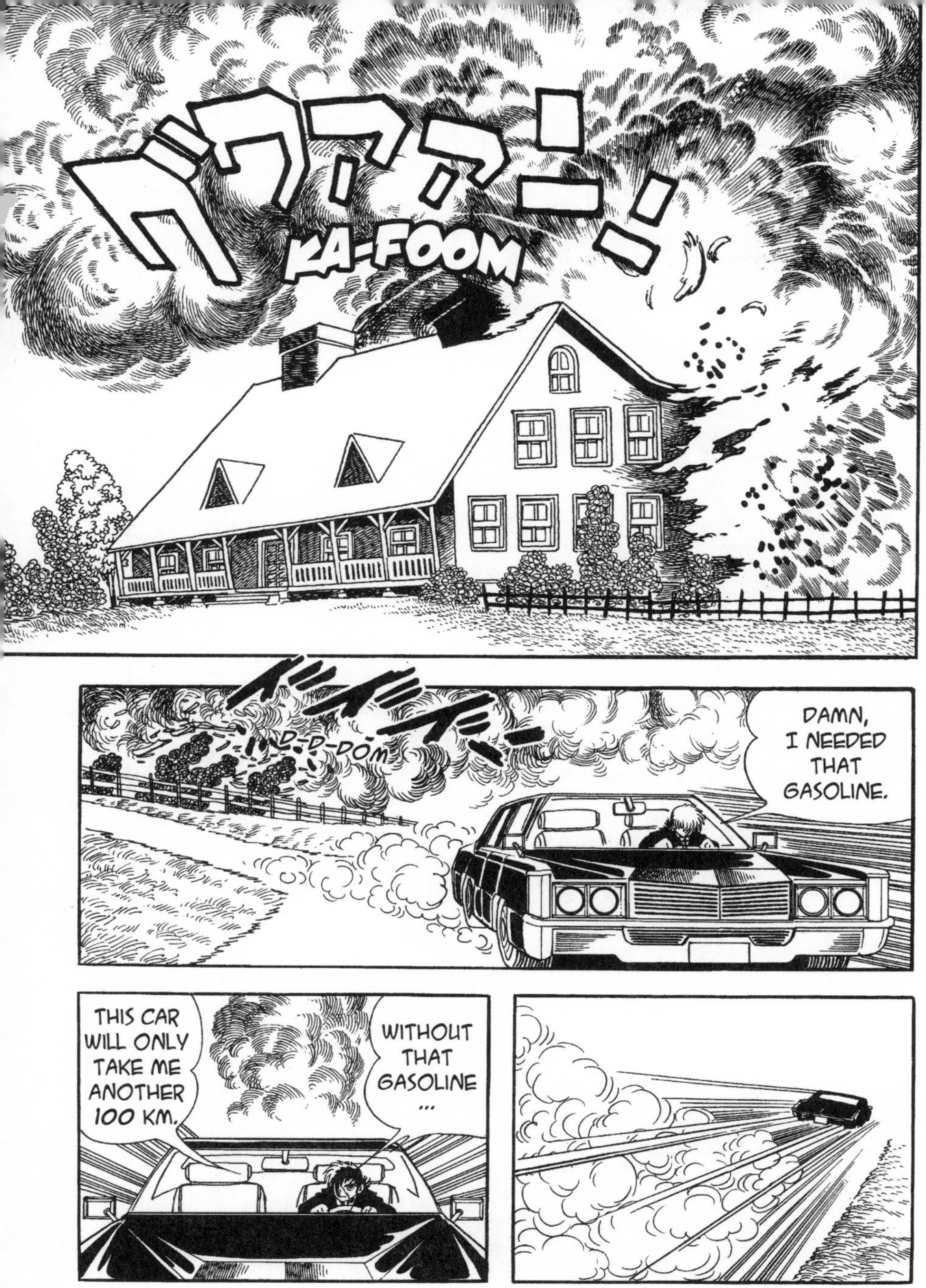
KA-FOOM
D-D-DOM
DAMN, I NEEDED THAT GASOLINE.
WITHOUT THAT GASOLINE ...
THIS CAR WILL ONLY TAKE ME ANOTHER 100 KM.

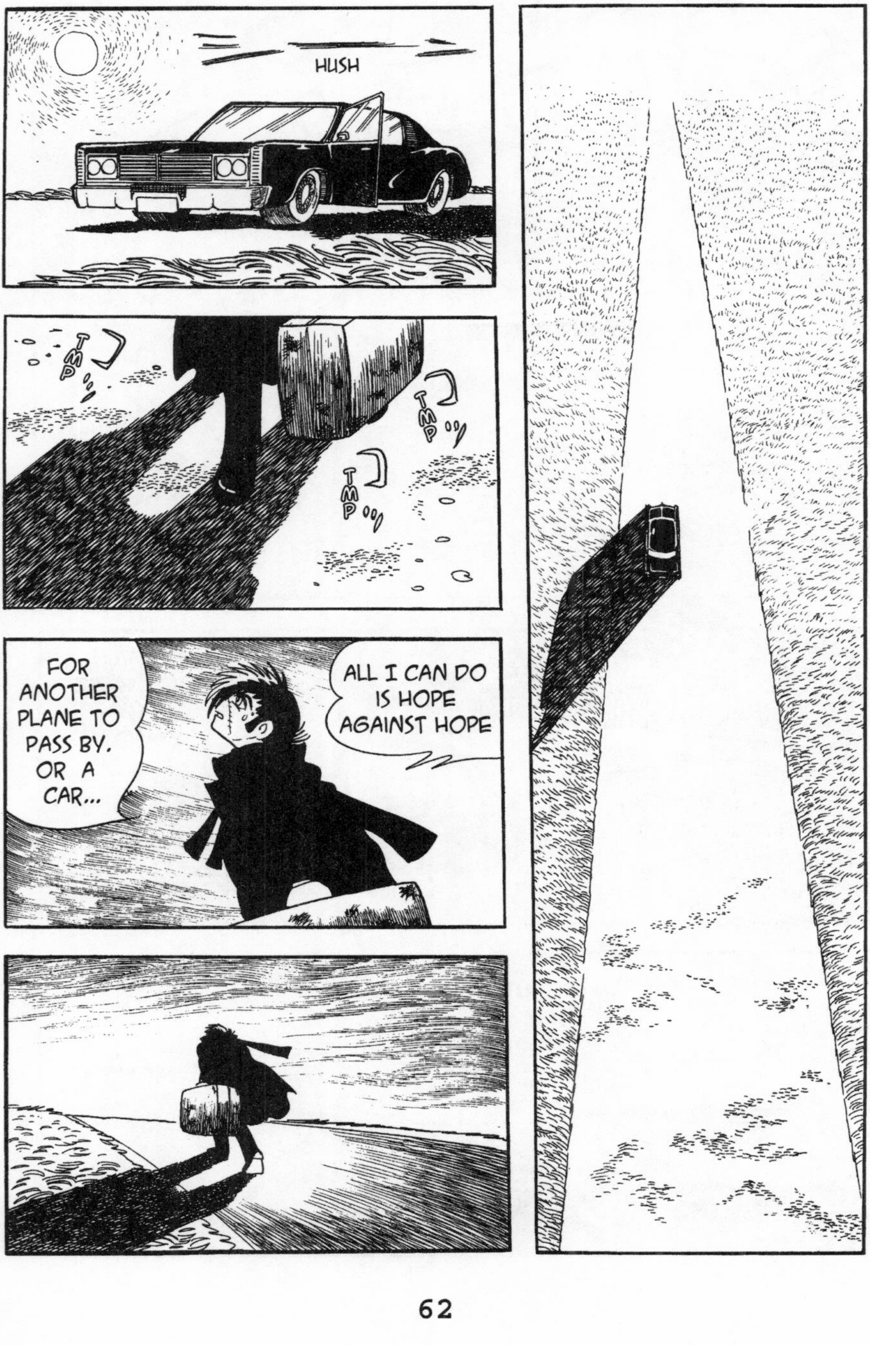
HUSH
TMP
TMP
TMP
ALL I CAN DO IS HOPE AGAINST HOPE
FOR ANOTHER PLANE TO PASS BY. OR A CAR...

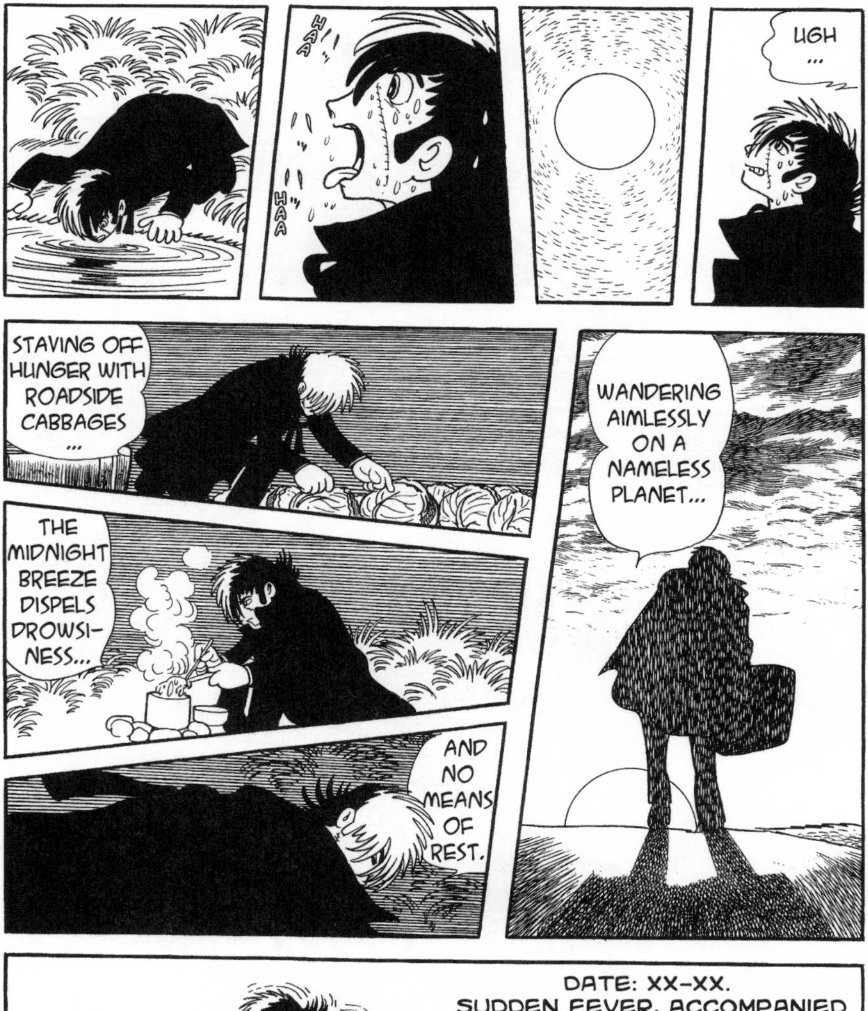
UGH ...
HAA HAA
WANDERING AIMLESSLY ON A NAMELESS PLANET...
STAVING OFF HUNGER WITH ROADSIDE CABBAGES ...
THE MIDNIGHT BREEZE DISPELS DROWSI-NESS...
AND NO MEANS OF REST.
DATE: XX-XX.
SUDDEN FEVER, ACCOMPANIED BY SHARP PAIN IN LOWER RIGHT ABDOMINAL AREA.
SUBSIDES AT NIGHT.

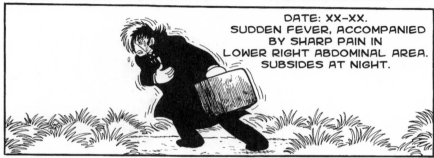

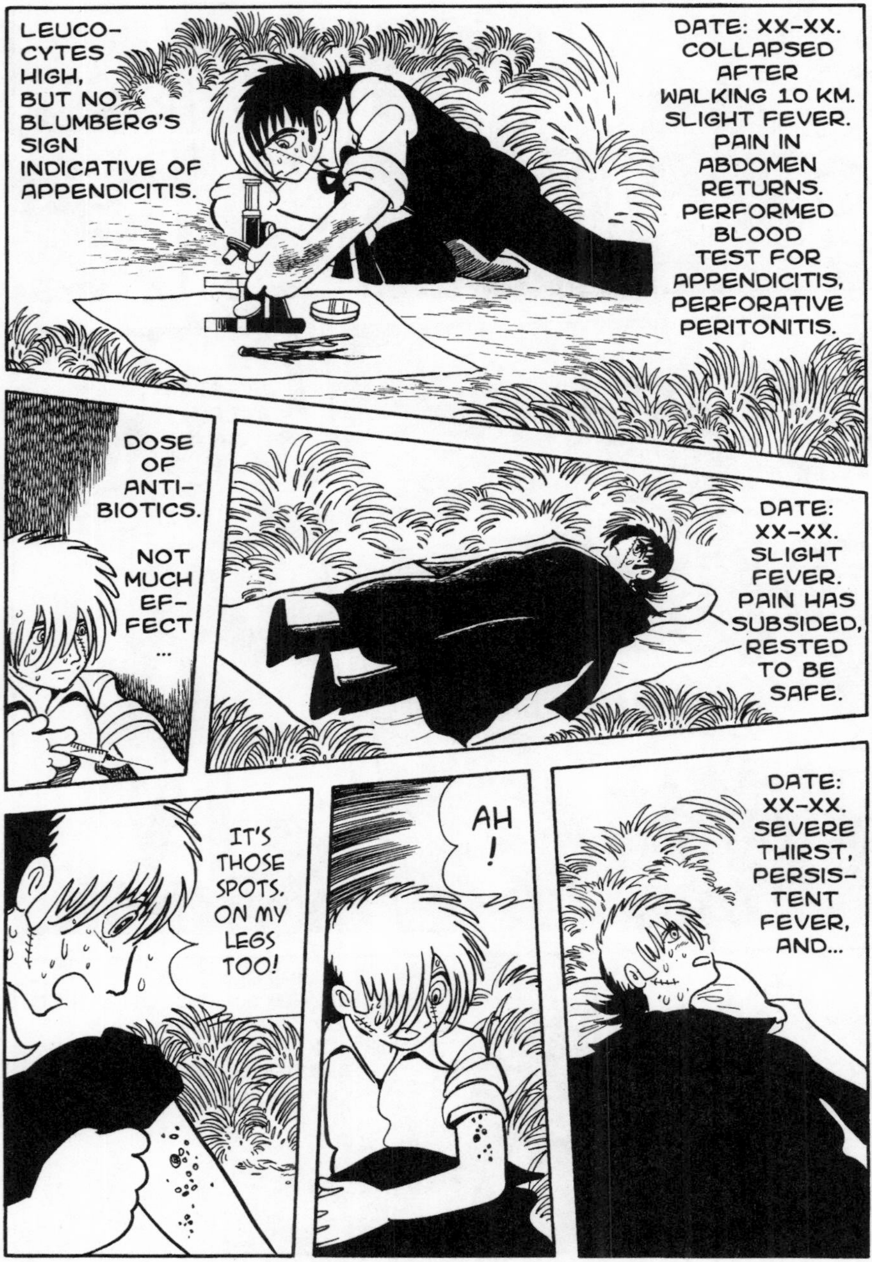
DATE: XX-XX. COLLAPSED AFTER WALKING 10 KM. SLIGHT FEVER. PAIN IN ABDOMEN RETURNS. PERFORMED BLOOD TEST FOR APPENDICITIS, PERFORATIVE PERITONITIS.
LEUCO-CYTES HIGH, BUT NO BLUMBERG'S SIGN INDICATIVE OF APPENDICITIS.
DATE: XX-XX. SLIGHT FEVER. PAIN HAS SUBSIDED, RESTED TO BE SAFE.
DOSE OF ANTI-BIOTICS.
NOT MUCH EF-FECT ...
DATE: XX-XX. SEVERE THIRST, PERSIS-TENT FEVER, AND...
AH !
IT'S THOSE SPOTS. ON MY LEGS TOO!

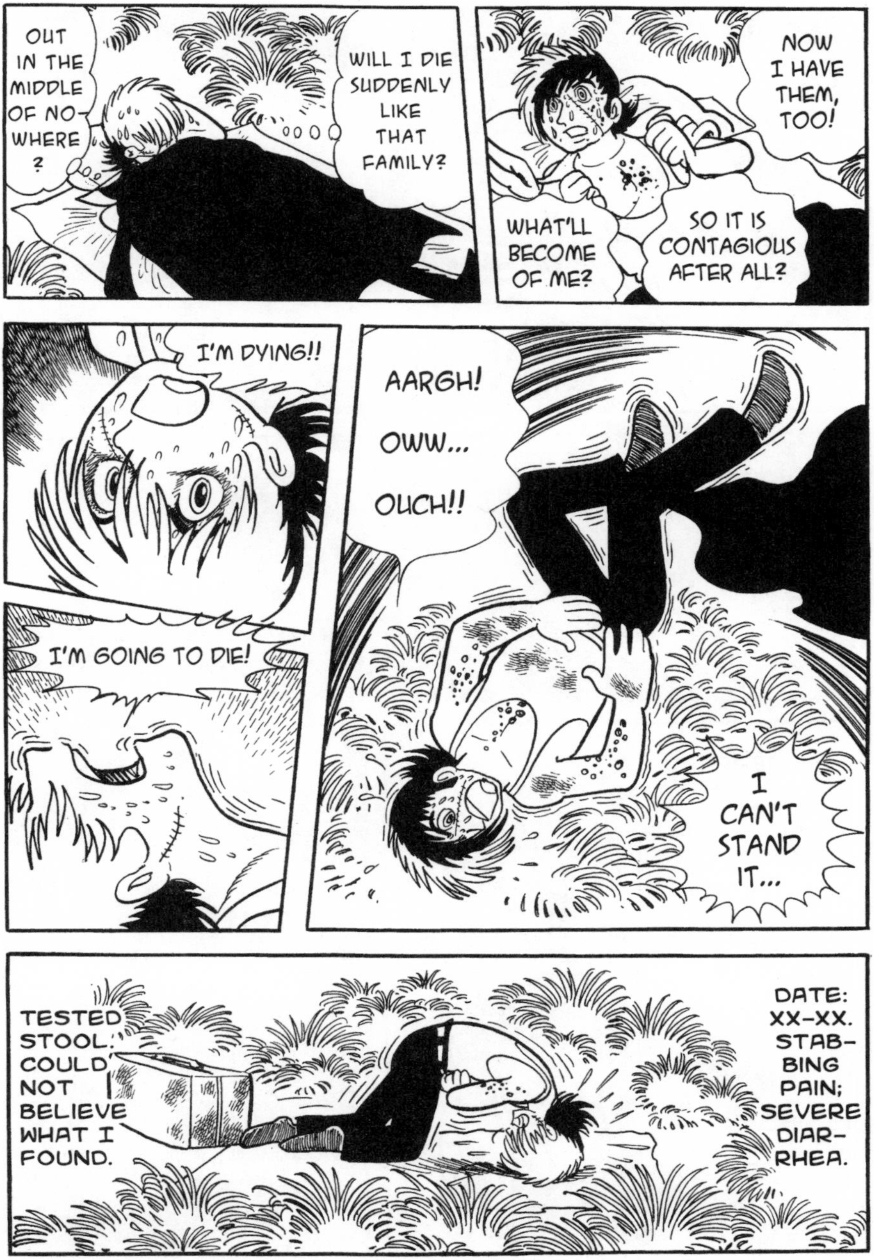
NOW I HAVE THEM, TOO!
SO IT IS CONTAGIOUS AFTER ALL?
WHAT'LL BECOME OF ME?
WILL I DIE SUDDENLY LIKE THAT FAMILY?
OUT IN THE MIDDLE OF NO-WHERE?
AARGH! OWW... OUCH!!
I CAN'T STAND IT...
I'M DYING!!
I'M GOING TO DIE!
DATE: XX-XX. STAB-BING PAIN; SEVERE DIAR-RHEA.
TESTED STOOL: COULD NOT BELIEVE WHAT I FOUND.

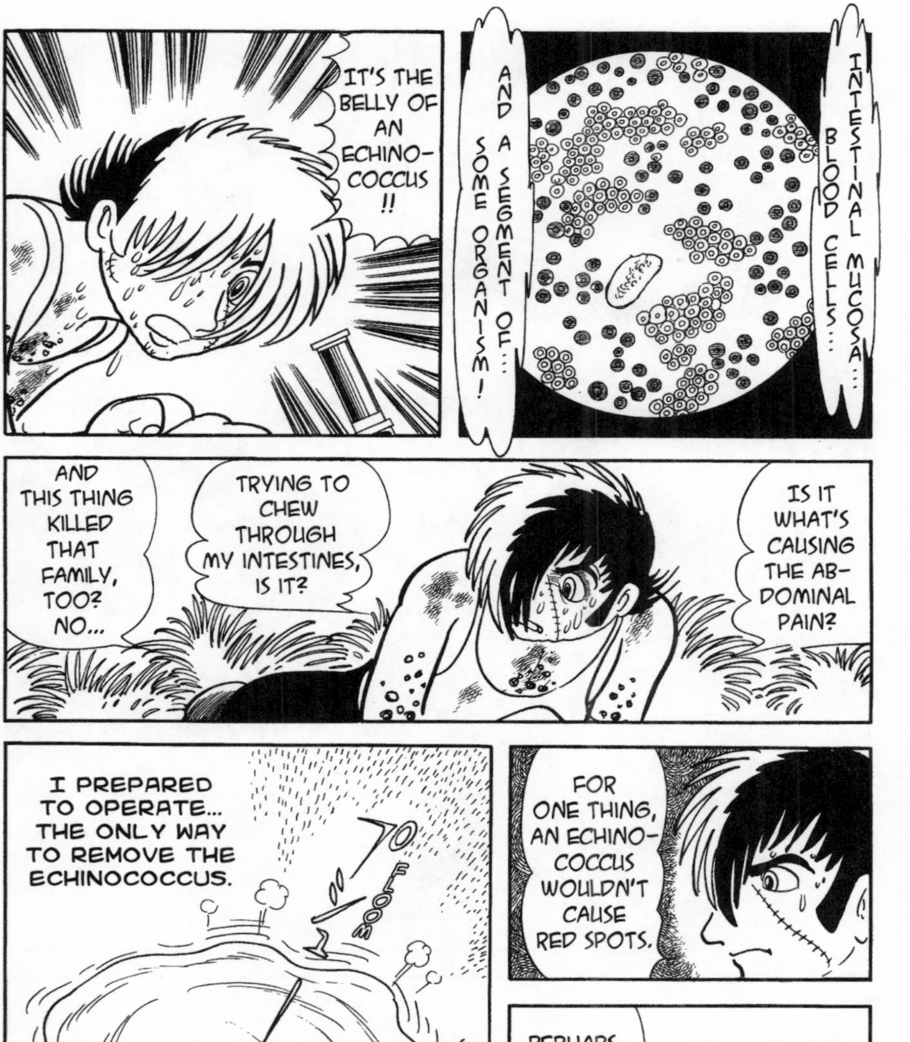

INTESTINAL MUCOSA... BLOOD CELLS...
AND A SEGMENT OF... SOME ORGANISM!
IT'S THE BELLY OF AN ECHINO-COCCUS !!
IS IT WHAT'S CAUSING THE AB-DOMINAL PAIN?
TRYING TO CHEW THROUGH MY INTESTINES, IS IT?
AND THIS THING KILLED THAT FAMILY, TOO? NO...
FOR ONE THING, AN ECHINO-COCCUS WOULDN'T CAUSE RED SPOTS.
PERHAPS IT'S AN UNKNOWN STRAIN OF ECHINO-COCCUS...
I PREPARED TO OPERATE... THE ONLY WAY TO REMOVE THE ECHINOCOCCUS.
FLOOM

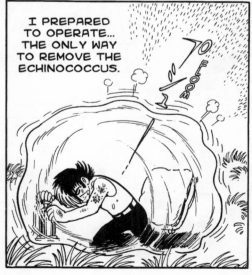

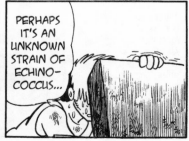

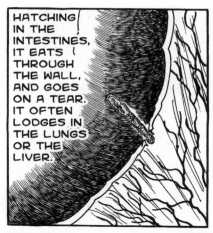

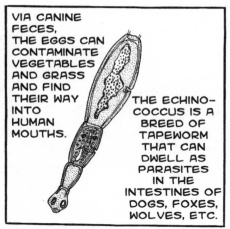

THE ECHINO-COCCUS IS A BREED OF TAPEWORM THAT CAN DWELL AS PARASITES IN THE INTESTINES OF DOGS, FOXES, WOLVES, ETC.
VIA CANINE FECES, THE EGGS CAN CONTAMINATE VEGETABLES AND GRASS AND FIND THEIR WAY INTO HUMAN MOUTHS.
HATCHING IN THE INTESTINES, IT EATS THROUGH THE WALL, AND GOES ON A TEAR. IT OFTEN LODGES IN THE LUNGS OR THE LIVER.
THE POISON IT EXCRETES OFTEN SENDS ITS HUMAN HOST INTO SHOCK.
PERHAPS THE RED SPOTS AND THE FAMILY'S DEMISE OWE TO A BRAND-NEW MUTANT STRAIN OF ECHINOCOCCUS.
FAR FROM STERILE. I HAVE NO CHOICE ...
LET US BEGIN !
LOCAL ANES-THETIC !
...

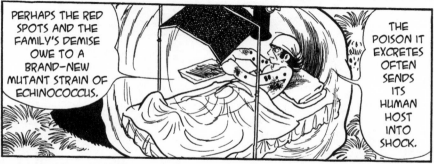

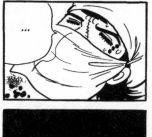

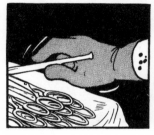

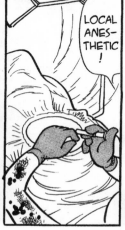

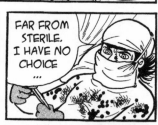

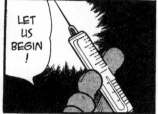

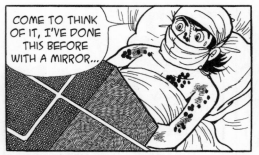

COME TO THINK OF IT, I'VE DONE THIS BEFORE WITH A MIRROR...
ギ
AGH !
I'M UNDER THE PERITONEUM ...
FUNNY. WHEN YOU'RE PREPARED TO DIE, FEAR AND PAIN VANISH.

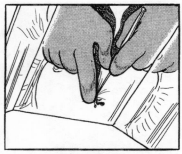

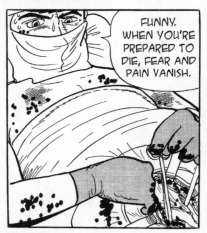

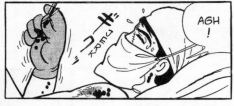

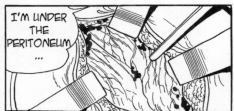

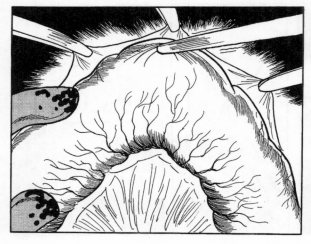

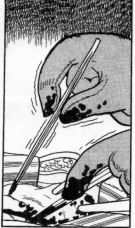

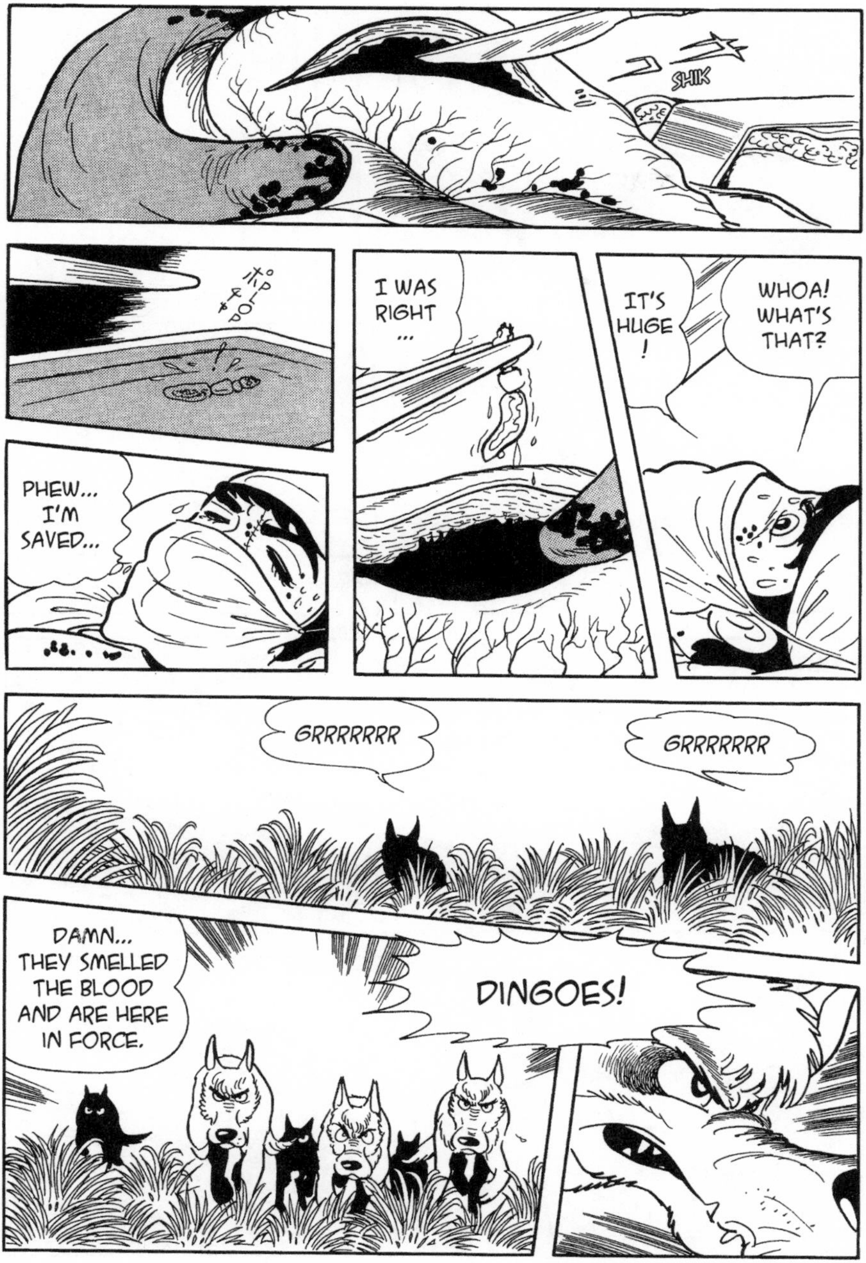
SHIK
WHOA! WHAT'S THAT?
IT'S HUGE!
I WAS RIGHT ...
PLOP
PHEW... I'M SAVED...
GRRRRRRR
GRRRRRRR
DINGOES!
DAMN... THEY SMELLED THE BLOOD AND ARE HERE IN FORCE.

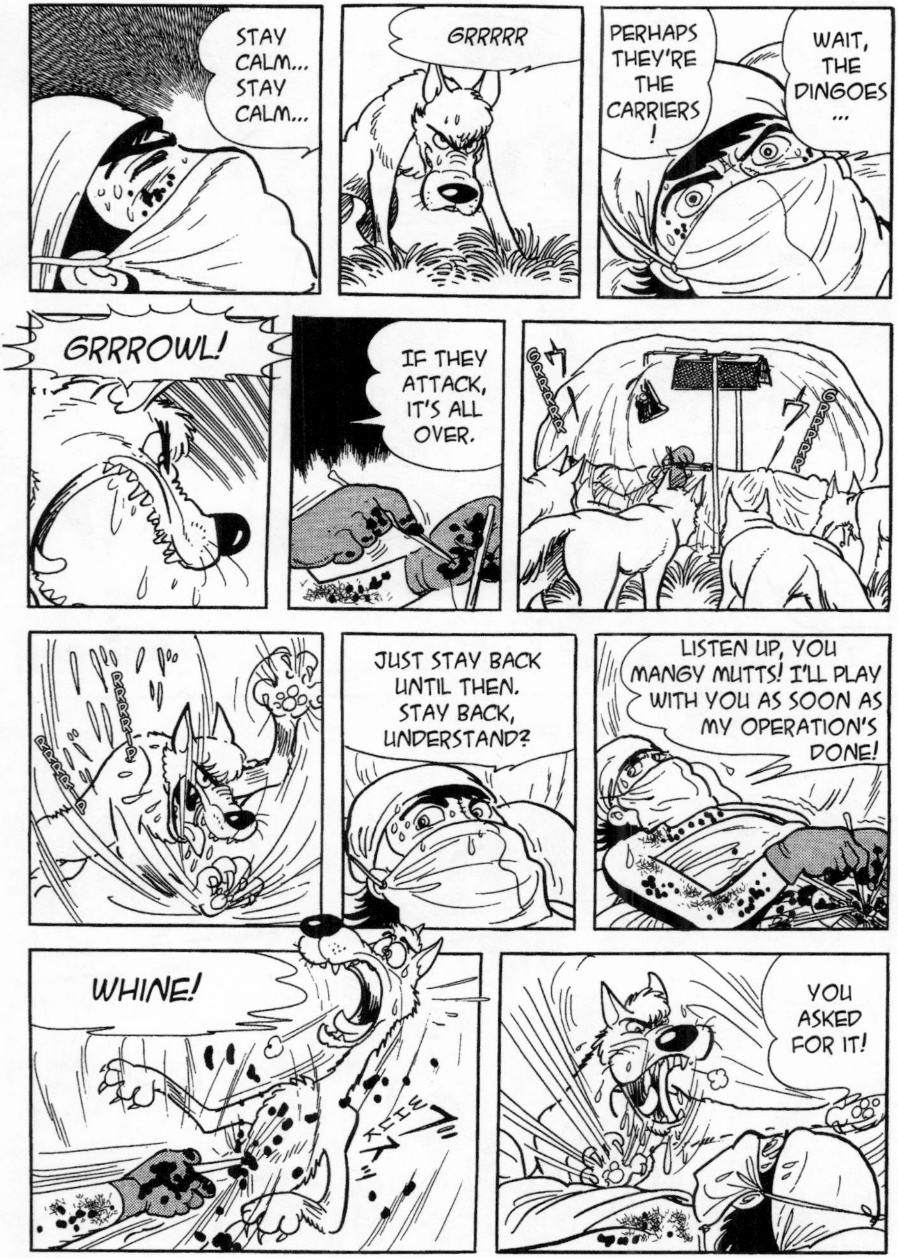
WAIT, THE DINGOES ...
PERHAPS THEY'RE THE CARRIERS !
GRRRRR
STAY CALM... STAY CALM...
IF THEY ATTACK, IT'S ALL OVER.
GRRROWL!
LISTEN UP, YOU MANGY MUTTS! I'LL PLAY WITH YOU AS SOON AS MY OPERATION'S DONE!
JUST STAY BACK UNTIL THEN. STAY BACK, UNDERSTAND?
YOU ASKED FOR IT!
WHINE!

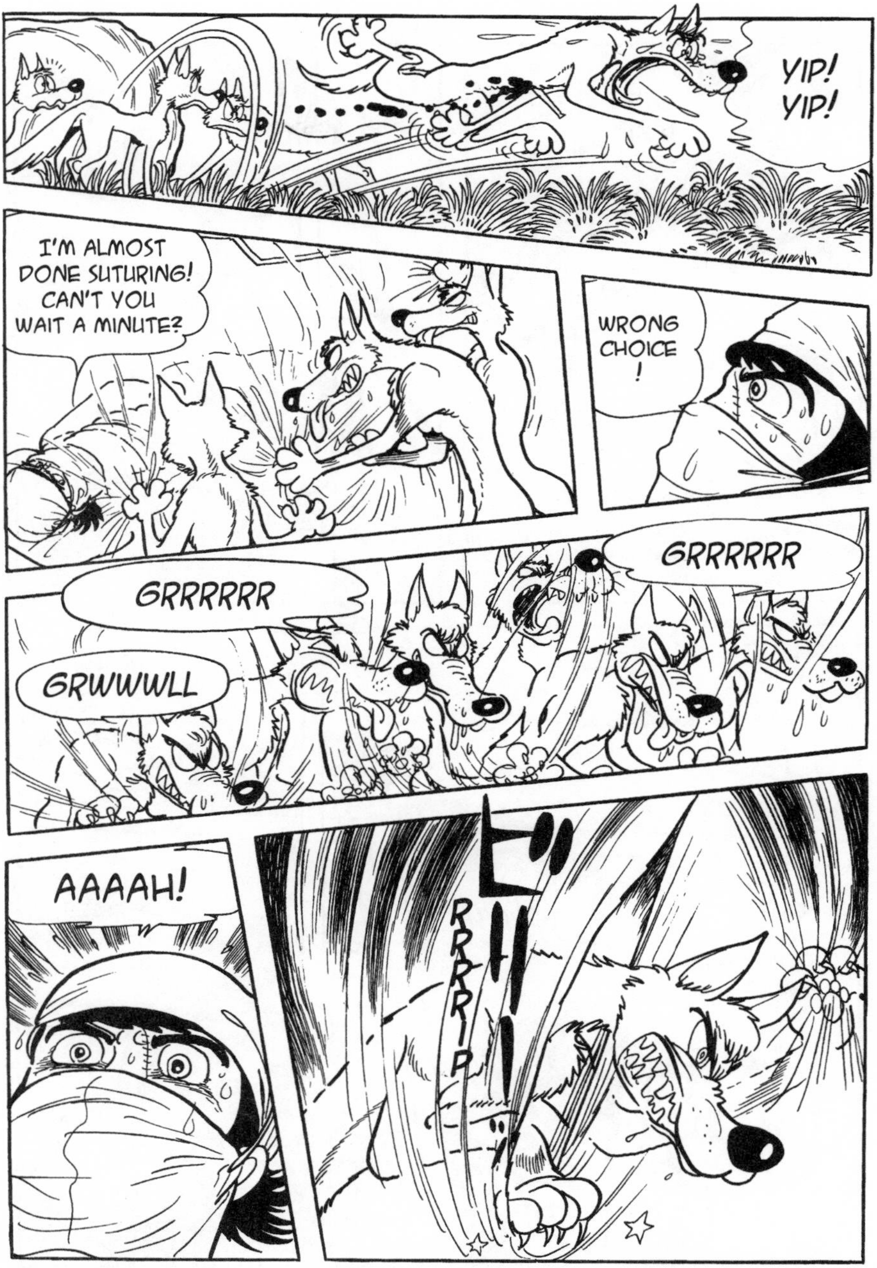
YIP! YIP!
WRONG CHOICE !
I'M ALMOST DONE SUTURING! CAN'T YOU WAIT A MINUTE?
GRRRRRR
GRRRRRR
GRWWWLL
RRRRRIP
AAAAH!

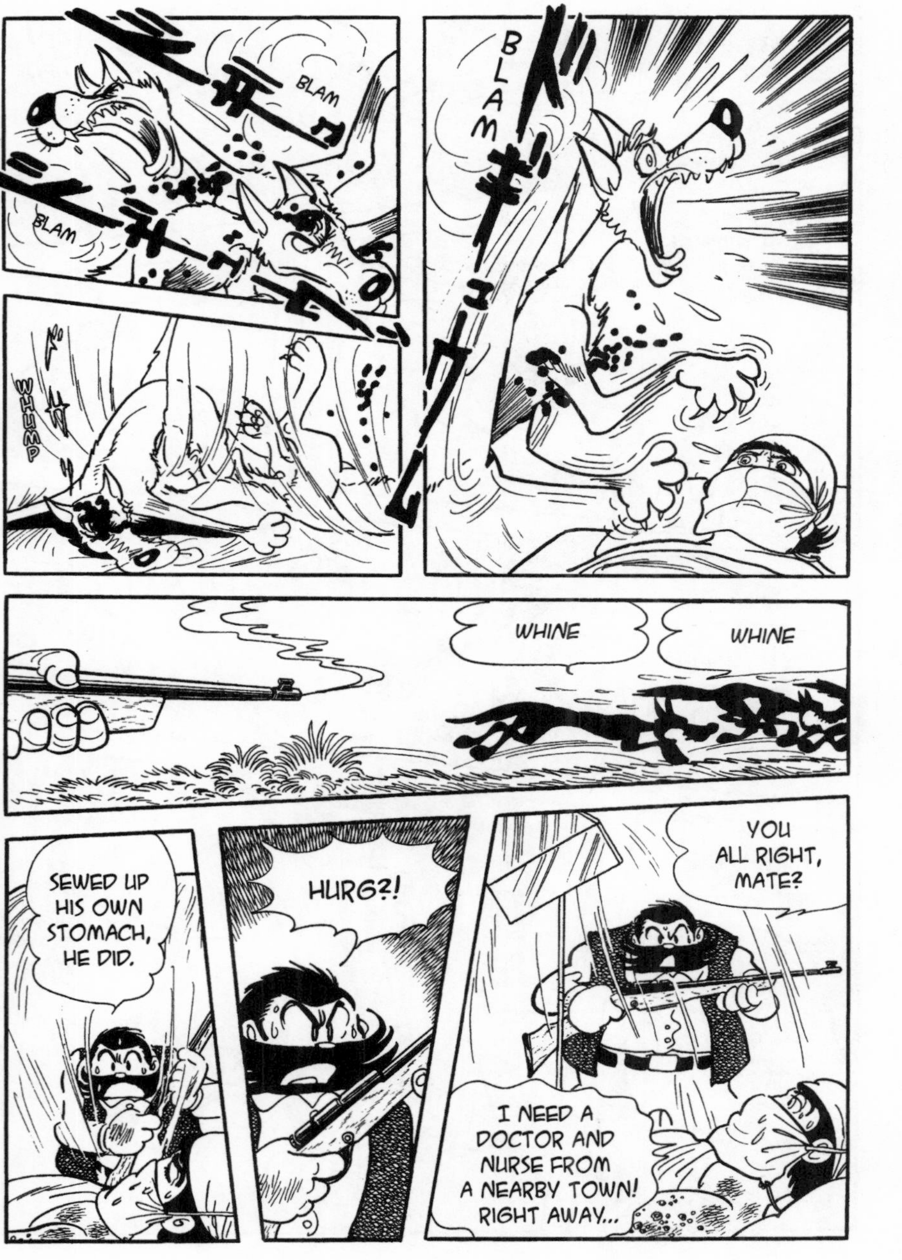
BLAM
BLAM
BLAM
WHUMP
WHINE
WHINE
YOU ALL RIGHT, MATE?
I NEED A DOCTOR AND NURSE FROM A NEARBY TOWN! RIGHT AWAY...
HURG?!
SEWED UP HIS OWN STOMACH, HE DID.

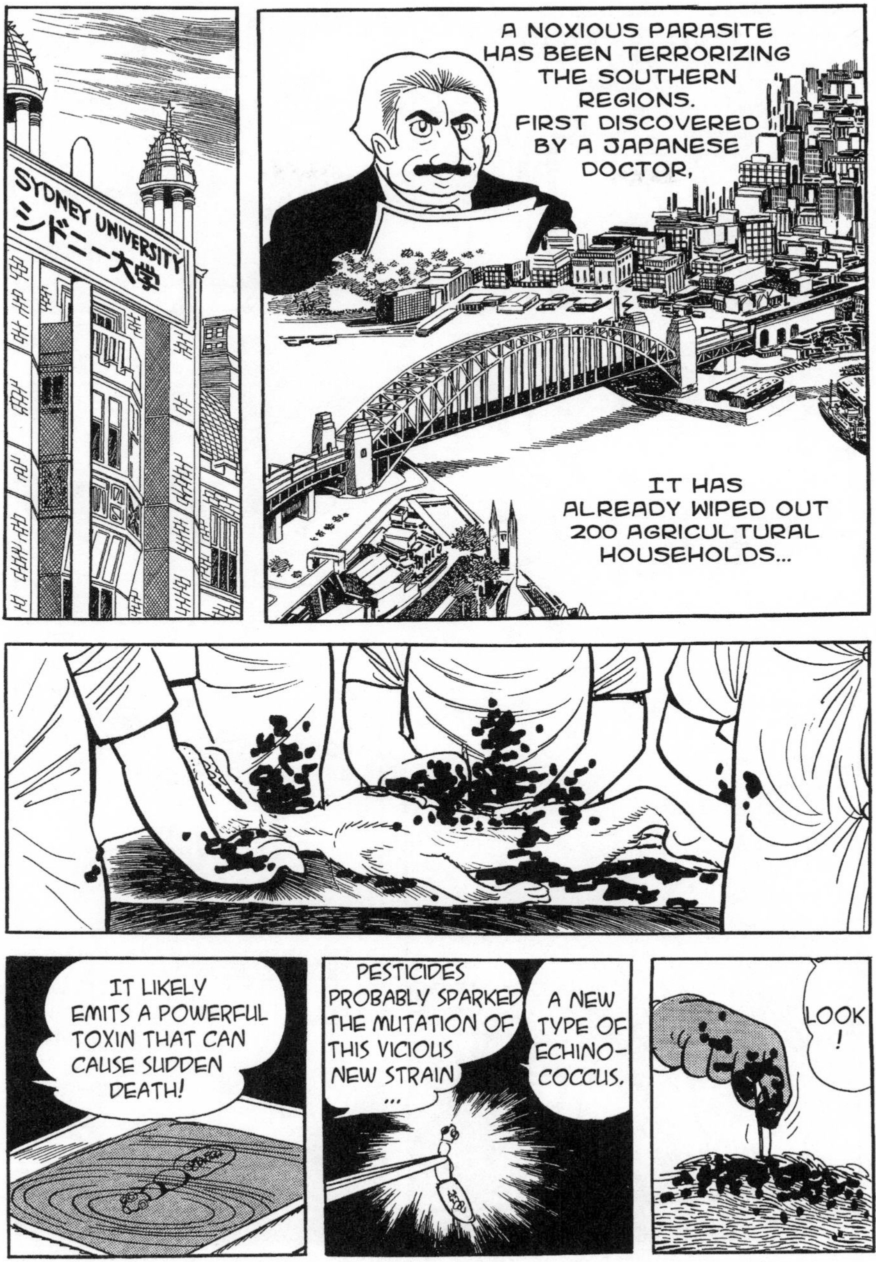
A NOXIOUS PARASITE HAS BEEN TERRORIZING THE SOUTHERN REGIONS. FIRST DISCOVERED BY A JAPANESE DOCTOR,
IT HAS ALREADY WIPED OUT 200 AGRICULTURAL HOUSEHOLDS...
SYDNEY UNIVERSITY
シドニー大学
LOOK!
A NEW TYPE OF ECHINO-COCCUS.
PESTICIDES PROBABLY SPARKED THE MUTATION OF THIS VICIOUS NEW STRAIN...
IT LIKELY EMITS A POWERFUL TOXIN THAT CAN CAUSE SUDDEN DEATH!

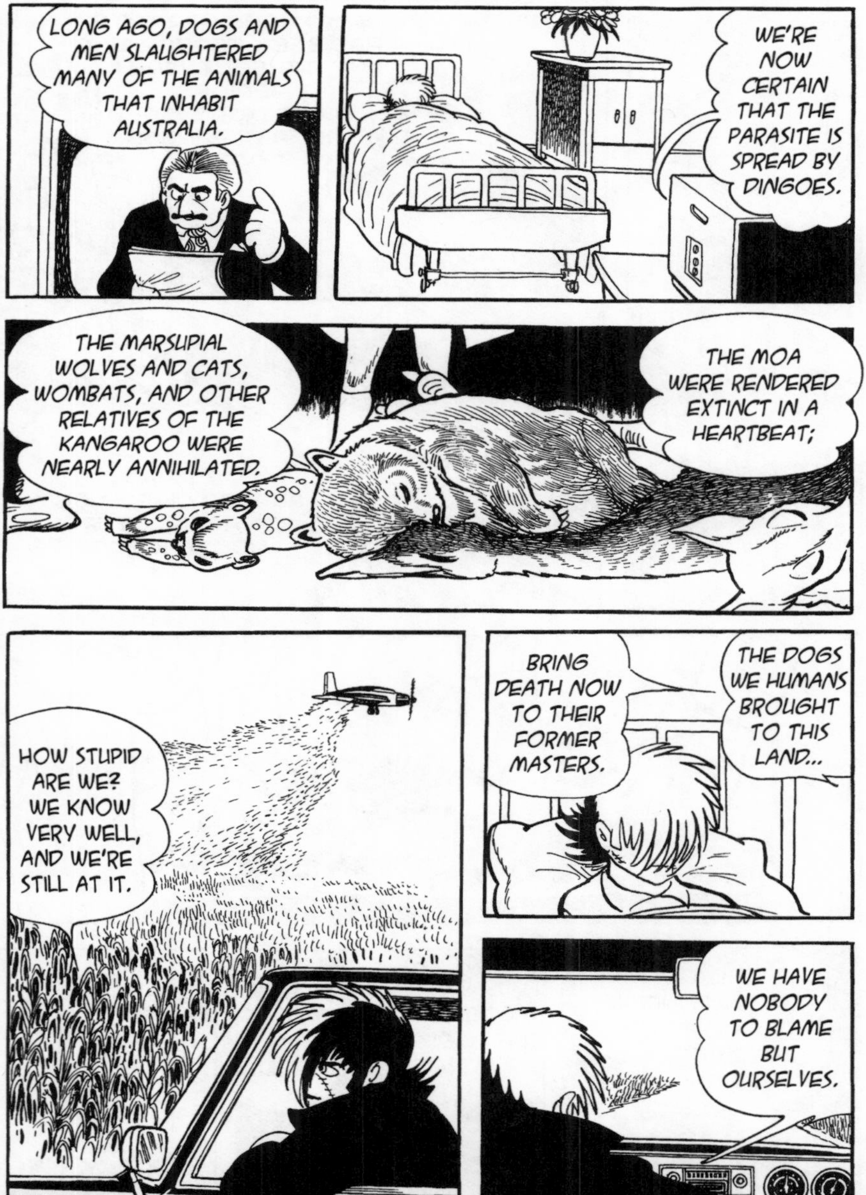
WE'RE NOW CERTAIN THAT THE PARASITE IS SPREAD BY DINGOES.
LONG AGO, DOGS AND MEN SLAUGHTERED MANY OF THE ANIMALS THAT INHABIT AUSTRALIA.
THE MOA WERE RENDERED EXTINCT IN A HEARTBEAT;
THE MARSUPIAL WOLVES AND CATS, WOMBATS, AND OTHER RELATIVES OF THE KANGAROO WERE NEARLY ANNIHILATED.
THE DOGS WE HUMANS BROUGHT TO THIS LAND...
BRING DEATH NOW TO THEIR FORMER MASTERS.
WE HAVE NOBODY TO BLAME BUT OURSELVES.
HOW STUPID ARE WE? WE KNOW VERY WELL, AND WE'RE STILL AT IT.

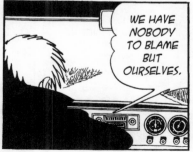

YOUR MISTAKE!

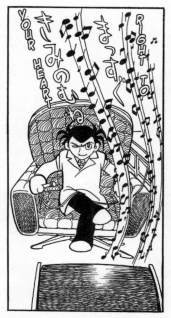

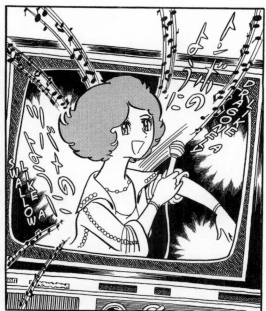

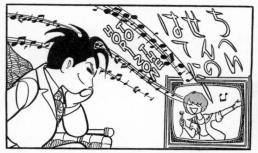

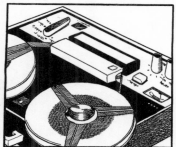

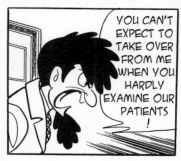

LIKE A DRAGONFLY
LIKE A SWALLOW
RIGHT TO YOUR HEART
SON! INSTEAD OF MAKING YOUR ROUNDS, YOU'RE LISTENING TO THAT SINGER AGAIN?
YOU CAN'T EXPECT TO TAKE OVER FROM ME WHEN YOU HARDLY EXAMINE OUR PATIENTS!

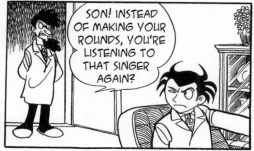

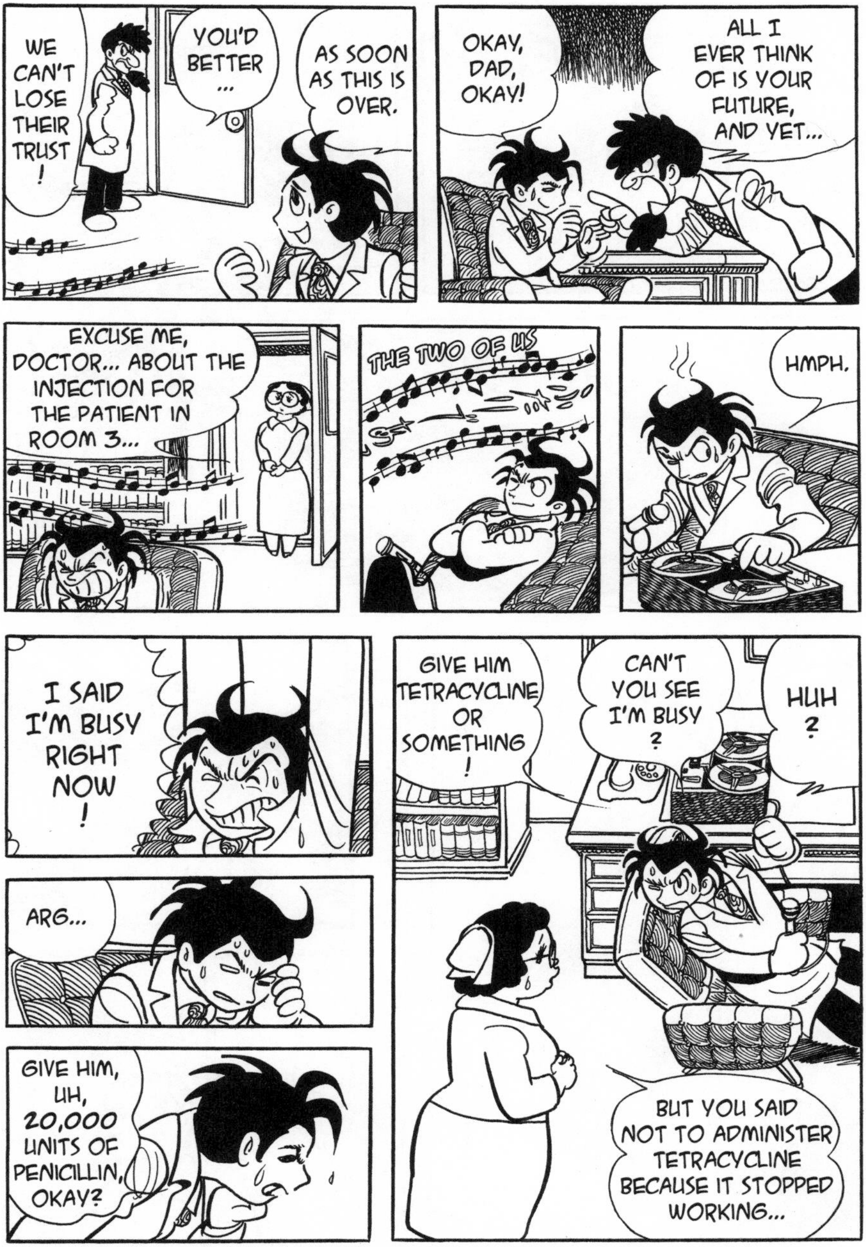
ALL I EVER THINK OF IS YOUR FUTURE, AND YET...
OKAY, DAD, OKAY!
AS SOON AS THIS IS OVER.
YOU'D BETTER ...
WE CAN'T LOSE THEIR TRUST!
HMPH.
THE TWO OF US
EXCUSE ME, DOCTOR... ABOUT THE INJECTION FOR THE PATIENT IN ROOM 3...
HUH?
CAN'T YOU SEE I'M BUSY?
GIVE HIM TETRACYCLINE OR SOMETHING!
BUT YOU SAID NOT TO ADMINISTER TETRACYCLINE BECAUSE IT STOPPED WORKING...
I SAID I'M BUSY RIGHT NOW!
ARG...
GIVE HIM, UH, 20,000 UNITS OF PENICILLIN, OKAY?

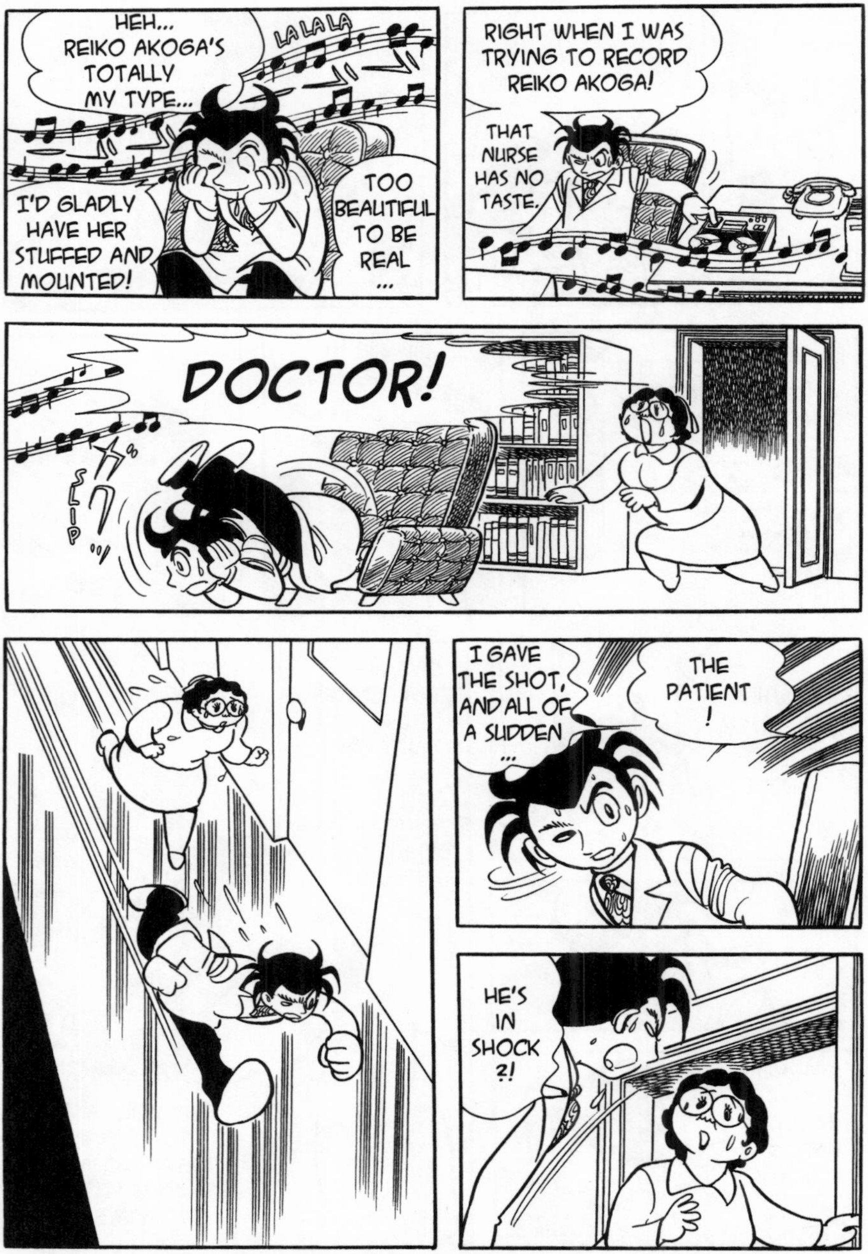
RIGHT WHEN I WAS TRYING TO RECORD REIKO AKOGA!
THAT NURSE HAS NO TASTE.
LA LA LA
HEH... REIKO AKOGA'S TOTALLY MY TYPE...
TOO BEAUTIFUL TO BE REAL ...
I'D GLADLY HAVE HER STUFFED AND MOUNTED!
DOCTOR!
SLIP
THE PATIENT !
I GAVE THE SHOT, AND ALL OF A SUDDEN ...
HE'S IN SHOCK ?!

NOTE: REIKO AKOGA, FAMILY NAME FIRST IN THE ORIGINAL, PUNS ON THE JAPANESE WORD "AKOGARE" (LONGING OR YEARNING).

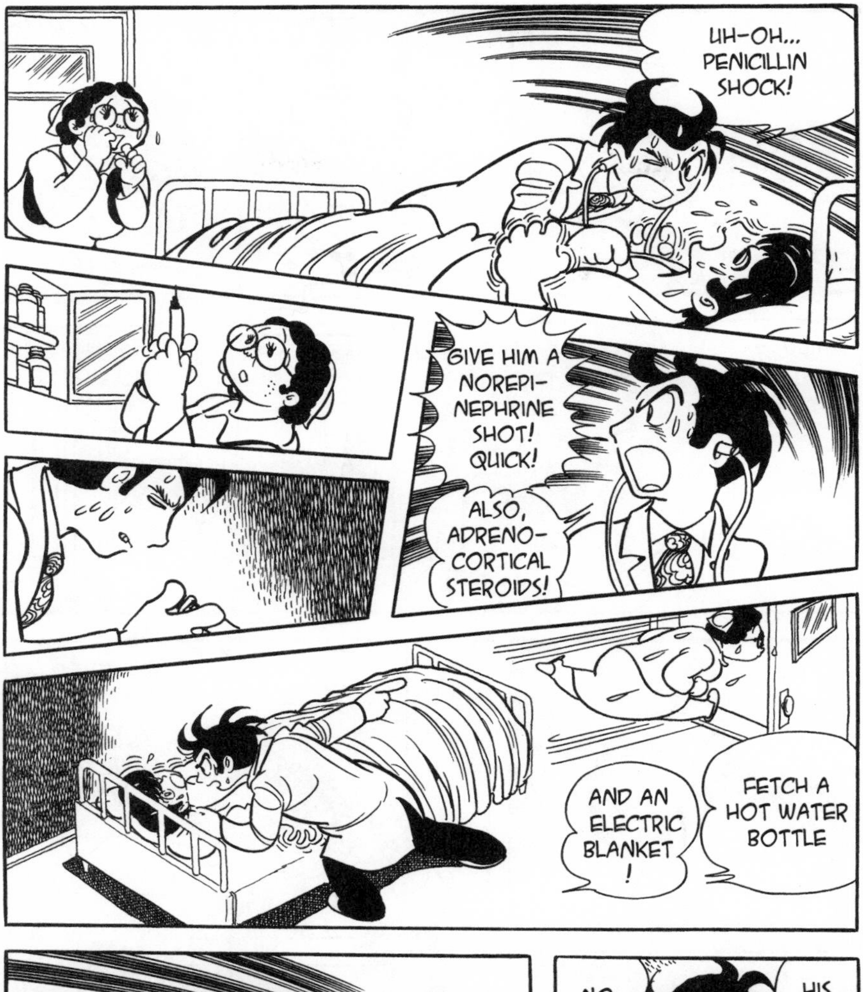
UH-OH... PENICILLIN SHOCK!
GIVE HIM A NOREPI-NEPHRINE SHOT! QUICK!
ALSO, ADRENO-CORTICAL STEROIDS!
FETCH A HOT WATER BOTTLE
AND AN ELECTRIC BLANKET !
HIS HEART ...
NO PULSE ...

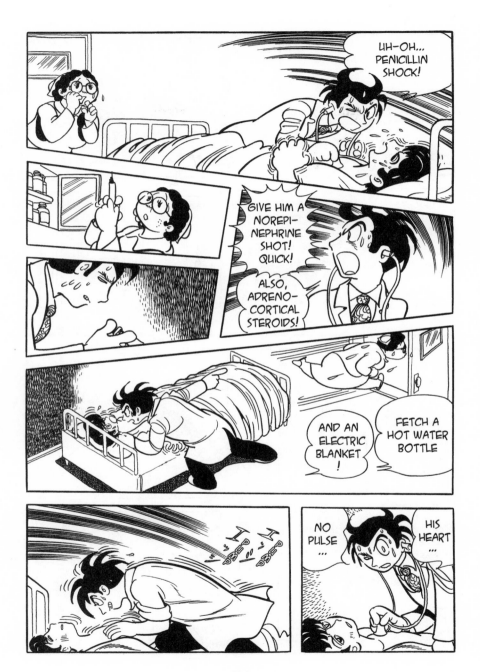

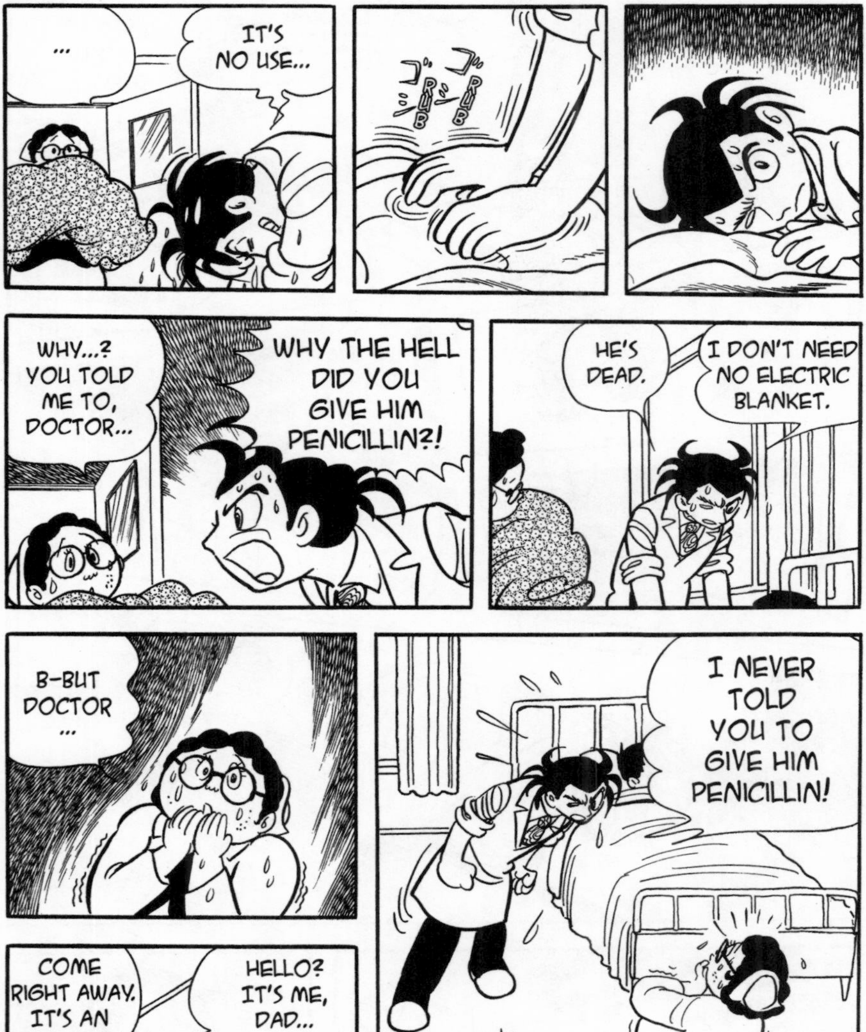
RUB
RUB
IT'S NO USE...
...
I DON'T NEED NO ELECTRIC BLANKET.
HE'S DEAD.
WHY THE HELL DID YOU GIVE HIM PENICILLIN?!
WHY...? YOU TOLD ME TO, DOCTOR...
I NEVER TOLD YOU TO GIVE HIM PENICILLIN!
I MOST DEFINITELY DID NOT! YOU ACTED ON YOUR OWN!
B-BUT DOCTOR ...
HELLO? IT'S ME, DAD... I MEAN, DIRECTOR!
COME RIGHT AWAY. IT'S AN EMERGENCY!

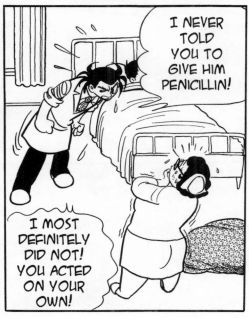

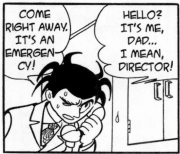

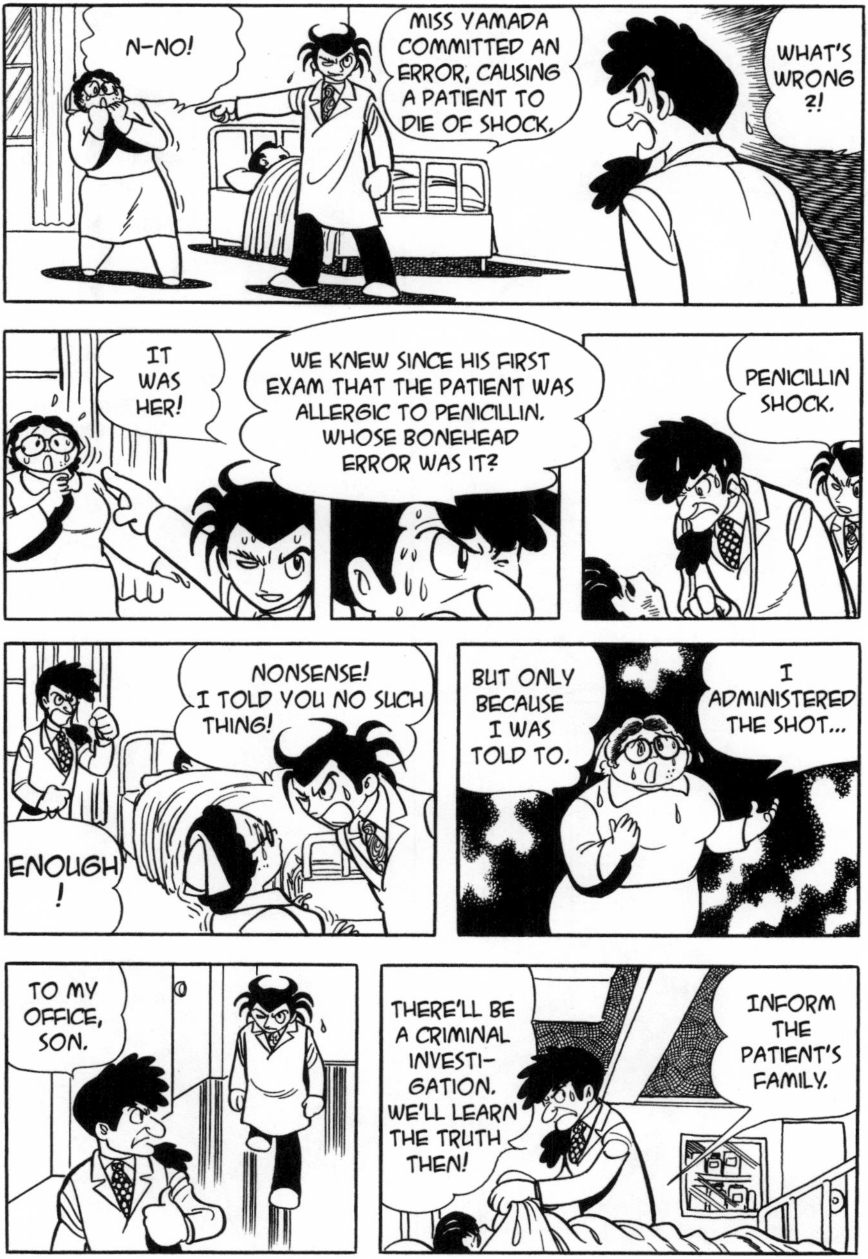
WHAT'S WRONG ?!
MISS YAMADA COMMITTED AN ERROR, CAUSING A PATIENT TO DIE OF SHOCK.
N-NO!
PENICILLIN SHOCK.
WE KNEW SINCE HIS FIRST EXAM THAT THE PATIENT WAS ALLERGIC TO PENICILLIN. WHOSE BONEHEAD ERROR WAS IT?
IT WAS HER!
I ADMINISTERED THE SHOT...
BUT ONLY BECAUSE I WAS TOLD TO.
NONSENSE! I TOLD YOU NO SUCH THING!
ENOUGH!
INFORM THE PATIENT'S FAMILY.
THERE'LL BE A CRIMINAL INVESTI-GATION. WE'LL LEARN THE TRUTH THEN!
TO MY OFFICE, SON.

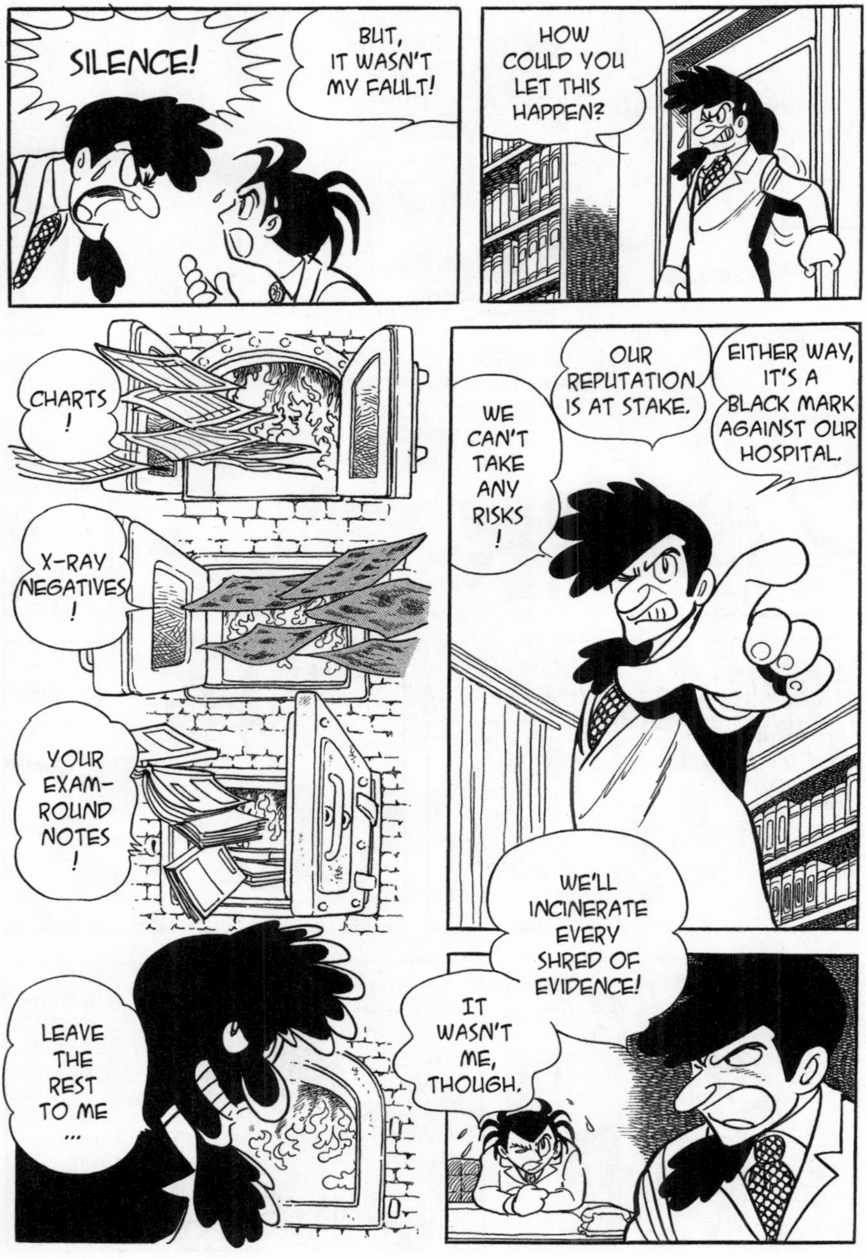
HOW COULD YOU LET THIS HAPPEN?
BUT, IT WASN'T MY FAULT!
SILENCE!
EITHER WAY, IT'S A BLACK MARK AGAINST OUR HOSPITAL.
OUR REPUTATION IS AT STAKE.
WE CAN'T TAKE ANY RISKS!
CHARTS!
X-RAY NEGATIVES!
YOUR EXAM-ROUND NOTES!
WE'LL INCINERATE EVERY SHRED OF EVIDENCE!
IT WASN'T ME, THOUGH.
LEAVE THE REST TO ME ...

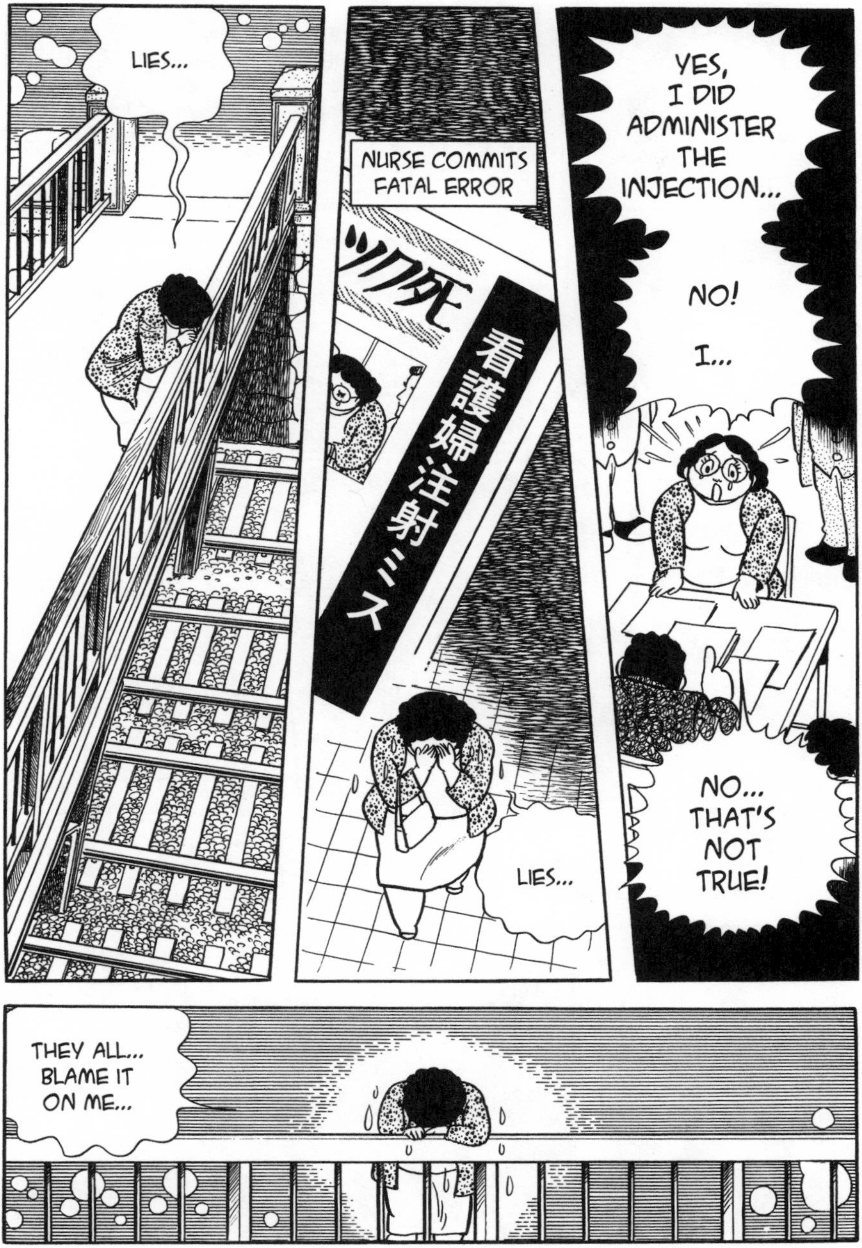
YES, I DID ADMINISTER THE INJECTION...
NO!
I...
NO... THAT'S NOT TRUE!
NURSE COMMITS FATAL ERROR
看護婦注射ミス
LIES...
LIES...
THEY ALL... BLAME IT ON ME...

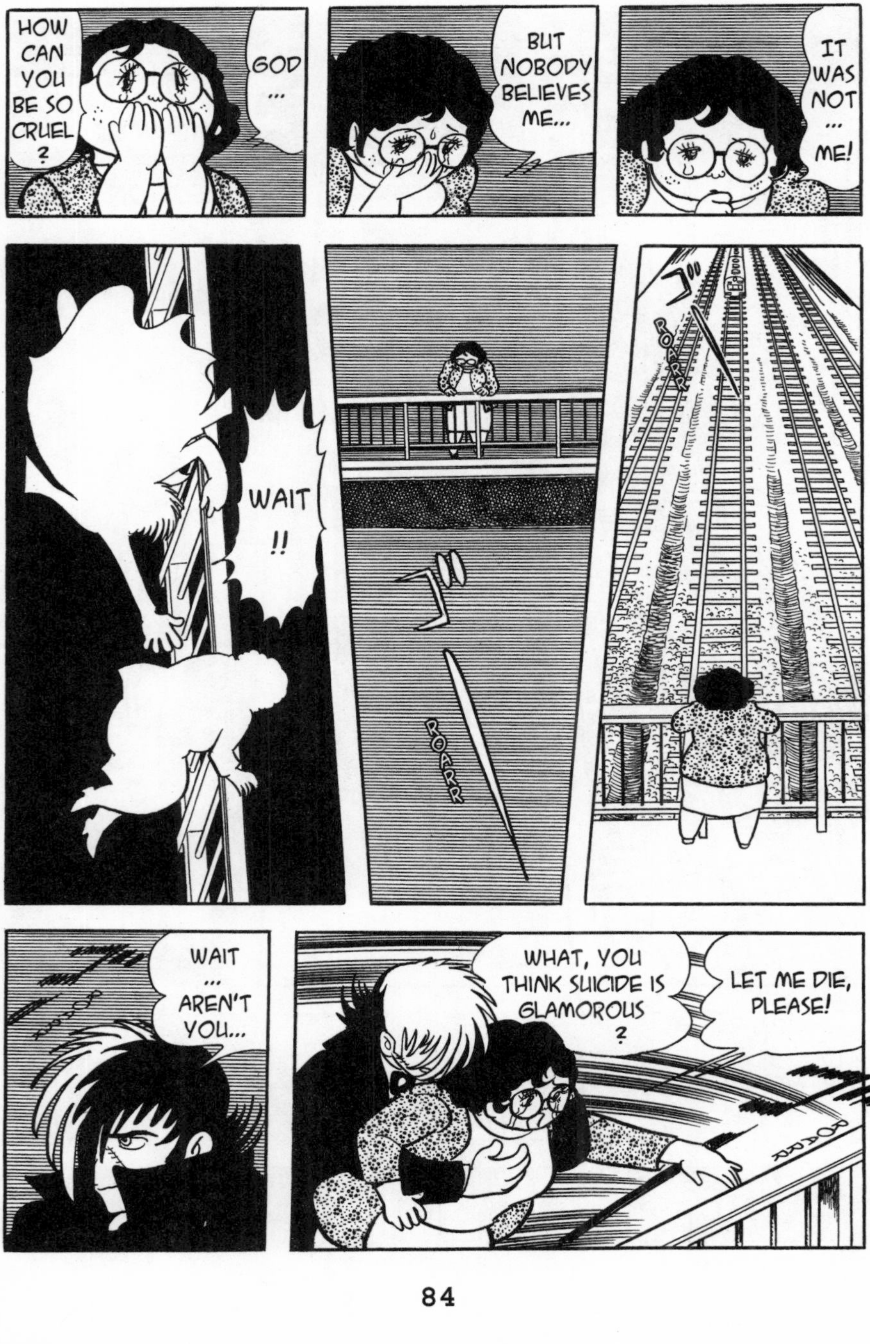
IT WAS NOT ... ME!
BUT NOBODY BELIEVES ME...
GOD ...
HOW CAN YOU BE SO CRUEL ?
ROARR
ROARR
WAIT !!
LET ME DIE, PLEASE!
WHAT, YOU THINK SUICIDE IS GLAMOROUS ?
ROARR
WAIT ... AREN'T YOU...

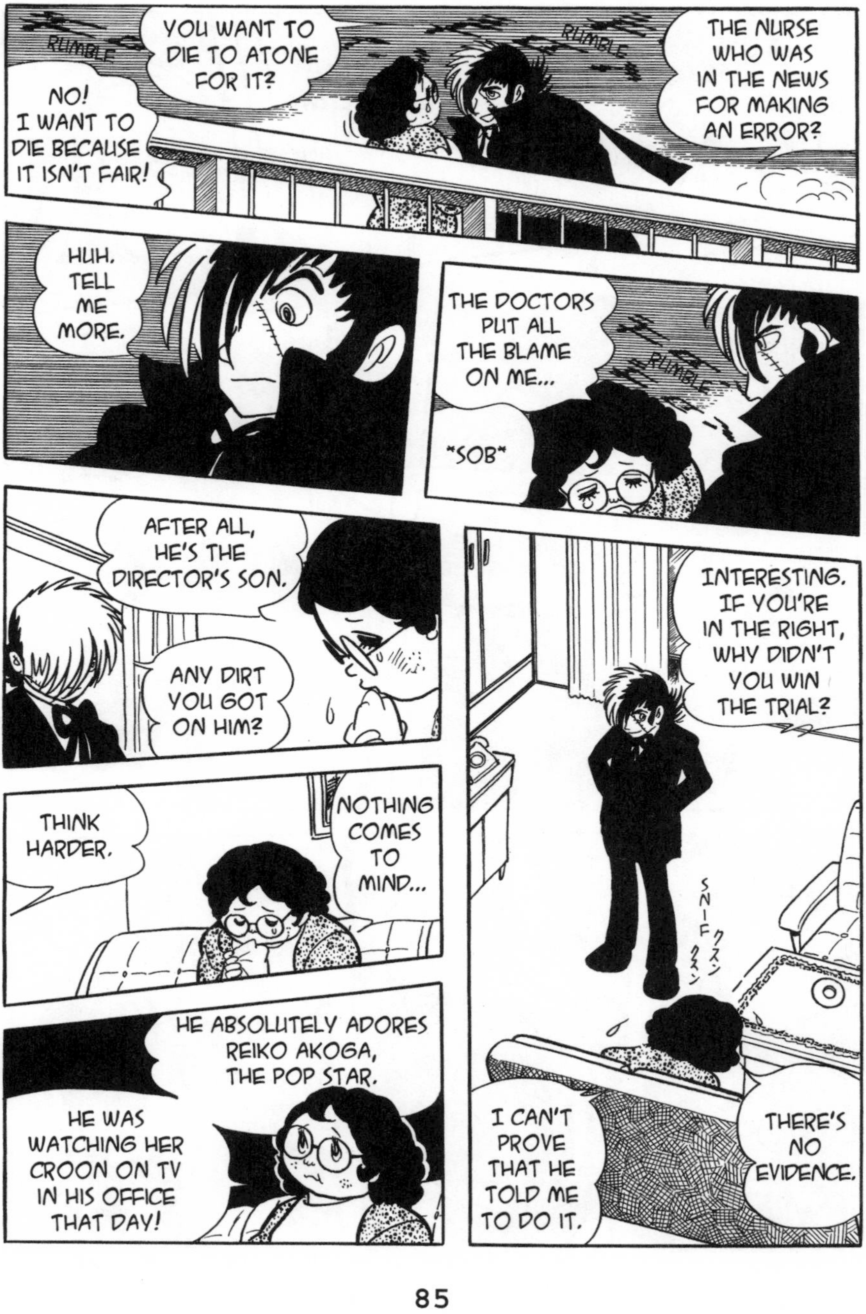
THE NURSE WHO WAS IN THE NEWS FOR MAKING AN ERROR?
RUMBLE
YOU WANT TO DIE TO ATONE FOR IT?
RUMBLE
NO! I WANT TO DIE BECAUSE IT ISN'T FAIR!
THE DOCTORS PUT ALL THE BLAME ON ME...
RUMBLE
SOB
HUH. TELL ME MORE.
INTERESTING. IF YOU'RE IN THE RIGHT, WHY DIDN'T YOU WIN THE TRIAL?
SNIFF
クスン クスン
THERE'S NO EVIDENCE.
I CAN'T PROVE THAT HE TOLD ME TO DO IT.
AFTER ALL, HE'S THE DIRECTOR'S SON.
ANY DIRT YOU GOT ON HIM?
NOTHING COMES TO MIND...
THINK HARDER.
HE ABSOLUTELY ADORES REIKO AKOGA, THE POP STAR.
HE WAS WATCHING HER CROON ON TV IN HIS OFFICE THAT DAY!

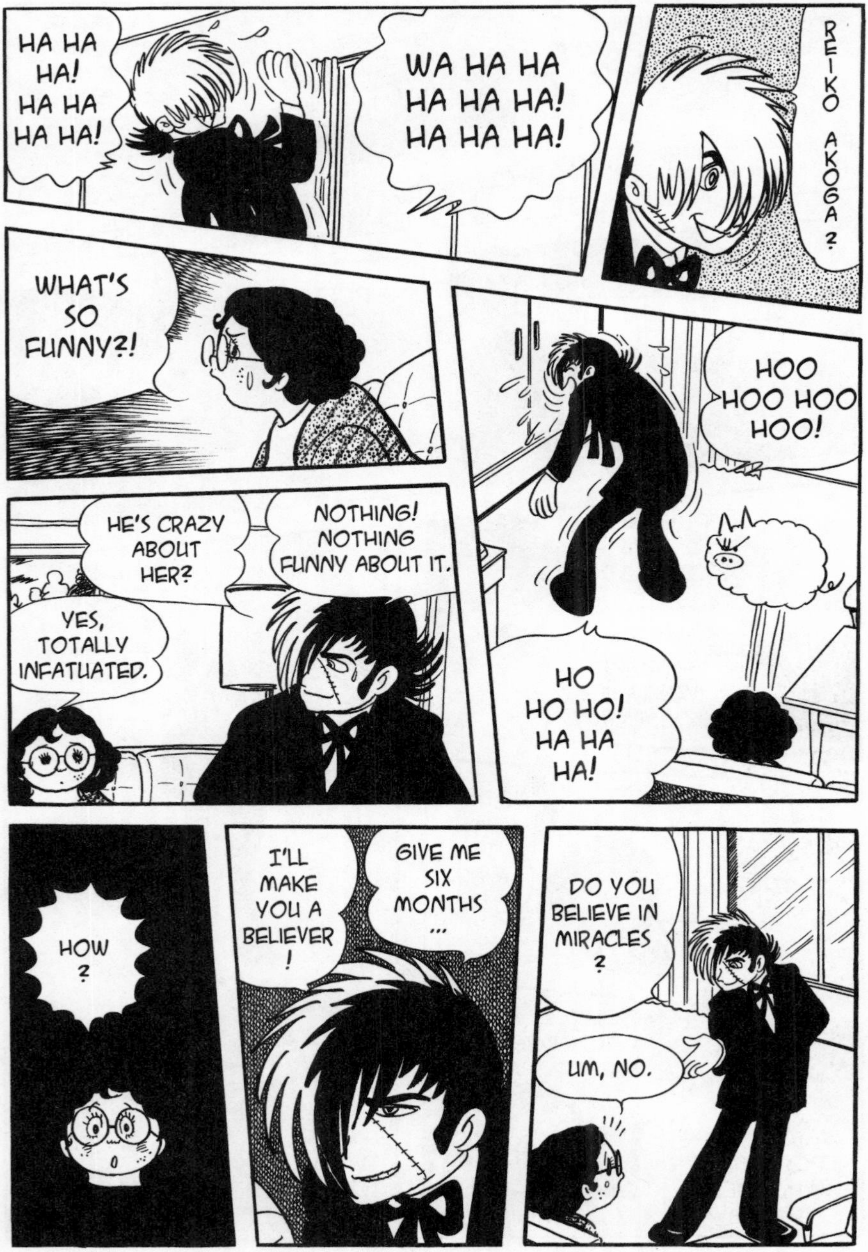

REIKO AKOGA?
WA HA HA HA HA HA! HA HA HA!
HA HA HA! HA HA HA HA!
HOO HOO HOO HOO!
HO HO HO! HA HA HA!
WHAT'S SO FUNNY?!
NOTHING! NOTHING FUNNY ABOUT IT.
HE'S CRAZY ABOUT HER?
YES, TOTALLY INFATUATED.
DO YOU BELIEVE IN MIRACLES?
UM, NO.
GIVE ME SIX MONTHS ...
I'LL MAKE YOU A BELIEVER!
HOW?

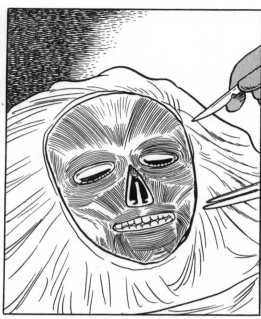

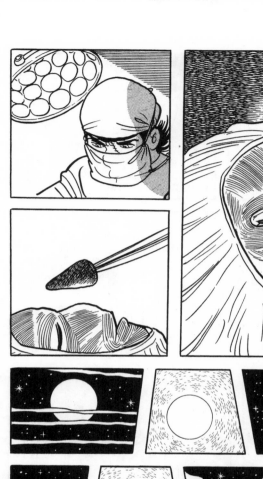

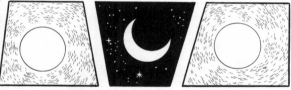

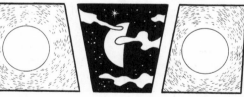

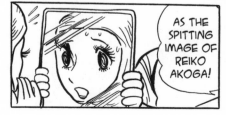

SIX MONTHS, AS PROMISED.
YOU'VE BEEN MIRACUL-OUSLY REBORN
AS THE SPITTING IMAGE OF REIKO AKOGA!

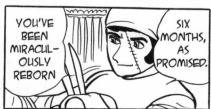

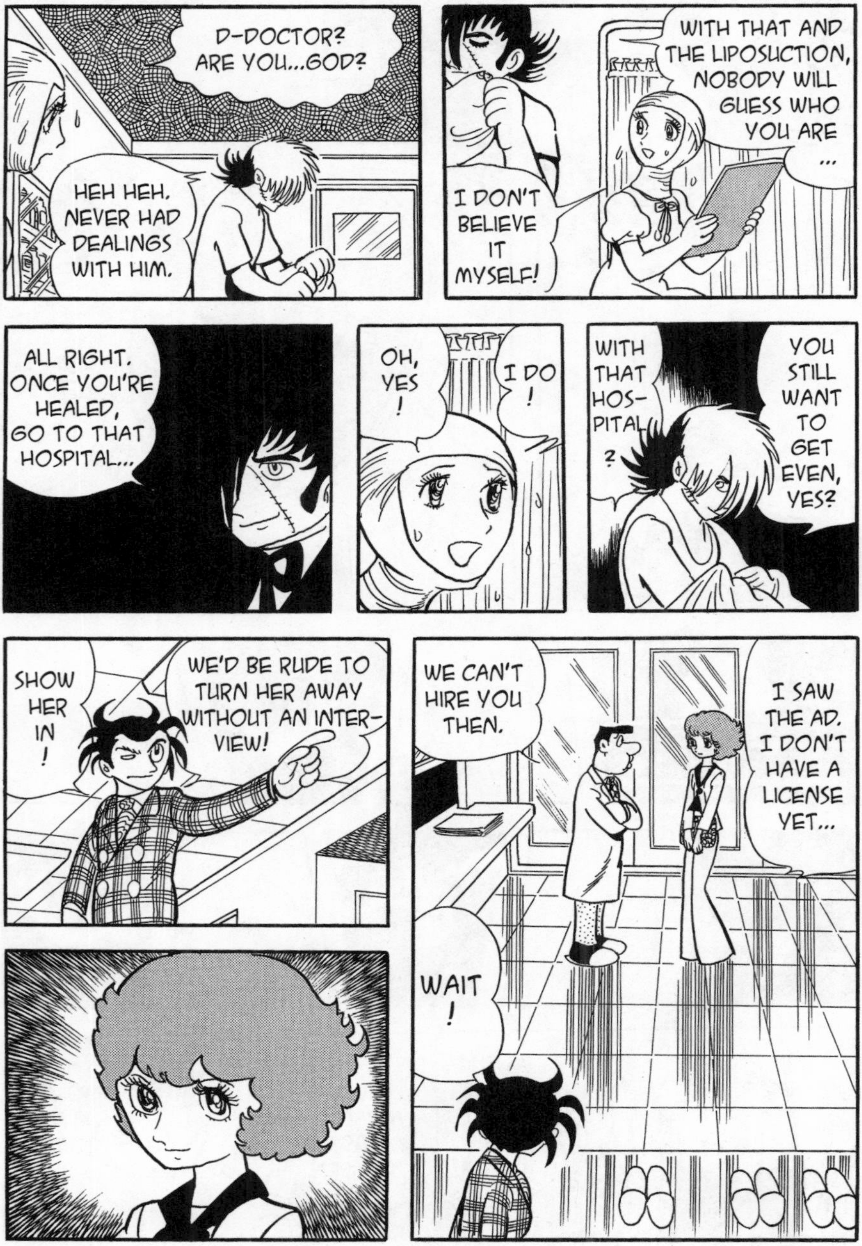
WITH THAT AND THE LIPOSUCTION, NOBODY WILL GUESS WHO YOU ARE ...
I DON'T BELIEVE IT MYSELF!
D-DOCTOR? ARE YOU...GOD?
HEH HEH. NEVER HAD DEALINGS WITH HIM.
YOU STILL WANT TO GET EVEN, YES?
WITH THAT HOS-PITAL?
I DO!
OH, YES!
ALL RIGHT. ONCE YOU'RE HEALED, GO TO THAT HOSPITAL...
I SAW THE AD. I DON'T HAVE A LICENSE YET...
WE CAN'T HIRE YOU THEN.
WAIT!
WE'D BE RUDE TO TURN HER AWAY WITHOUT AN INTER-VIEW!
SHOW HER IN!

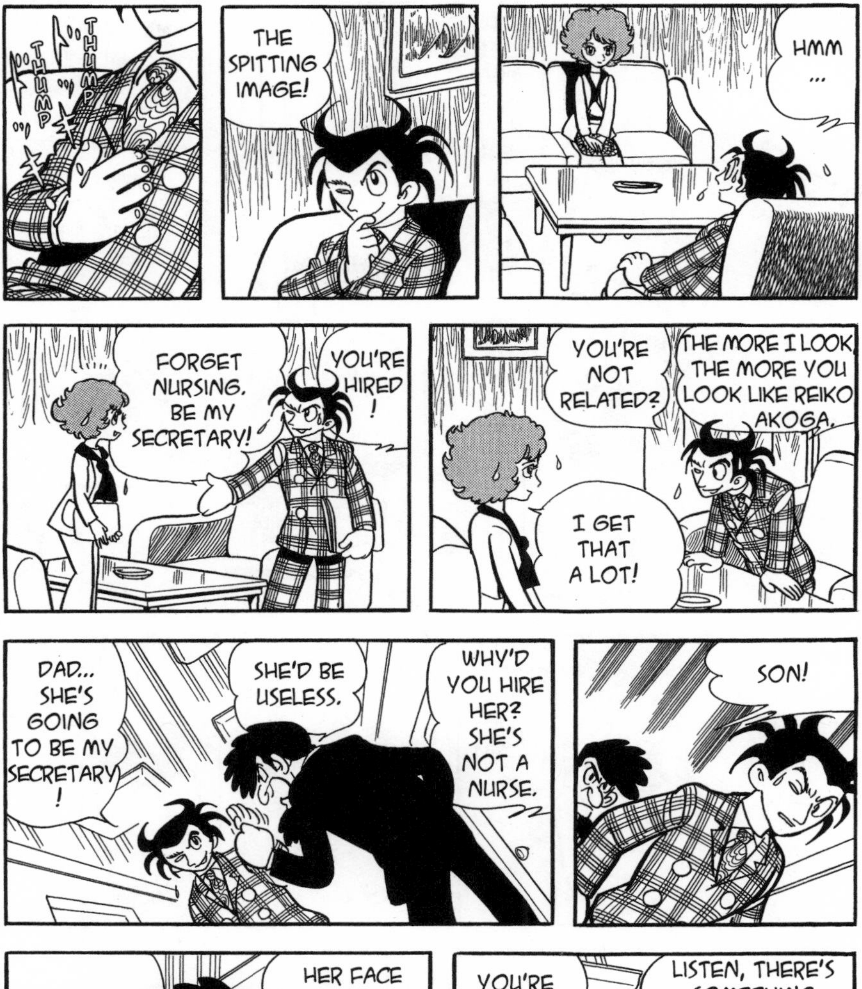
HMM ...
THE SPITTING IMAGE!
THUMP
THUMP
THE MORE I LOOK THE MORE YOU LOOK LIKE REIKO AKOGA.
YOU'RE NOT RELATED?
I GET THAT A LOT!
YOU'RE HIRED!
FORGET NURSING. BE MY SECRETARY!
SON!
WHY'D YOU HIRE HER? SHE'S NOT A NURSE.
SHE'D BE USELESS.
DAD... SHE'S GOING TO BE MY SECRETARY!
LISTEN, THERE'S SOMETHING STRANGE ABOUT HER...
YOU'RE IMAGINING THINGS.
HER FACE LOOKS ALMOST FAKE.
SHE'S HAD PLASTIC SURGERY.

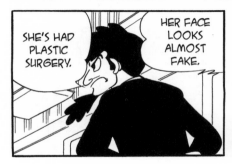

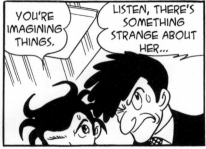

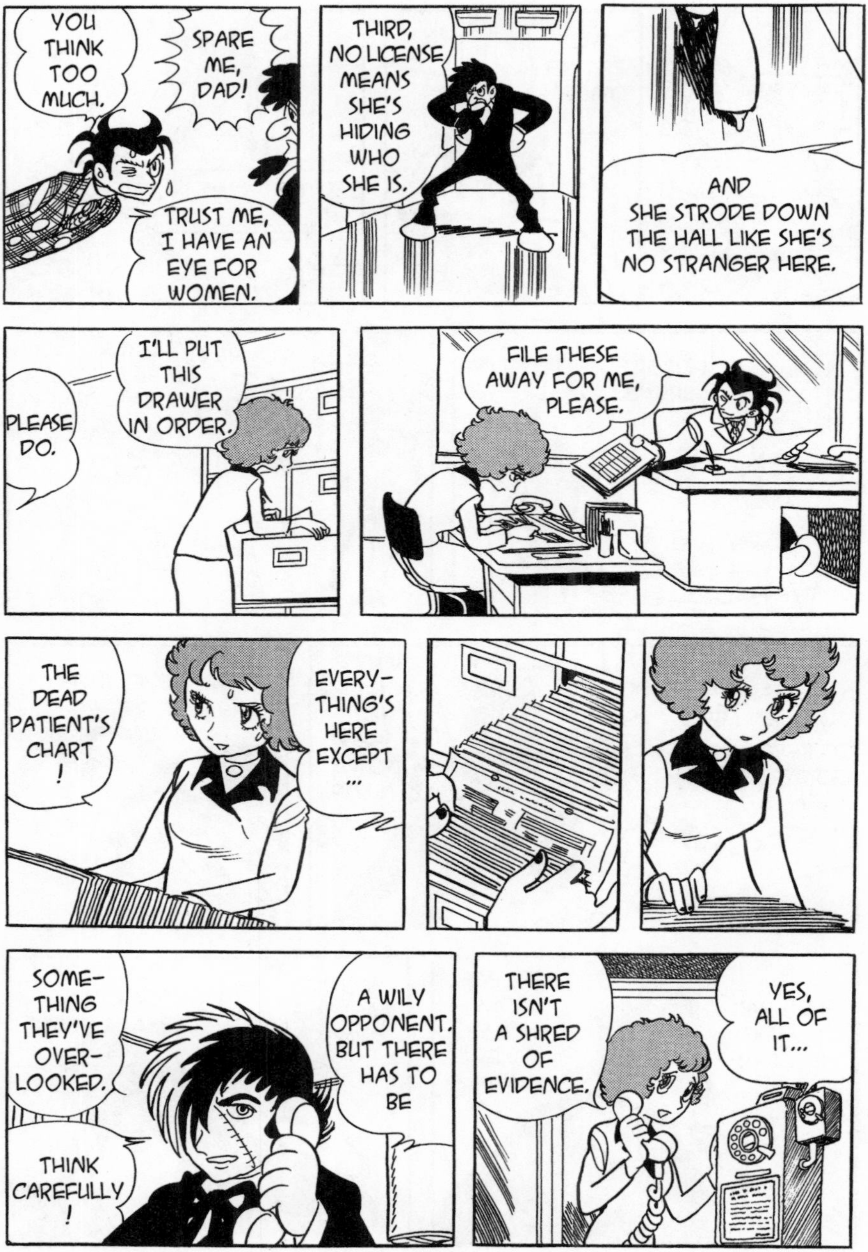
AND SHE STRODE DOWN THE HALL LIKE SHE'S NO STRANGER HERE.
THIRD, NO LICENSE MEANS SHE'S HIDING WHO SHE IS.
SPARE ME, DAD!
YOU THINK TOO MUCH.
TRUST ME, I HAVE AN EYE FOR WOMEN.
FILE THESE AWAY FOR ME, PLEASE.
I'LL PUT THIS DRAWER IN ORDER.
PLEASE DO.
EVERY-THING'S HERE EXCEPT ...
THE DEAD PATIENT'S CHART !
YES, ALL OF IT...
THERE ISN'T A SHRED OF EVIDENCE.
A WILY OPPONENT. BUT THERE HAS TO BE
SOME-THING THEY'VE OVER-LOOKED.
THINK CAREFULLY !

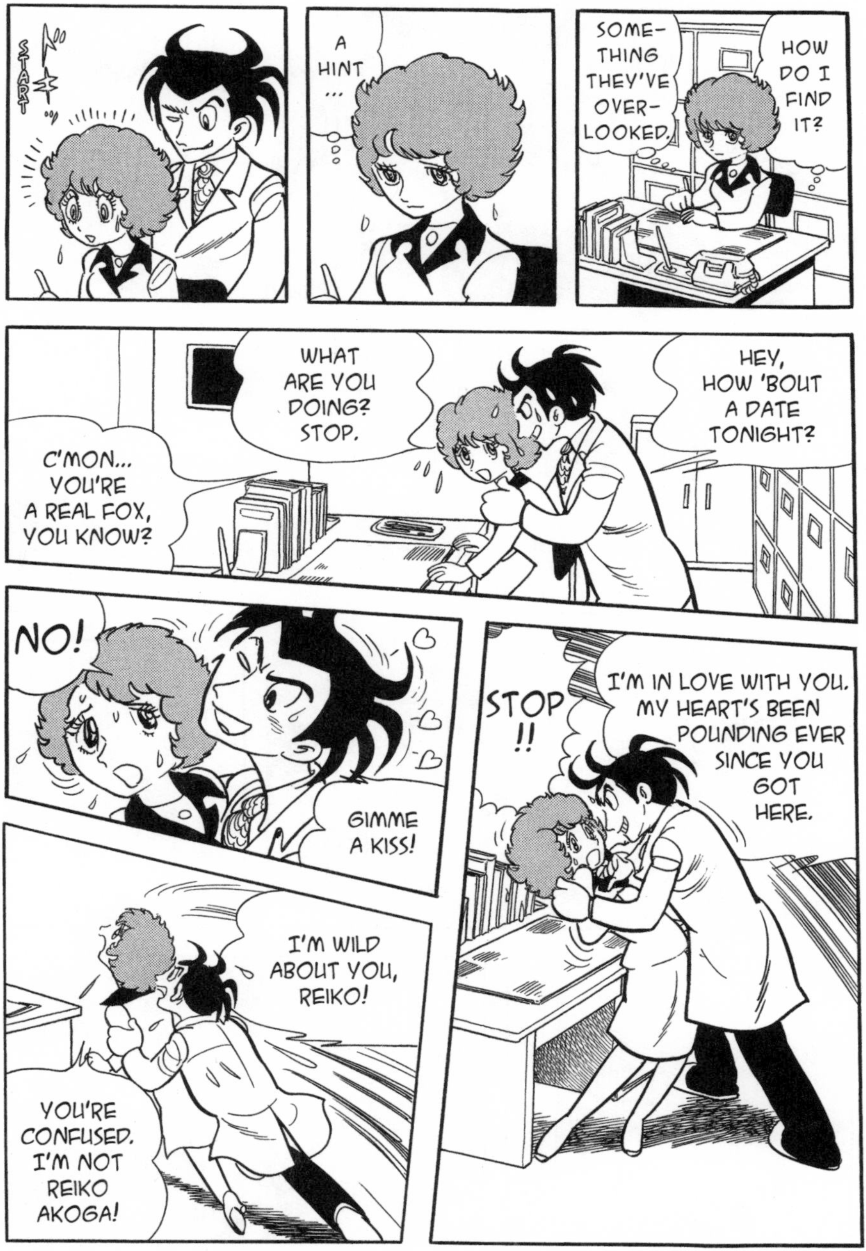
HOW DO I FIND IT?
SOMETHING THEY'VE OVERLOOKED.
A HINT...
START
HEY, HOW 'BOUT A DATE TONIGHT?
WHAT ARE YOU DOING? STOP.
C'MON... YOU'RE A REAL FOX, YOU KNOW?
I'M IN LOVE WITH YOU. MY HEART'S BEEN POUNDING EVER SINCE YOU GOT HERE.
STOP!!
NO!
GIMME A KISS!
I'M WILD ABOUT YOU, REIKO!
YOU'RE CONFUSED. I'M NOT REIKO AKOGA!

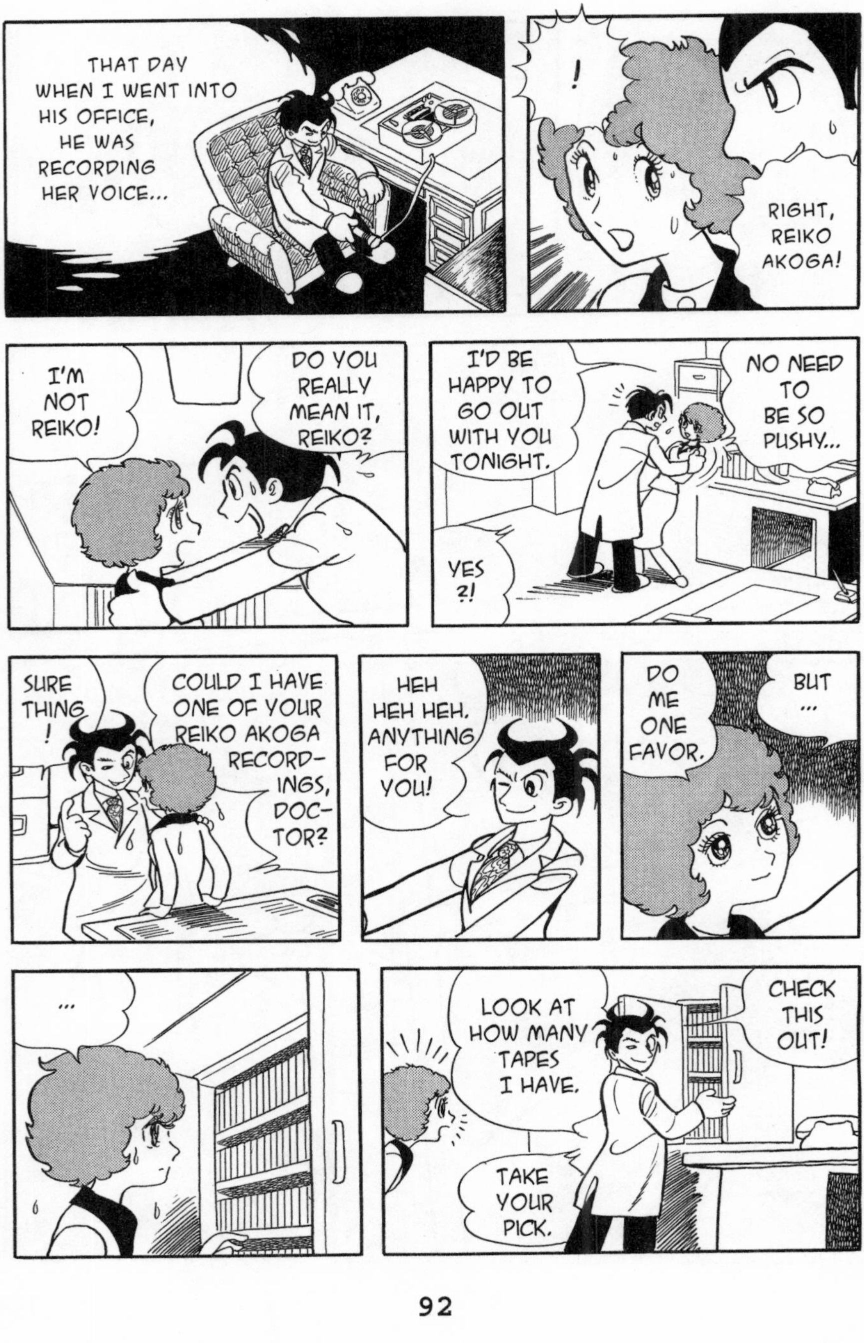
!
RIGHT, REIKO AKOGA!
THAT DAY WHEN I WENT INTO HIS OFFICE, HE WAS RECORDING HER VOICE...
NO NEED TO BE SO PUSHY...
I'D BE HAPPY TO GO OUT WITH YOU TONIGHT.
YES ?!
DO YOU REALLY MEAN IT, REIKO?
I'M NOT REIKO!
BUT ...
DO ME ONE FAVOR.
HEH HEH HEH. ANYTHING FOR YOU!
COULD I HAVE ONE OF YOUR REIKO AKOGA RECORD-INGS, DOC-TOR?
SURE THING!
CHECK THIS OUT!
LOOK AT HOW MANY TAPES I HAVE.
TAKE YOUR PICK.
...

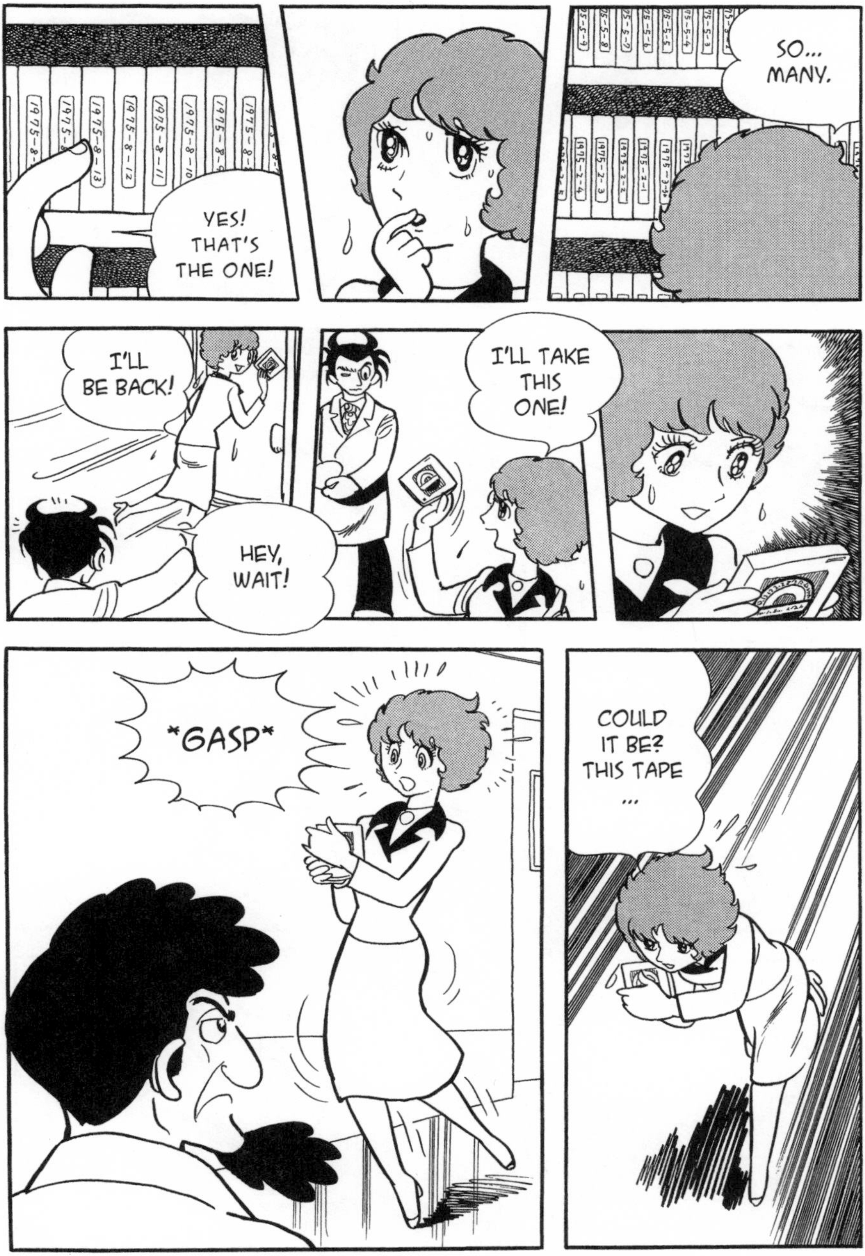
SO... MANY.
YES! THAT'S THE ONE!
I'LL TAKE THIS ONE!
I'LL BE BACK!
HEY, WAIT!
COULD IT BE? THIS TAPE ...
GASP

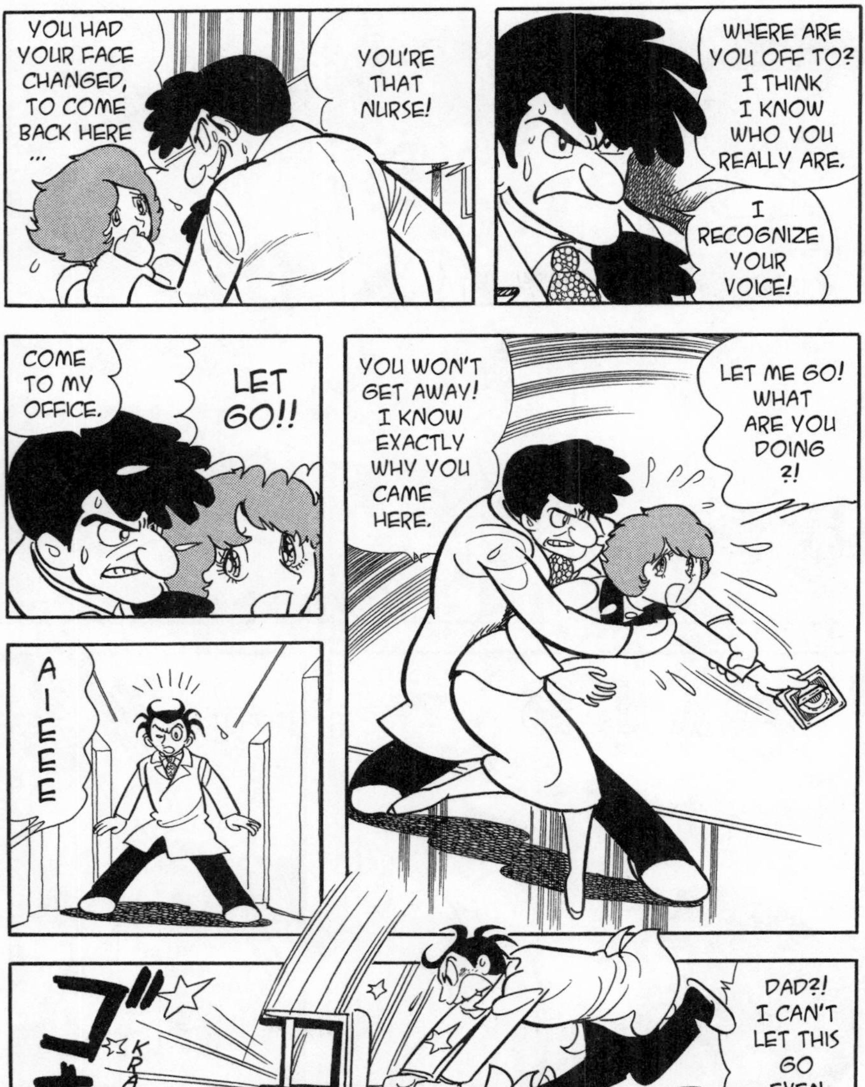
WHERE ARE YOU OFF TO? I THINK I KNOW WHO YOU REALLY ARE.
I RECOGNIZE YOUR VOICE!
YOU'RE THAT NURSE!
YOU HAD YOUR FACE CHANGED, TO COME BACK HERE ...
LET ME GO! WHAT ARE YOU DOING ?!
YOU WON'T GET AWAY! I KNOW EXACTLY WHY YOU CAME HERE.
LET GO!!
COME TO MY OFFICE.
AIEEE
DAD?! I CAN'T LET THIS GO EVEN IF IT'S YOU!
KRAK
ゴキーン

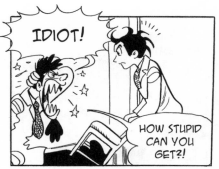

SHE'S MY GIRL— HANDS OFF!
HURRY, GO!
IDIOT!
HOW STUPID CAN YOU GET?!
LIKE A SWALLOW
ツバメのように
DRAGON
EXCUSE ME, DOCTOR... ABOUT THE INJECTION FOR THE PATIENT IN ROOM 3...
HUH? CAN'T YOU SEE I'M BUSY? GIVE HIM TETRACYCLINE OR SOMETHING!
BUT YOU SAID NOT TO ADMINISTER TETRACYCLINE BECAUSE IT STOPPED WORKING...
I SAID I'M BUSY RIGHT NOW! ARG... GIVE HIM, UH, 20,000 UNITS OF PENICILLIN, OKAY?
SOLID EVIDENCE ...
YOU DID IT, MISS YAMADA.
135

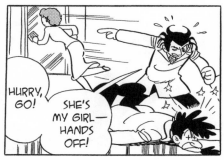

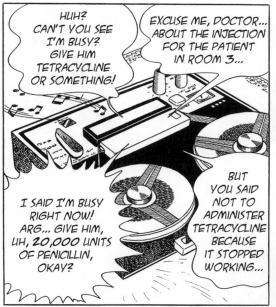

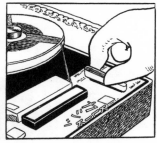

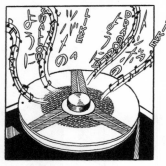

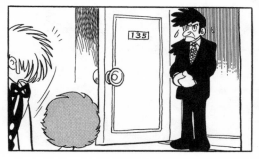

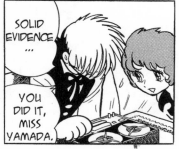

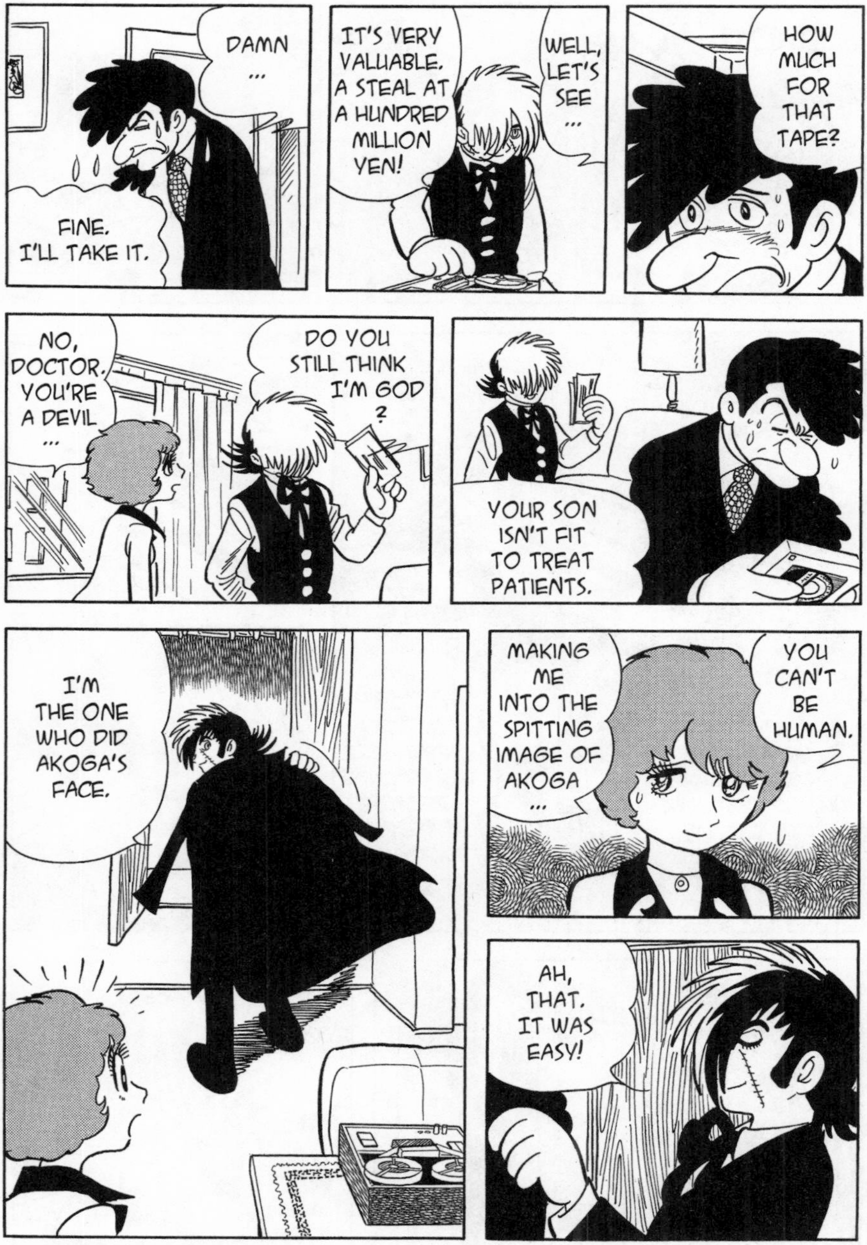
HOW MUCH FOR THAT TAPE?
WELL, LET'S SEE ...
IT'S VERY VALUABLE. A STEAL AT A HUNDRED MILLION YEN!
DAMN ...
FINE. I'LL TAKE IT.
YOUR SON ISN'T FIT TO TREAT PATIENTS.
DO YOU STILL THINK I'M GOD ?
NO, DOCTOR. YOU'RE A DEVIL ...
YOU CAN'T BE HUMAN.
MAKING ME INTO THE SPITTING IMAGE OF AKOGA ...
AH, THAT. IT WAS EASY!
I'M THE ONE WHO DID AKOGA'S FACE.

THE ROBIN AND THE BOY

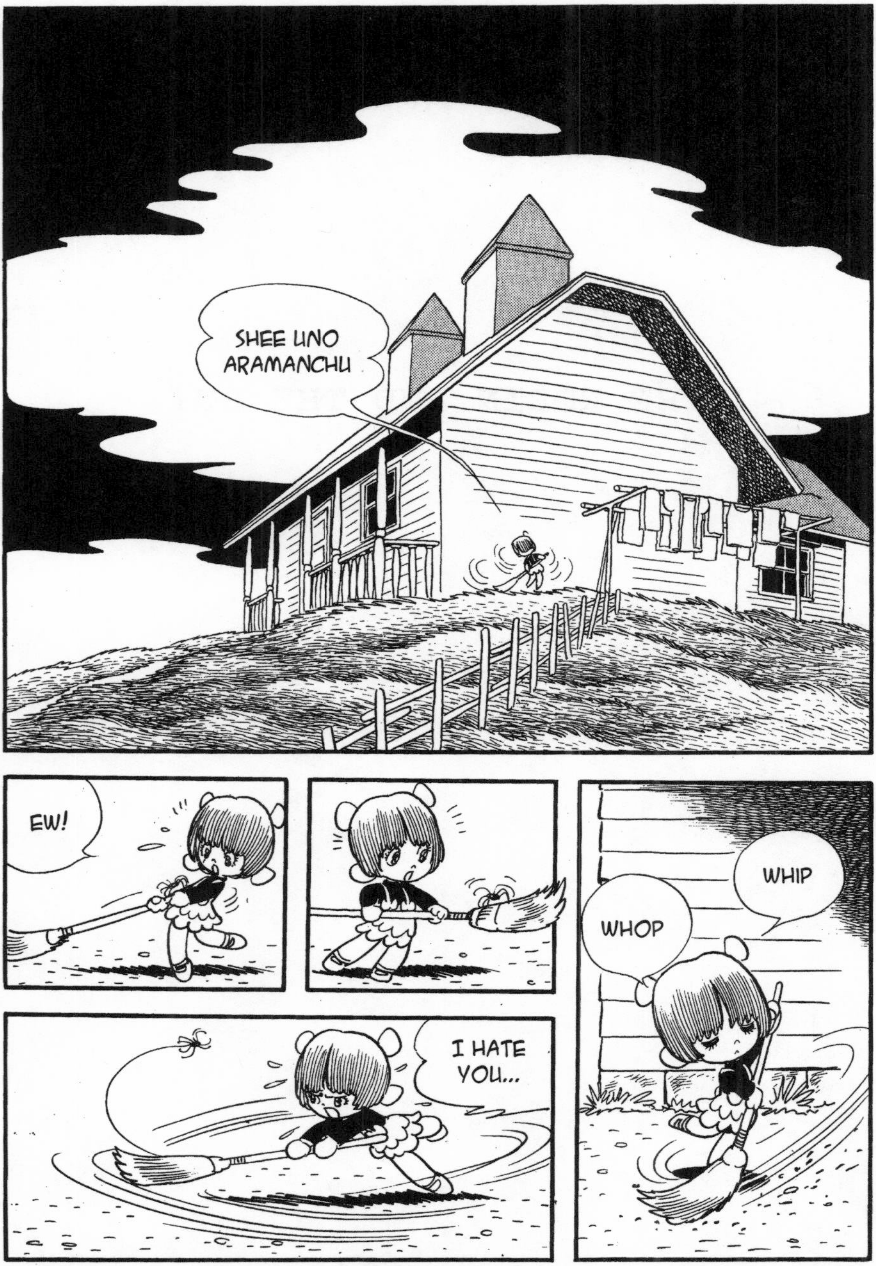
SHEE UNO ARAMANCHU
WHIP
WHOP
EW!
I HATE YOU...

NOTE: "SHEE UNO ARAMANCHU" = THE PINOKO-ISM IS SECOND ONLY TO "ACCHONBURIKE" IN NOTORIETY AND OPACITY OF MEANING

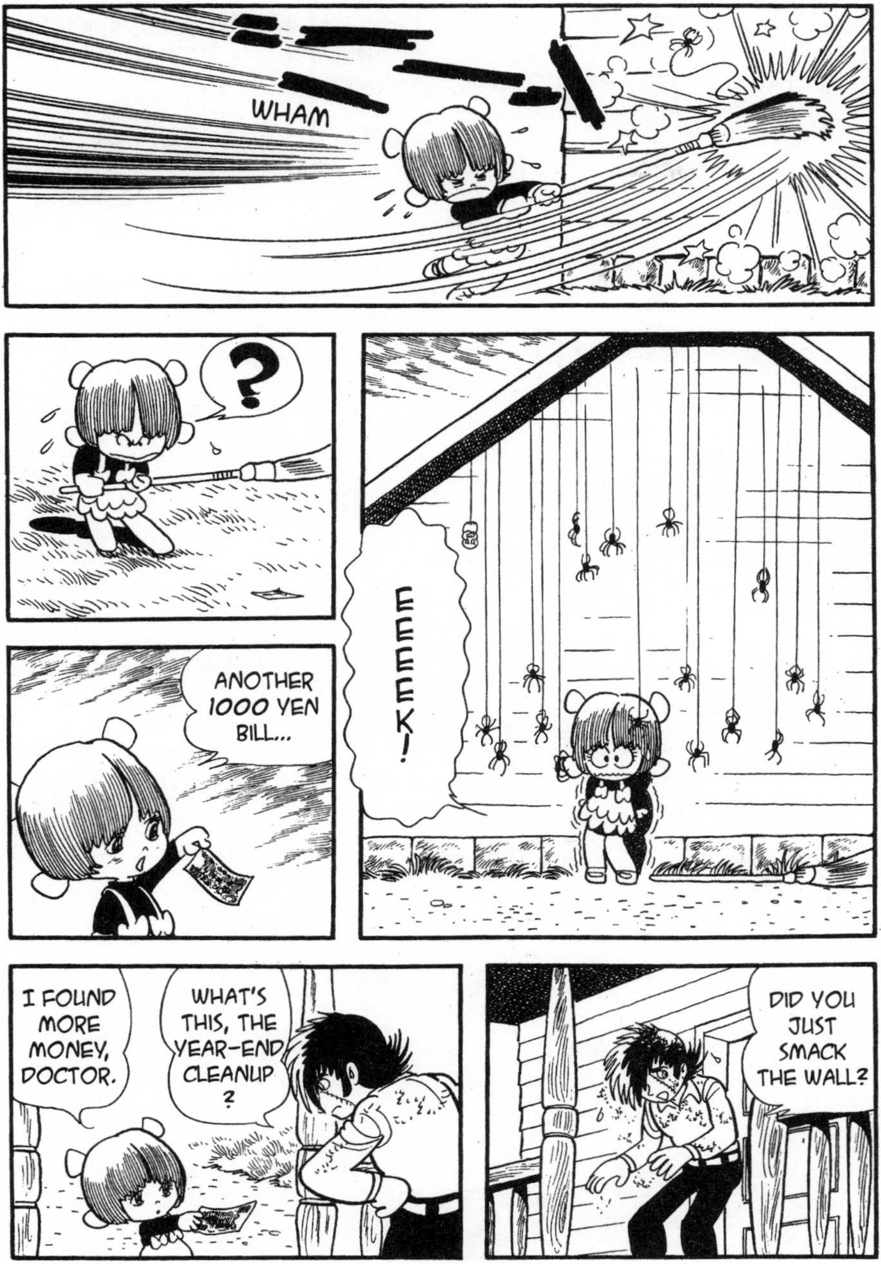
WHAM
EEEEEK!
?
ANOTHER 1000 YEN BILL...
DID YOU JUST SMACK THE WALL?
WHAT'S THIS, THE YEAR-END CLEANUP?
I FOUND MORE MONEY, DOCTOR.

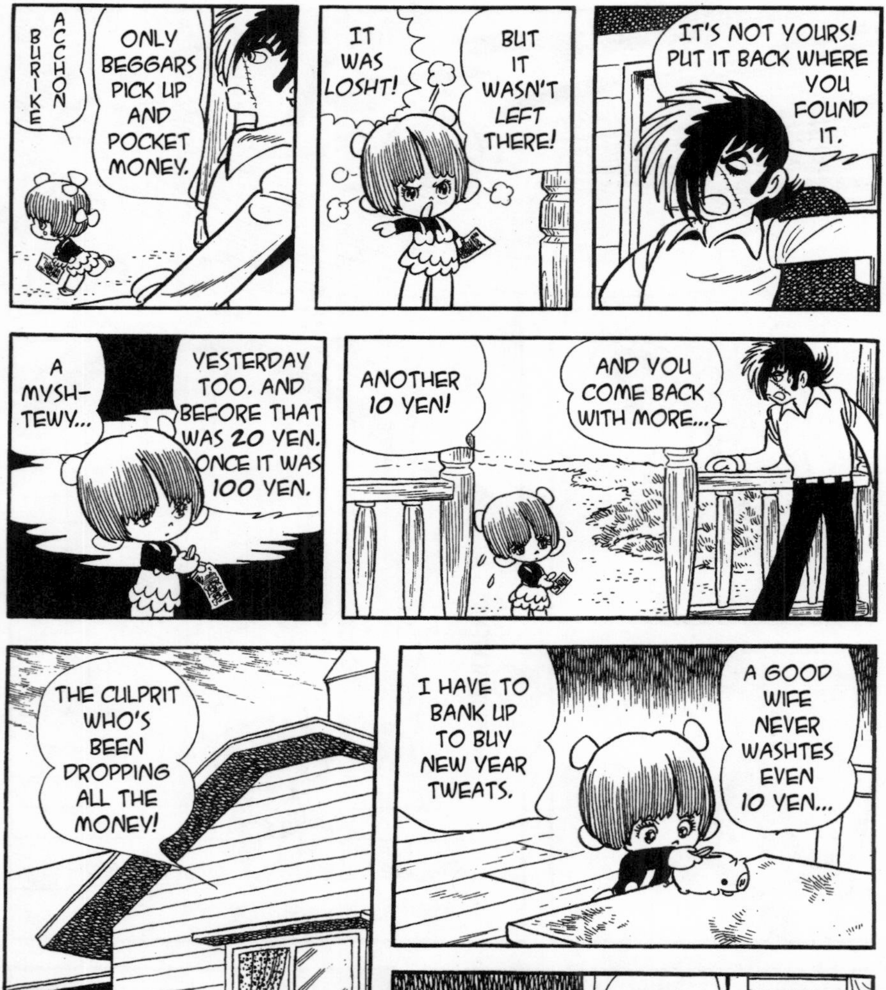
IT'S NOT YOURS! PUT IT BACK WHERE YOU FOUND IT.
BUT IT WASN'T LEFT THERE!
IT WAS LOSHT!
ONLY BEGGARS PICK UP AND POCKET MONEY.
ACCHON
BURIKE
AND YOU COME BACK WITH MORE...
ANOTHER 10 YEN!
YESTERDAY TOO. AND BEFORE THAT WAS 20 YEN. ONCE IT WAS 100 YEN.
A MYSH-TEWY...
A GOOD WIFE NEVER WASHTES EVEN 10 YEN...
I HAVE TO BANK UP TO BUY NEW YEAR TWEATS.
HEY, COME HERE AND SEE THIS!
THE CULPRIT WHO'S BEEN DROPPING ALL THE MONEY!

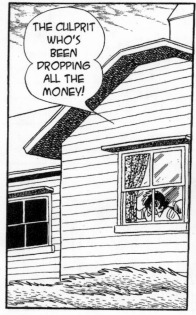

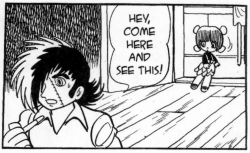

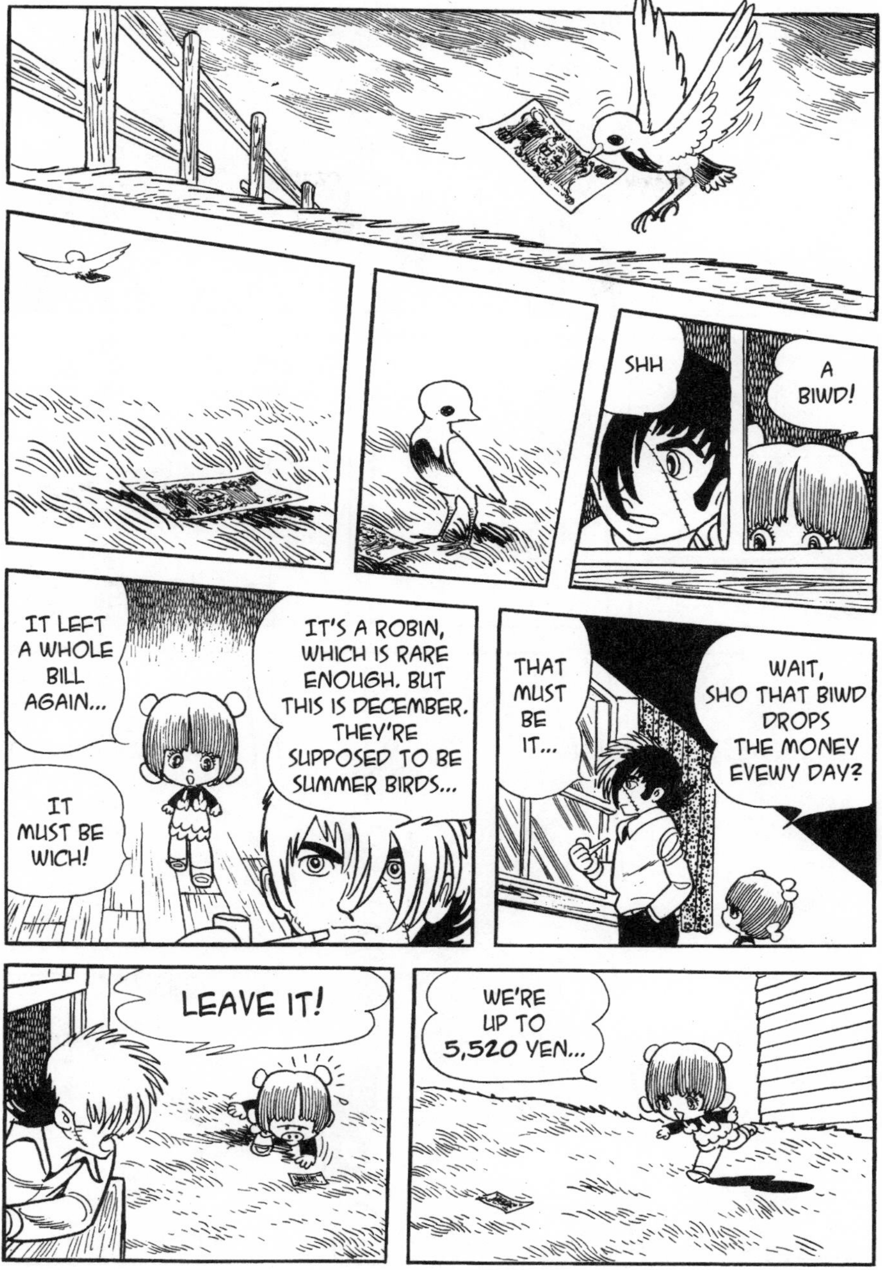
A BIWD!
SHH
WAIT, SHO THAT BIWD DROPS THE MONEY EVEWY DAY?
THAT MUST BE IT...
IT'S A ROBIN, WHICH IS RARE ENOUGH. BUT THIS IS DECEMBER. THEY'RE SUPPOSED TO BE SUMMER BIRDS...
IT LEFT A WHOLE BILL AGAIN...
IT MUST BE WICH!
WE'RE UP TO 5,520 YEN...
LEAVE IT!

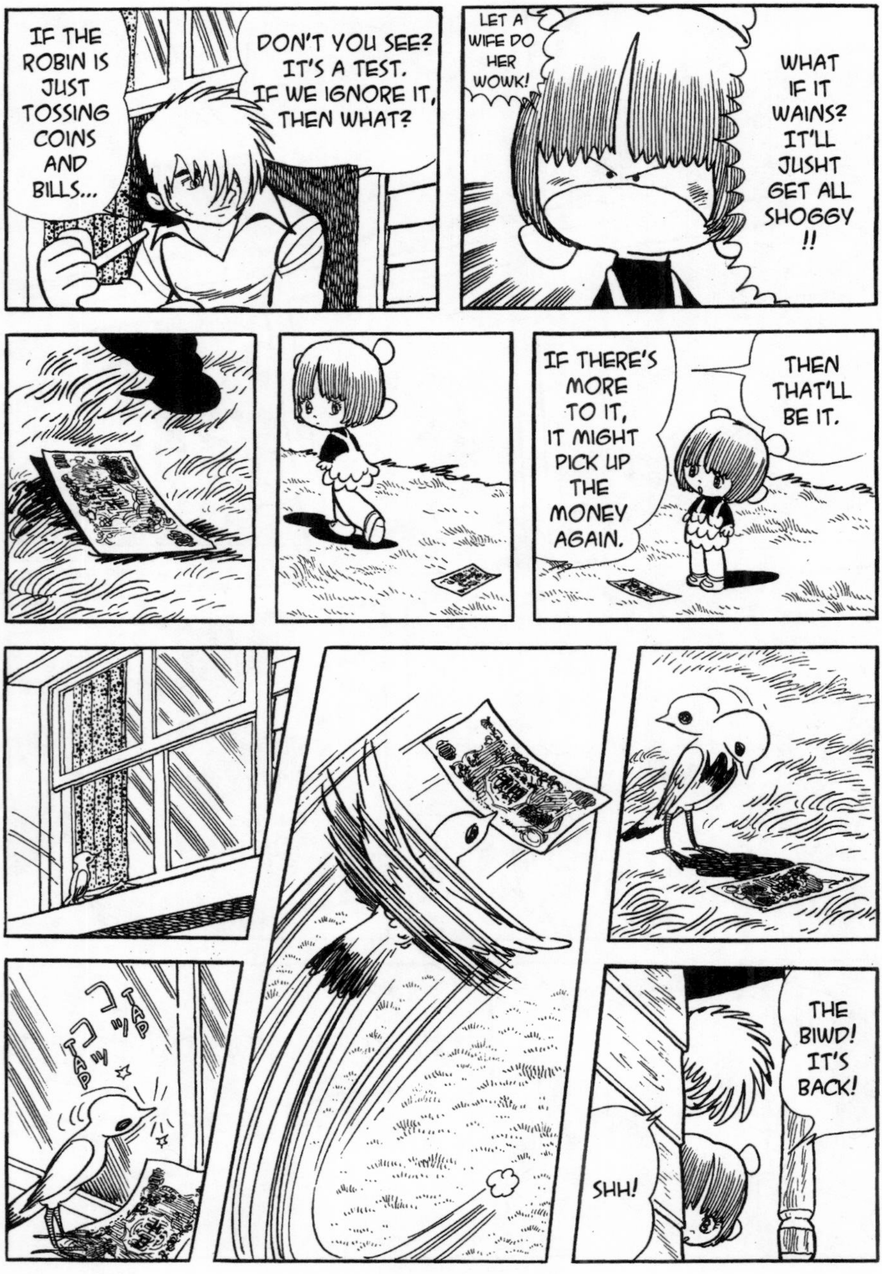
WHAT IF IT WAINS? IT'LL JUSHT GET ALL SHOGGY !!
LET A WIFE DO HER WOWK!
DON'T YOU SEE? IT'S A TEST. IF WE IGNORE IT, THEN WHAT?
IF THE ROBIN IS JUST TOSSING COINS AND BILLS...
THEN THAT'LL BE IT.
IF THERE'S MORE TO IT, IT MIGHT PICK UP THE MONEY AGAIN.
THE BIWD! IT'S BACK!
SHH!
コッ TAP
コッ TAP

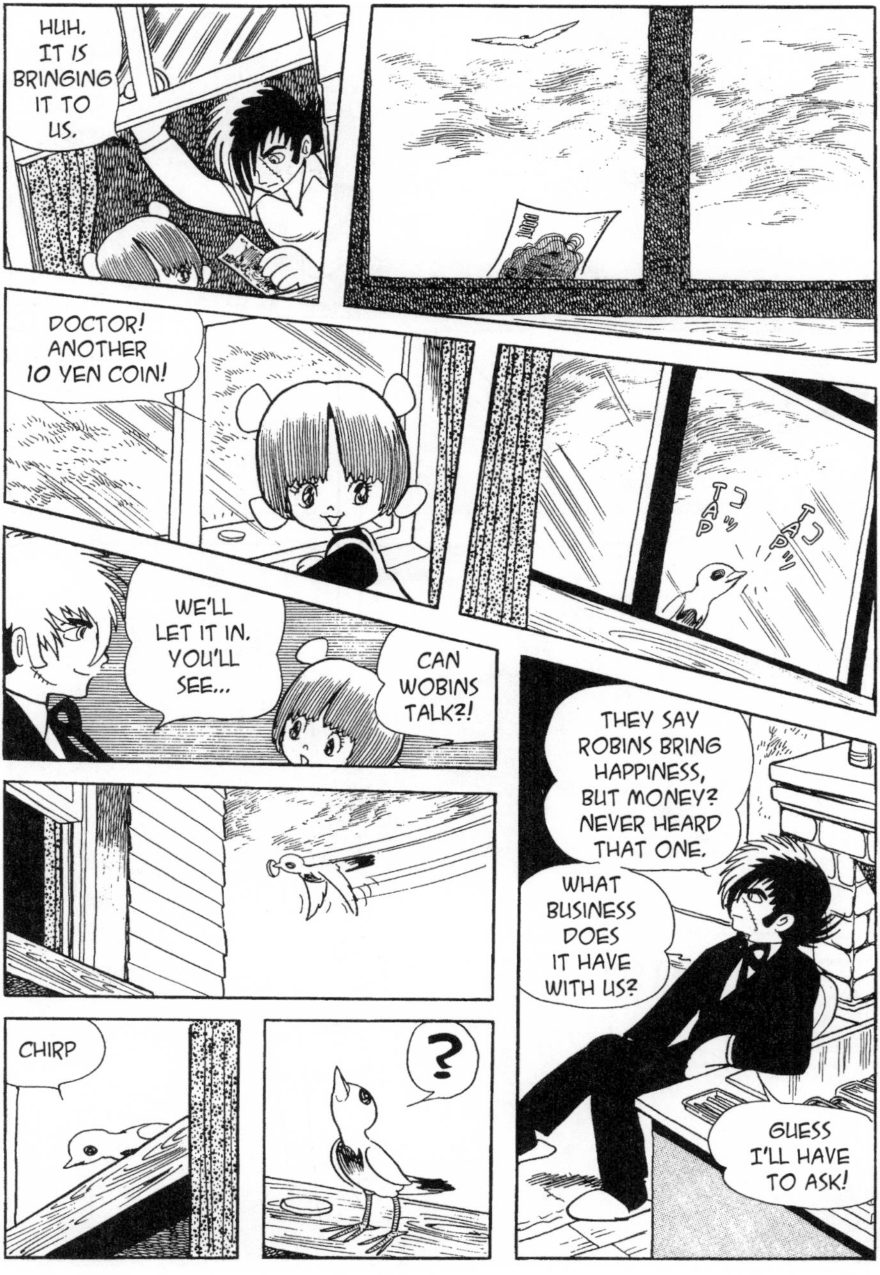
HUH. IT IS BRINGING IT TO US.
コツ TAP
コツ TAP
DOCTOR! ANOTHER 10 YEN COIN!
THEY SAY ROBINS BRING HAPPINESS, BUT MONEY? NEVER HEARD THAT ONE.
WHAT BUSINESS DOES IT HAVE WITH US?
GUESS I'LL HAVE TO ASK!
CAN WOBINS TALK?!
WE'LL LET IT IN. YOU'LL SEE...
?
CHIRP

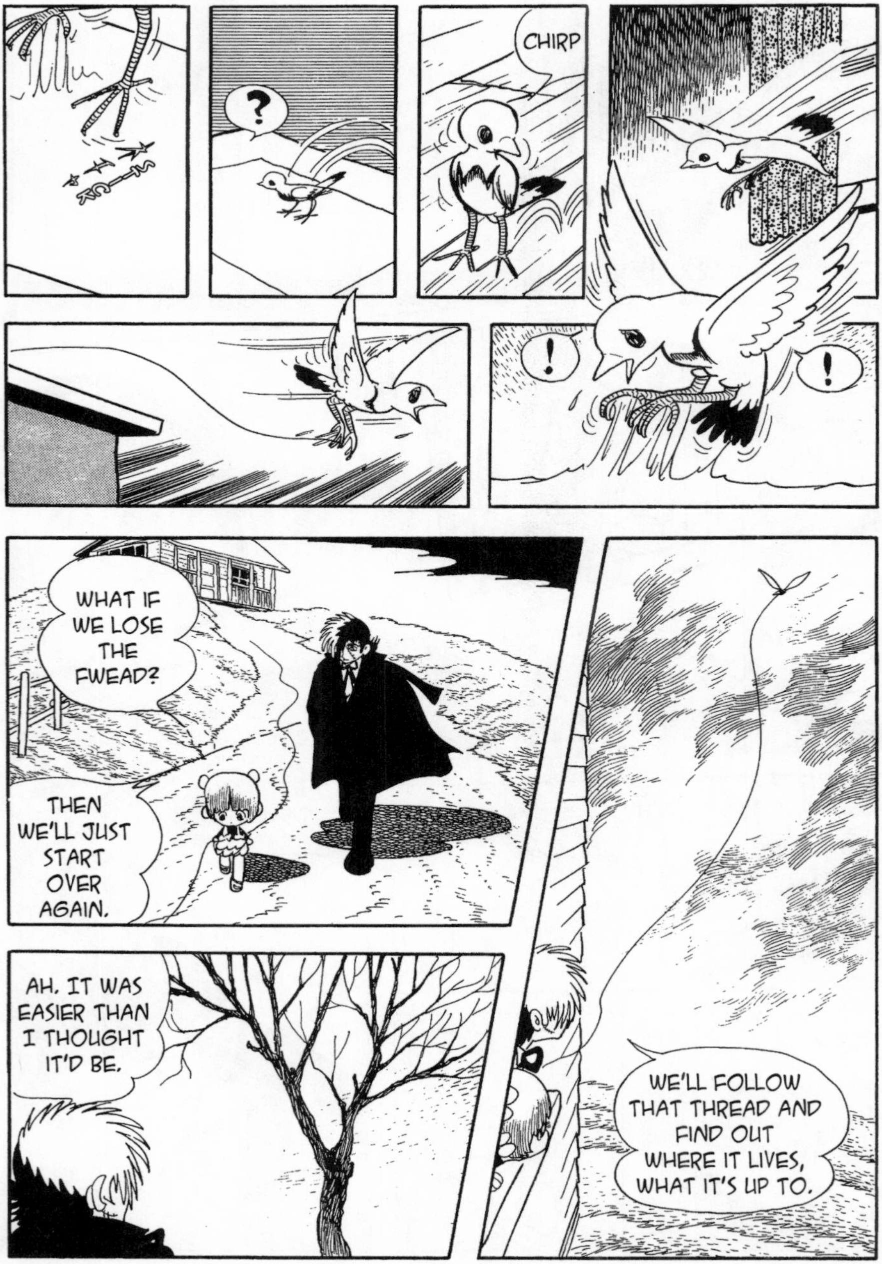
CHIRP
?
!
!
WE'LL FOLLOW THAT THREAD AND FIND OUT WHERE IT LIVES, WHAT IT'S UP TO.
WHAT IF WE LOSE THE FWEAD?
THEN WE'LL JUST START OVER AGAIN.
AH. IT WAS EASIER THAN I THOUGHT IT'D BE.

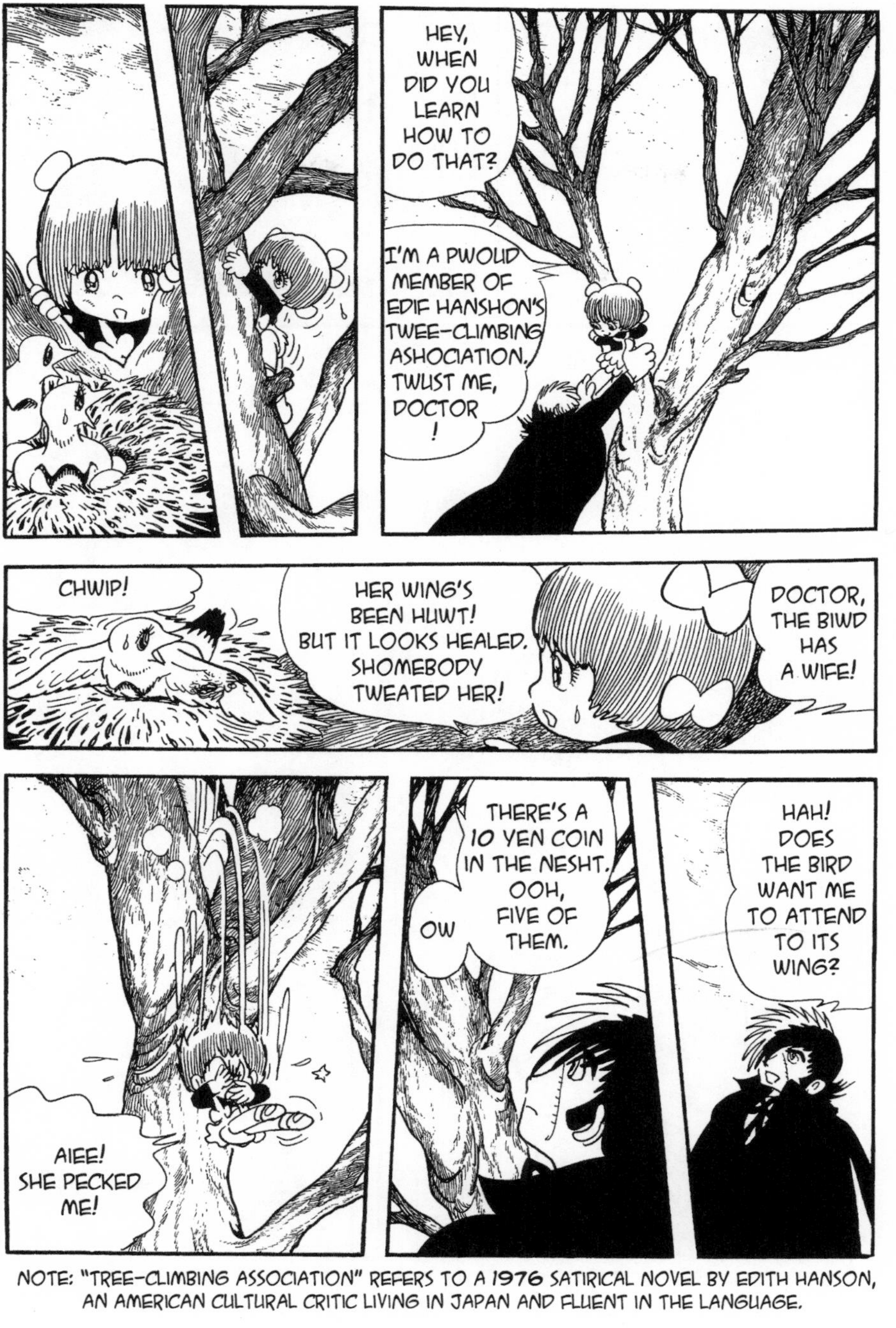
HEY, WHEN DID YOU LEARN HOW TO DO THAT?
I'M A PWOUD MEMBER OF EDIF HANSHON'S TWEE-CLIMBING ASHOCIATION, TWUST ME, DOCTOR!
DOCTOR, THE BIWD HAS A WIFE!
HER WING'S BEEN HUWT! BUT IT LOOKS HEALED. SHOMEBODY TWEATED HER!
CHWIP!
HAH! DOES THE BIRD WANT ME TO ATTEND TO ITS WING?
THERE'S A 10 YEN COIN IN THE NESHT. OOH, FIVE OF THEM.
OW
AIEE! SHE PECKED ME!

NOTE: "TREE-CLIMBING ASSOCIATION" REFERS TO A 1976 SATIRICAL NOVEL BY EDITH HANSON, AN AMERICAN CULTURAL CRITIC LIVING IN JAPAN AND FLUENT IN THE LANGUAGE.

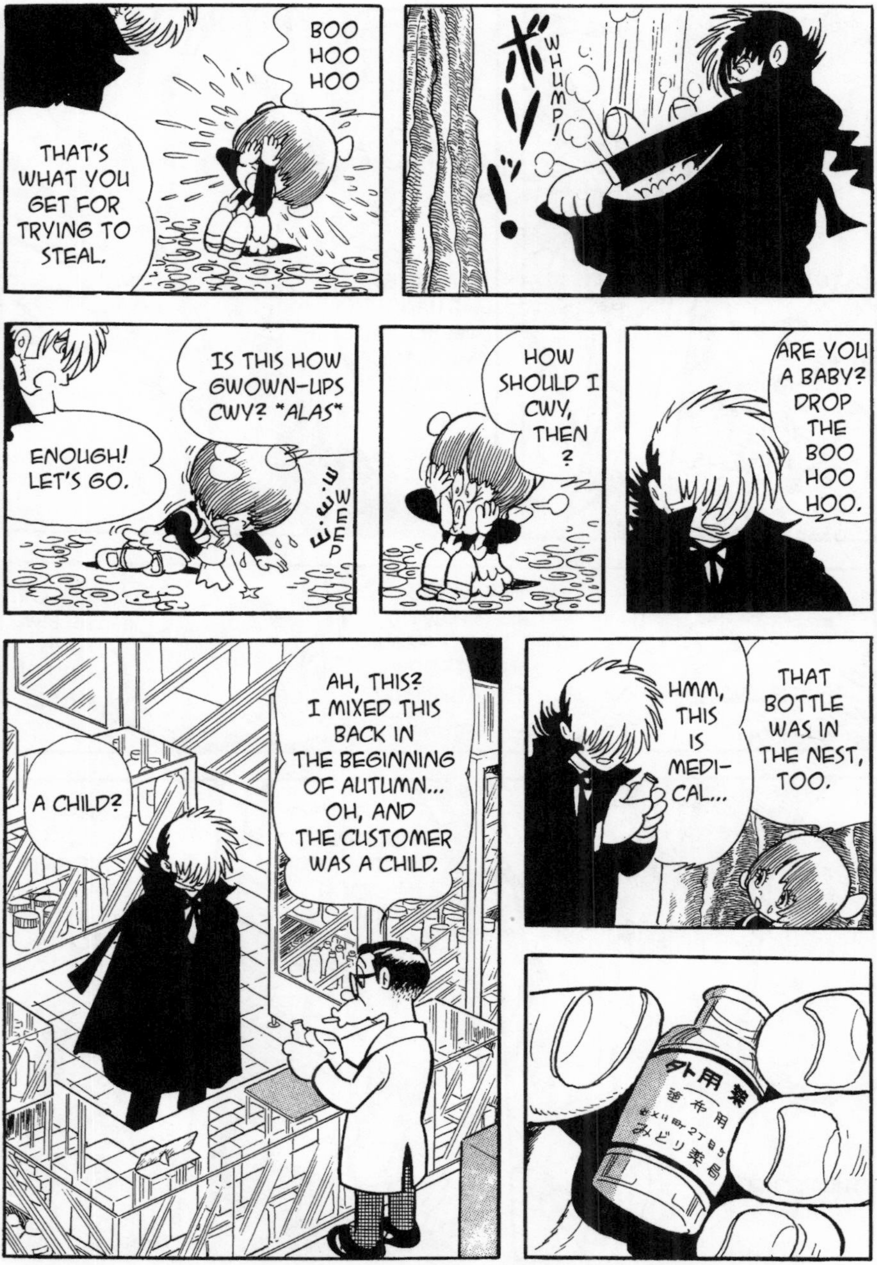
WHUMP!
BOO HOO HOO
THAT'S WHAT YOU GET FOR TRYING TO STEAL.
ARE YOU A BABY? DROP THE BOO HOO HOO.
HOW SHOULD I CWY, THEN?
IS THIS HOW GWOWN-UPS CWY? *ALAS*
ENOUGH! LET'S GO.
WEEP
THAT BOTTLE WAS IN THE NEST, TOO.
HMM, THIS IS MEDICAL...
外用薬
塗布用
みどり薬局
AH, THIS? I MIXED THIS BACK IN THE BEGINNING OF AUTUMN... OH, AND THE CUSTOMER WAS A CHILD.
A CHILD?

NOTE: BOTTLE LABEL = FOR EXTERNAL USE ONLY, LINIMENT; ADDRESS, MIDORI PHARMACY

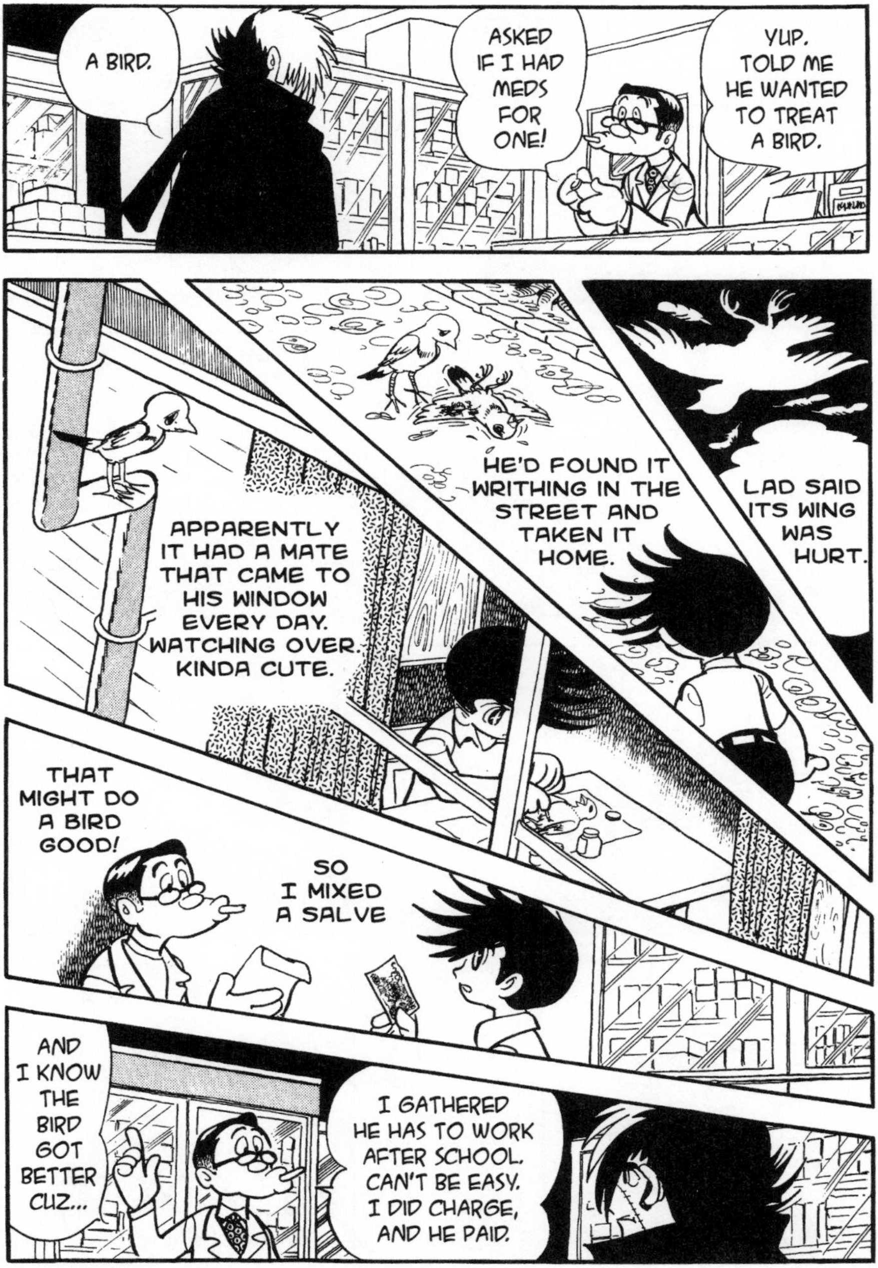
YUP. TOLD ME HE WANTED TO TREAT A BIRD.
ASKED IF I HAD MEDS FOR ONE!
A BIRD.
LAD SAID ITS WING WAS HURT.
HE'D FOUND IT WRITHING IN THE STREET AND TAKEN IT HOME.
APPARENTLY IT HAD A MATE THAT CAME TO HIS WINDOW EVERY DAY. WATCHING OVER. KINDA CUTE.
SO I MIXED A SALVE
THAT MIGHT DO A BIRD GOOD!
I GATHERED HE HAS TO WORK AFTER SCHOOL. CAN'T BE EASY. I DID CHARGE, AND HE PAID.
AND I KNOW THE BIRD GOT BETTER CUZ...

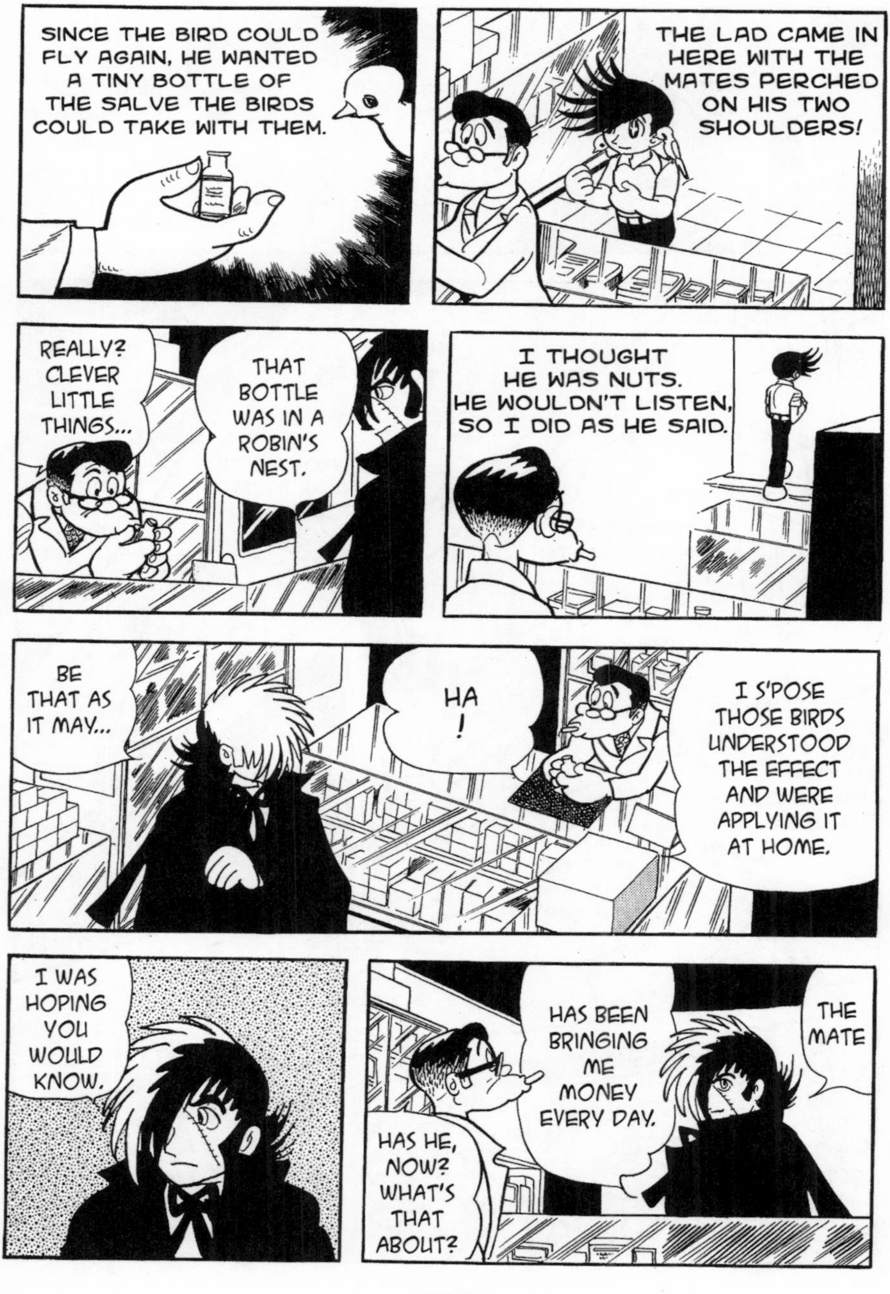
THE LAD CAME IN HERE WITH THE MATES PERCHED ON HIS TWO SHOULDERS!
SINCE THE BIRD COULD FLY AGAIN, HE WANTED A TINY BOTTLE OF THE SALVE THE BIRDS COULD TAKE WITH THEM.
I THOUGHT HE WAS NUTS. HE WOULDN'T LISTEN, SO I DID AS HE SAID.
THAT BOTTLE WAS IN A ROBIN'S NEST.
REALLY? CLEVER LITTLE THINGS...
I S'POSE THOSE BIRDS UNDERSTOOD THE EFFECT AND WERE APPLYING IT AT HOME.
HA!
BE THAT AS IT MAY...
THE MATE
HAS BEEN BRINGING ME MONEY EVERY DAY.
HAS HE, NOW? WHAT'S THAT ABOUT?
I WAS HOPING YOU WOULD KNOW.

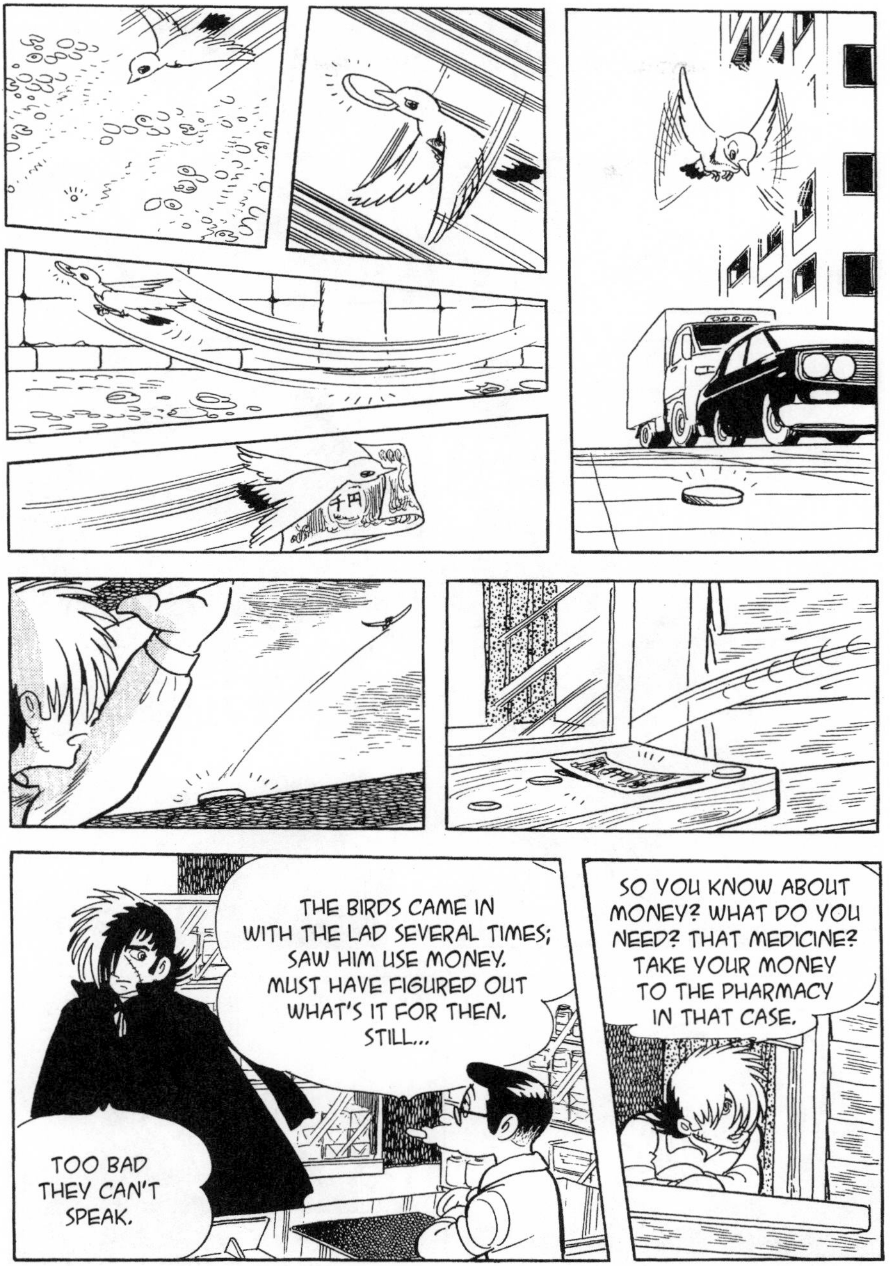
千円
SO YOU KNOW ABOUT MONEY? WHAT DO YOU NEED? THAT MEDICINE? TAKE YOUR MONEY TO THE PHARMACY IN THAT CASE.
THE BIRDS CAME IN WITH THE LAD SEVERAL TIMES; SAW HIM USE MONEY. MUST HAVE FIGURED OUT WHAT'S IT FOR THEN. STILL...
TOO BAD THEY CAN'T SPEAK.

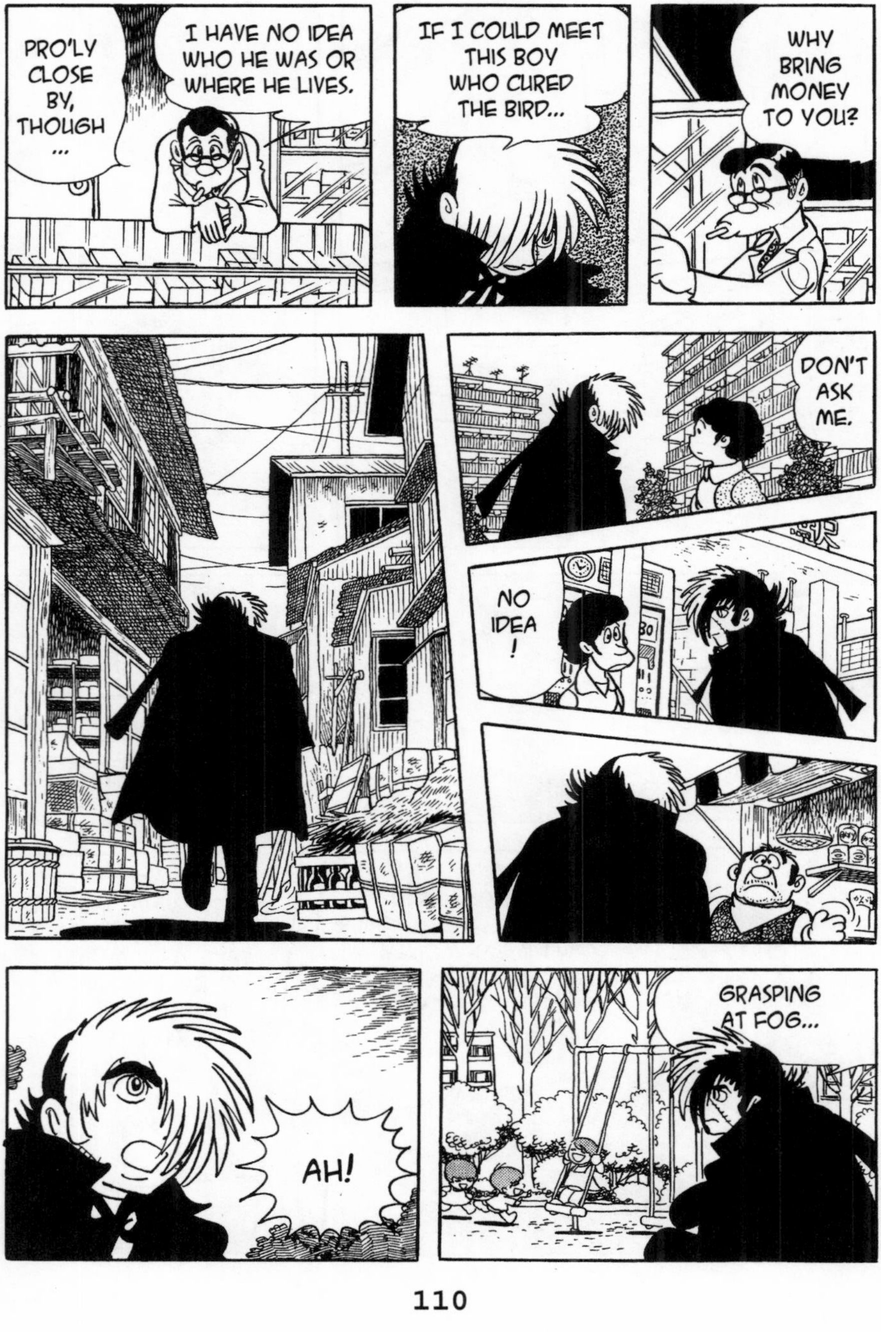
WHY BRING MONEY TO YOU?
IF I COULD MEET THIS BOY WHO CURED THE BIRD...
I HAVE NO IDEA WHO HE WAS OR WHERE HE LIVES.
PRO'LY CLOSE BY, THOUGH ...
DON'T ASK ME.
NO IDEA !
GRASPING AT FOG...
AH!

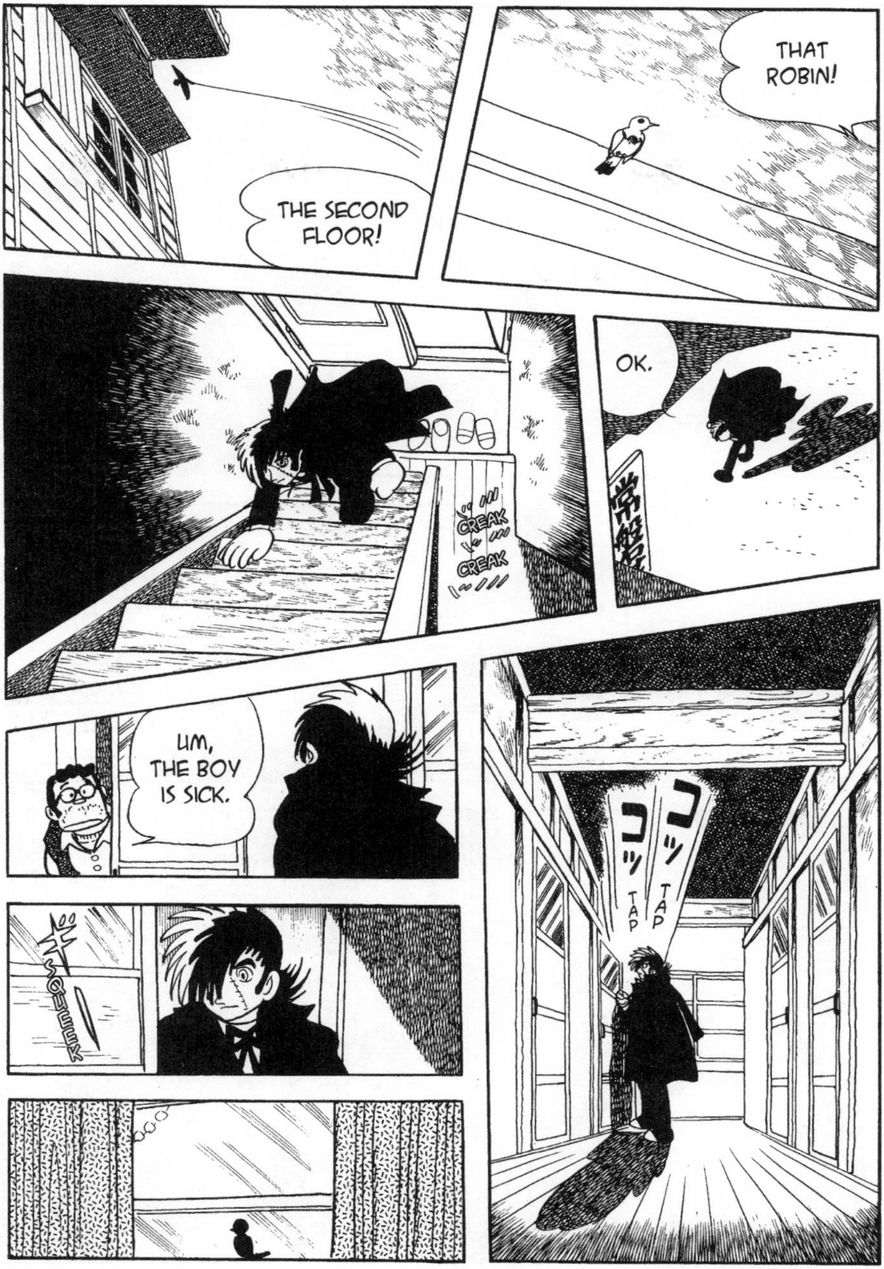
THAT ROBIN!
THE SECOND FLOOR!
OK.
常磐
CREAK
CREAK
コッ TAP
コッ TAP
UM, THE BOY IS SICK.
ギ SQUEEK

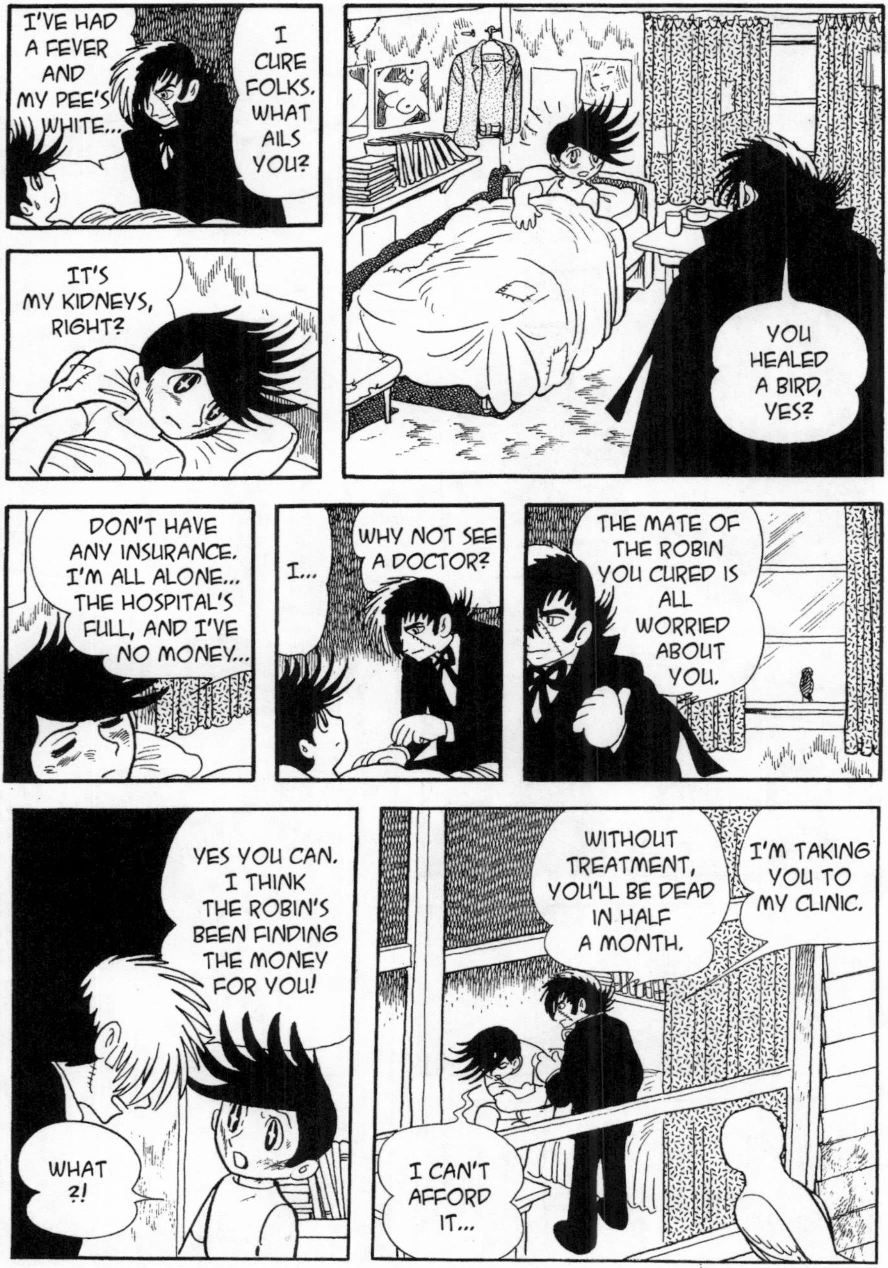
YOU HEALED A BIRD, YES?
I CURE FOLKS. WHAT AILS YOU?
I'VE HAD A FEVER AND MY PEE'S WHITE...
IT'S MY KIDNEYS, RIGHT?
THE MATE OF THE ROBIN YOU CURED IS ALL WORRIED ABOUT YOU.
WHY NOT SEE A DOCTOR?
I...
DON'T HAVE ANY INSURANCE. I'M ALL ALONE... THE HOSPITAL'S FULL, AND I'VE NO MONEY...
I'M TAKING YOU TO MY CLINIC.
WITHOUT TREATMENT, YOU'LL BE DEAD IN HALF A MONTH.
I CAN'T AFFORD IT...
YES YOU CAN. I THINK THE ROBIN'S BEEN FINDING THE MONEY FOR YOU!
WHAT ?!

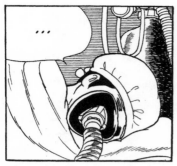

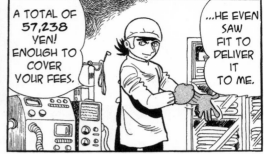

...HE EVEN SAW FIT TO DELIVER IT TO ME.
A TOTAL OF 57,238 YEN! ENOUGH TO COVER YOUR FEES.
...
THAT ROBIN, GLUED TO YOUR WINDOW, WAS HOW I FOUND YOU.
HE FIGURED OUT I'M A DOCTOR AND COURTED MY AID. AN AMAZING FELLOW, EH?
AND TO GATHER MONEY, HE STAYED IN JAPAN FOR THE WINTER!

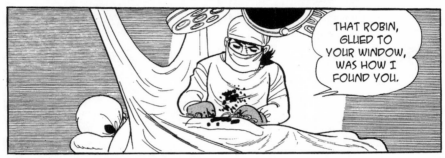

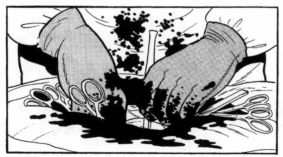

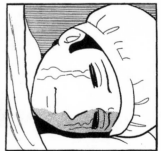

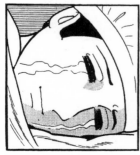

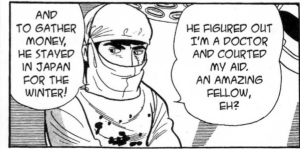

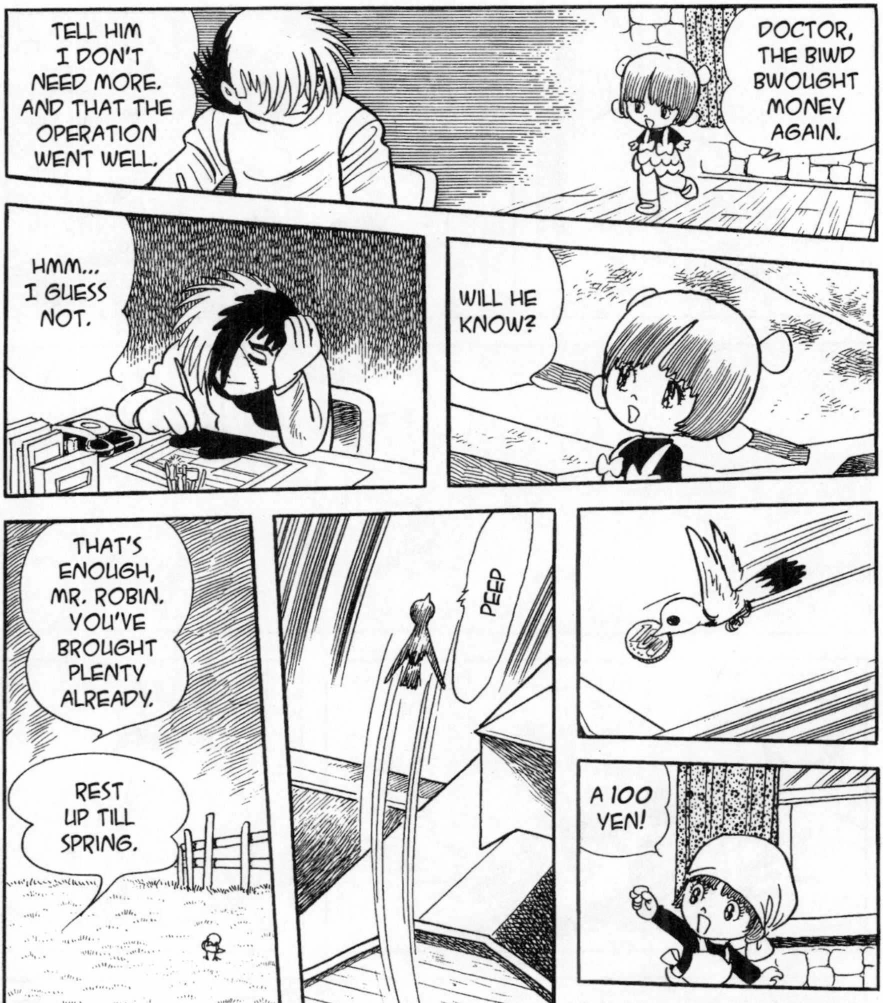
DOCTOR, THE BIWD BWOUGHT MONEY AGAIN.
TELL HIM I DON'T NEED MORE. AND THAT THE OPERATION WENT WELL.
WILL HE KNOW?
HMM... I GUESS NOT.
A 100 YEN!
A 1000 YEN!
PEEP
THAT'S ENOUGH, MR. ROBIN. YOU'VE BROUGHT PLENTY ALREADY.
REST UP TILL SPRING.

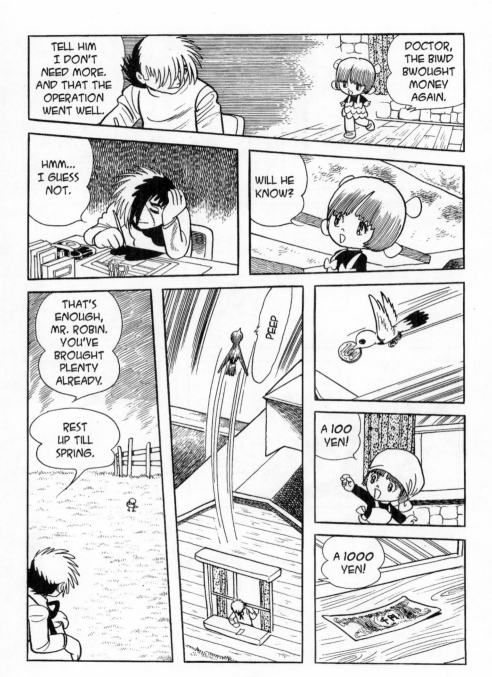

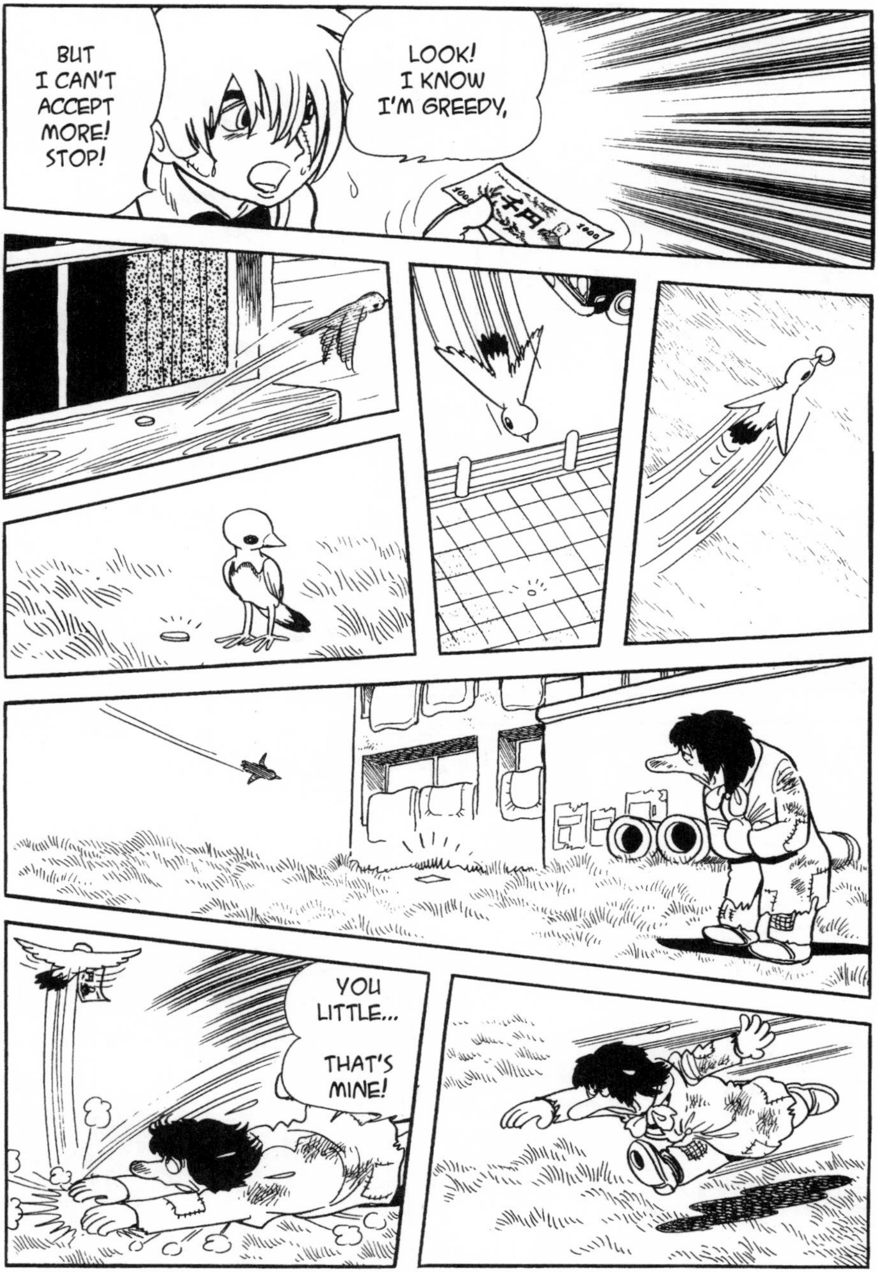
LOOK! I KNOW I'M GREEDY,
BUT I CAN'T ACCEPT MORE! STOP!
YOU LITTLE...
THAT'S MINE!

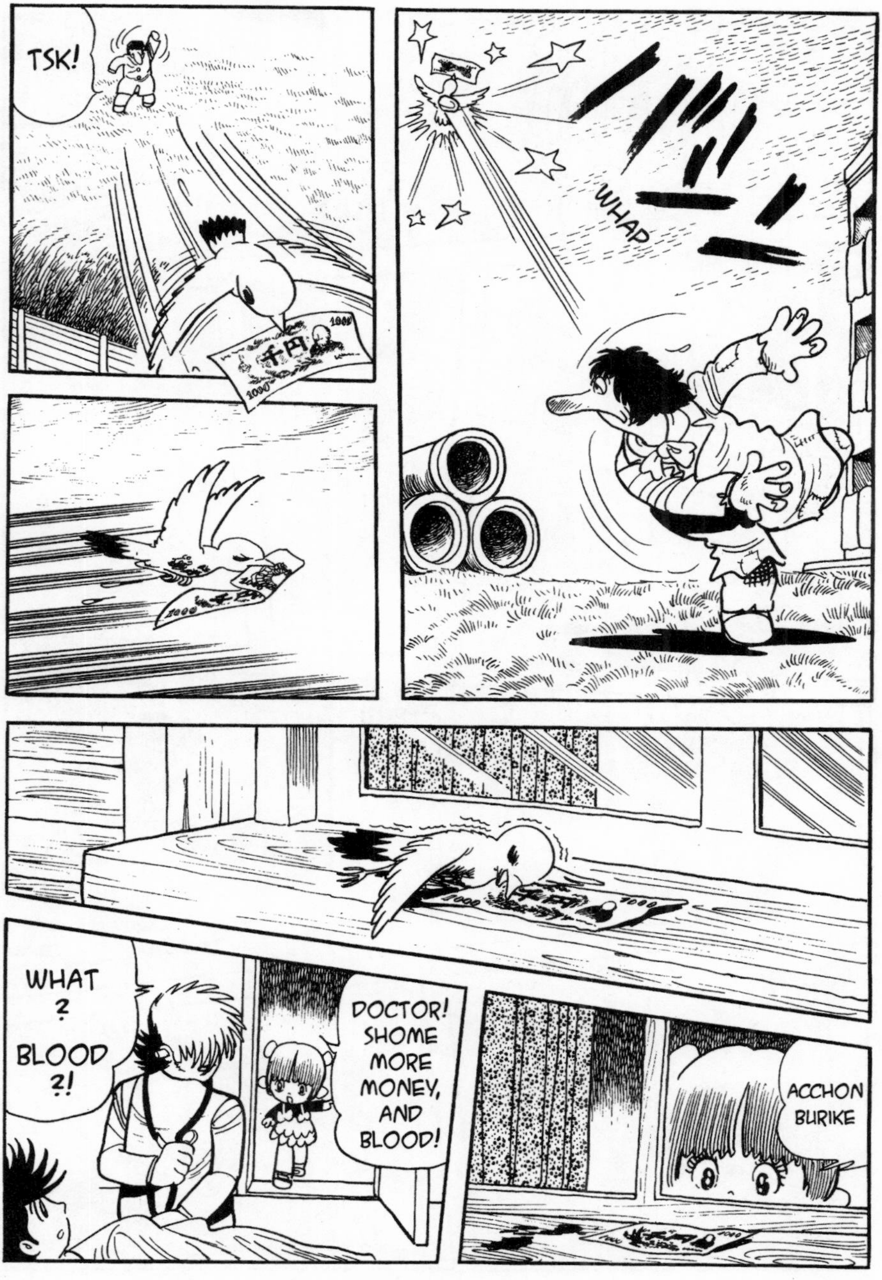
WHAP
TSK!
ACCHON BURIKE
DOCTOR! SHOME MORE MONEY, AND BLOOD!
WHAT? BLOOD?!

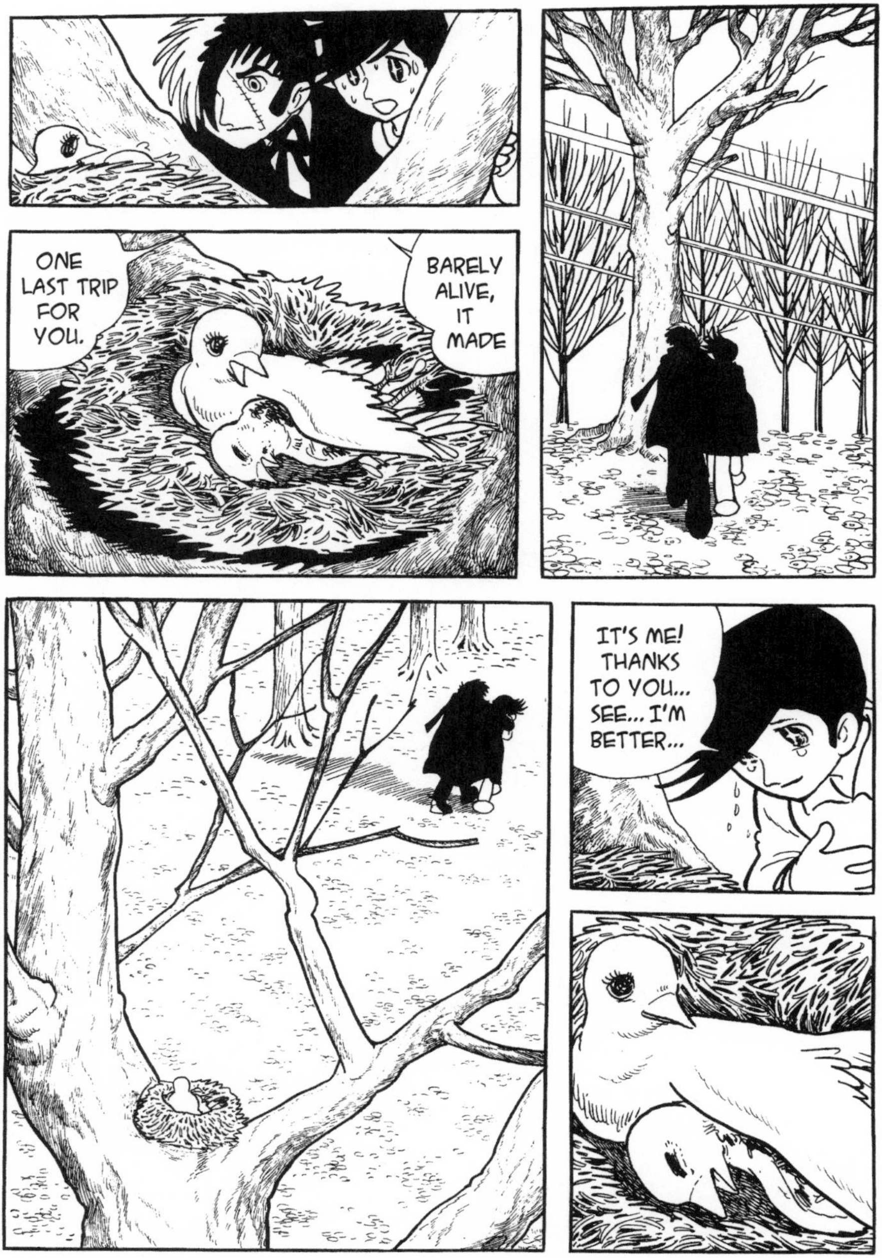
BARELY ALIVE, IT MADE
ONE LAST TRIP FOR YOU.
IT'S ME! THANKS TO YOU... SEE... I'M BETTER...

THE BOY WHO CAME FROM THE SKY

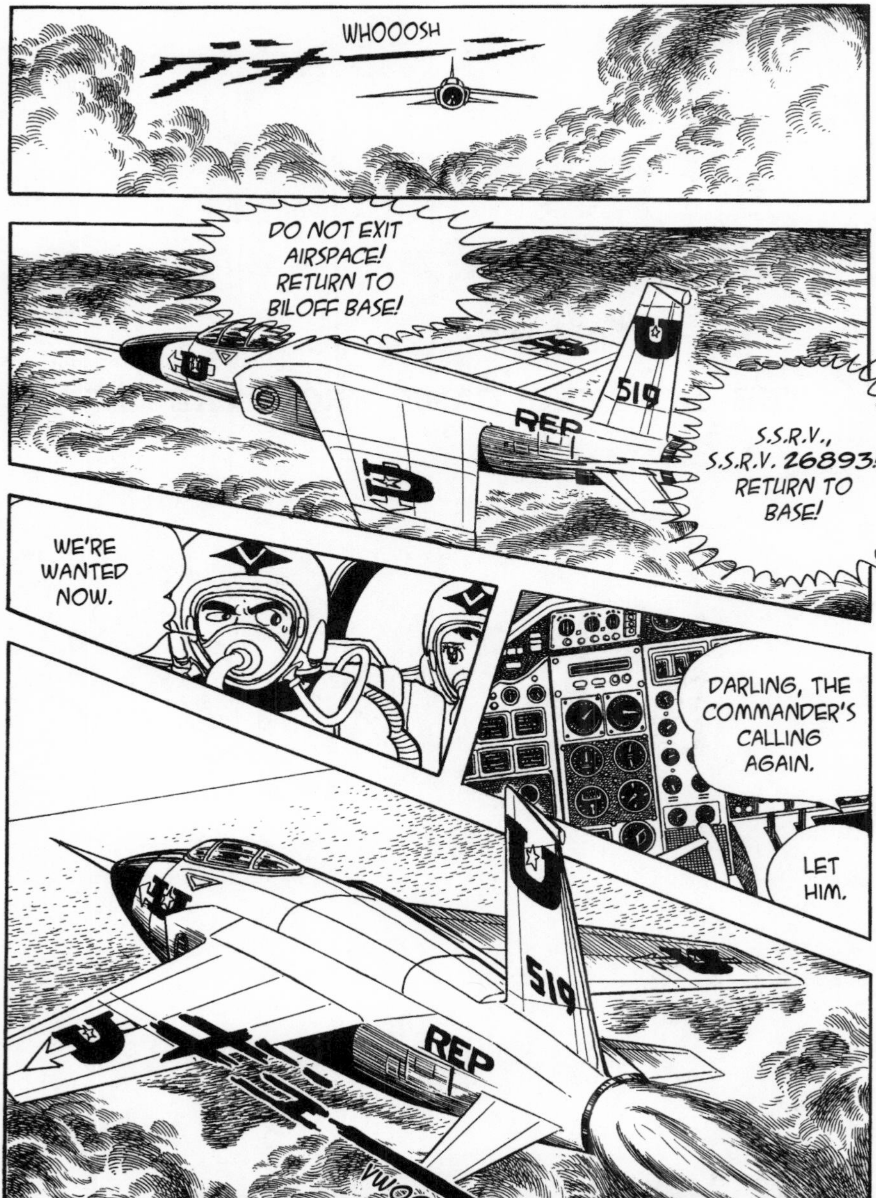
WHOOOSH
DO NOT EXIT AIRSPACE! RETURN TO BILOFF BASE!
S.S.R.V., S.S.R.V. 26893! RETURN TO BASE!
DARLING, THE COMMANDER'S CALLING AGAIN.
LET HIM.
WE'RE WANTED NOW.
VWOOOSH

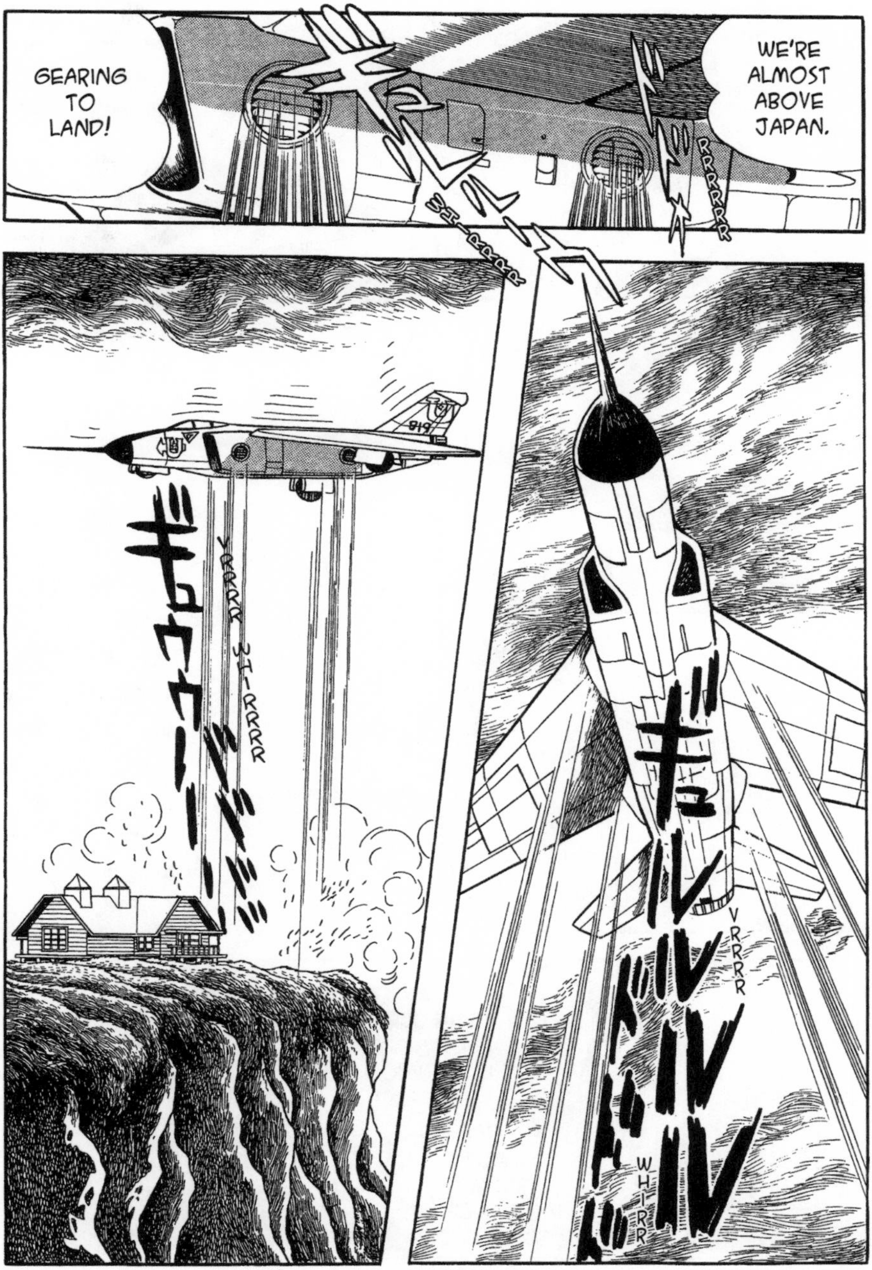
WE'RE ALMOST ABOVE JAPAN.
GEARING TO LAND!
RRRRRRR
VRRRR
WHIRR
VRRRR
WHIRRRR

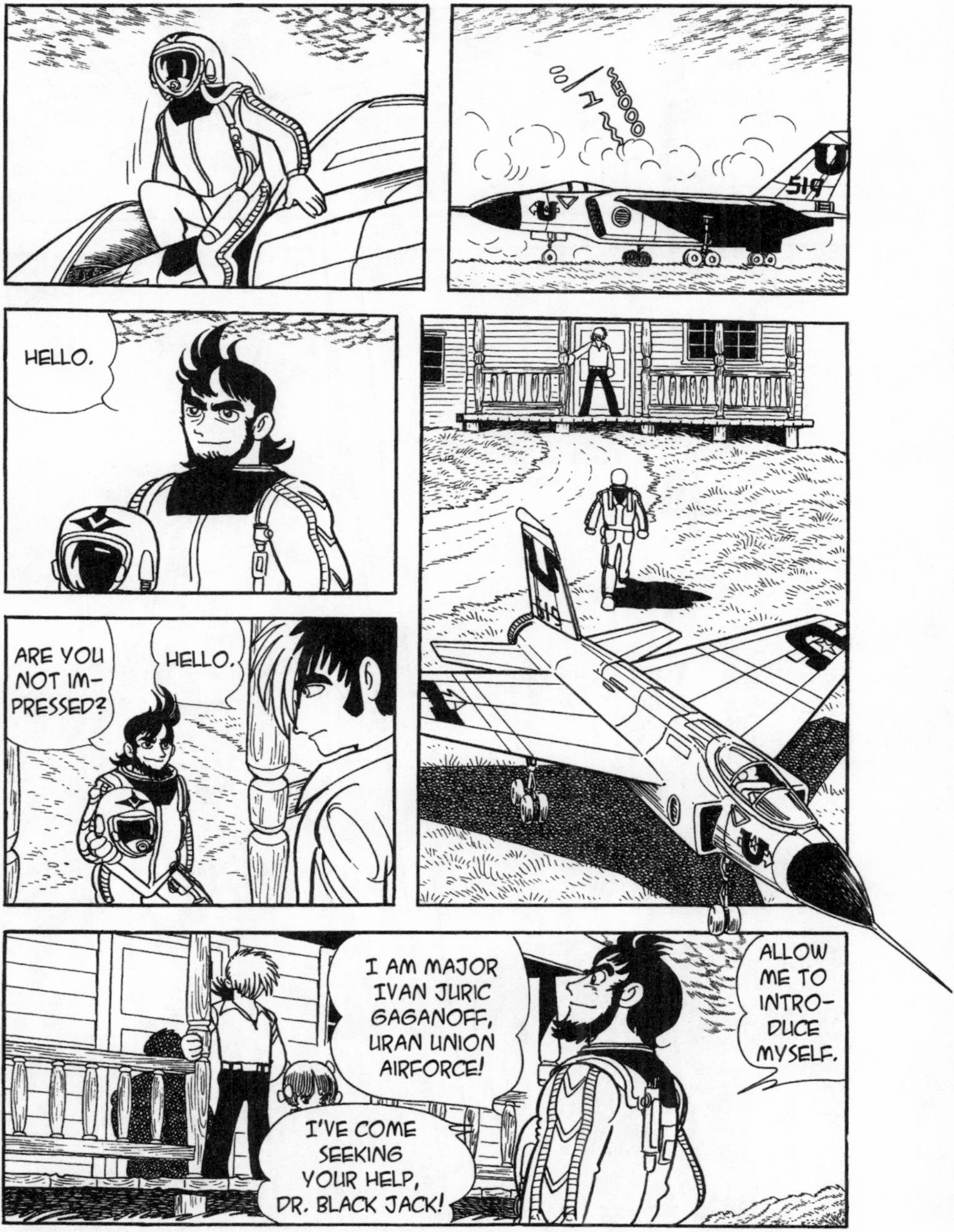
HELLO.
HELLO.
ARE YOU NOT IMPRESSED?
ALLOW ME TO INTRODUCE MYSELF.
I AM MAJOR IVAN JURIC GAGANOFF, URAN UNION AIRFORCE!
I'VE COME SEEKING YOUR HELP, DR. BLACK JACK!

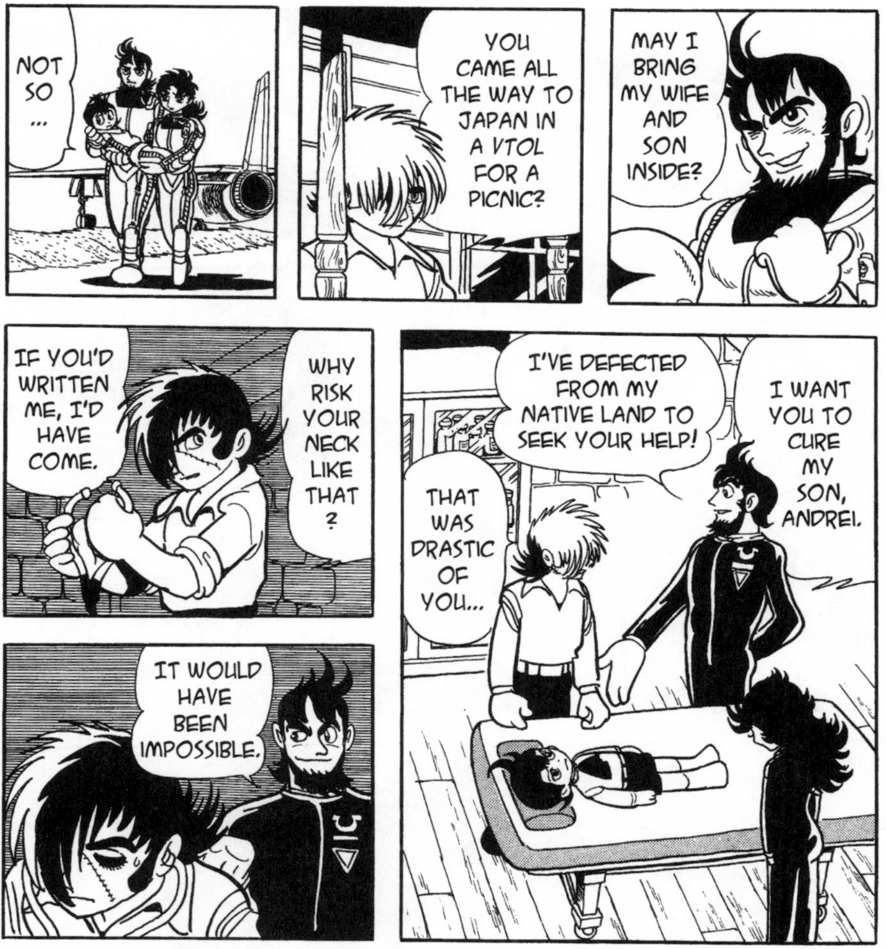
MAY I BRING MY WIFE AND SON INSIDE?
YOU CAME ALL THE WAY TO JAPAN IN A VTOL FOR A PICNIC?
NOT SO ...
I WANT YOU TO CURE MY SON, ANDREI.
I'VE DEFECTED FROM MY NATIVE LAND TO SEEK YOUR HELP!
THAT WAS DRASTIC OF YOU...
WHY RISK YOUR NECK LIKE THAT?
IF YOU'D WRITTEN ME, I'D HAVE COME.
IT WOULD HAVE BEEN IMPOSSIBLE.
YOU SEE, I'M A MEMBER OF A SPECIALLY TRAINED UNIT.
WE'RE CONFINED TO A RESTRICTED ZONE AND FORBIDDEN ALL CONTACT WITH FOREIGNERS.

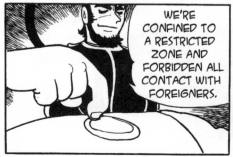

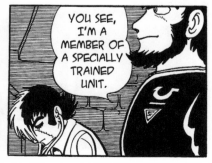

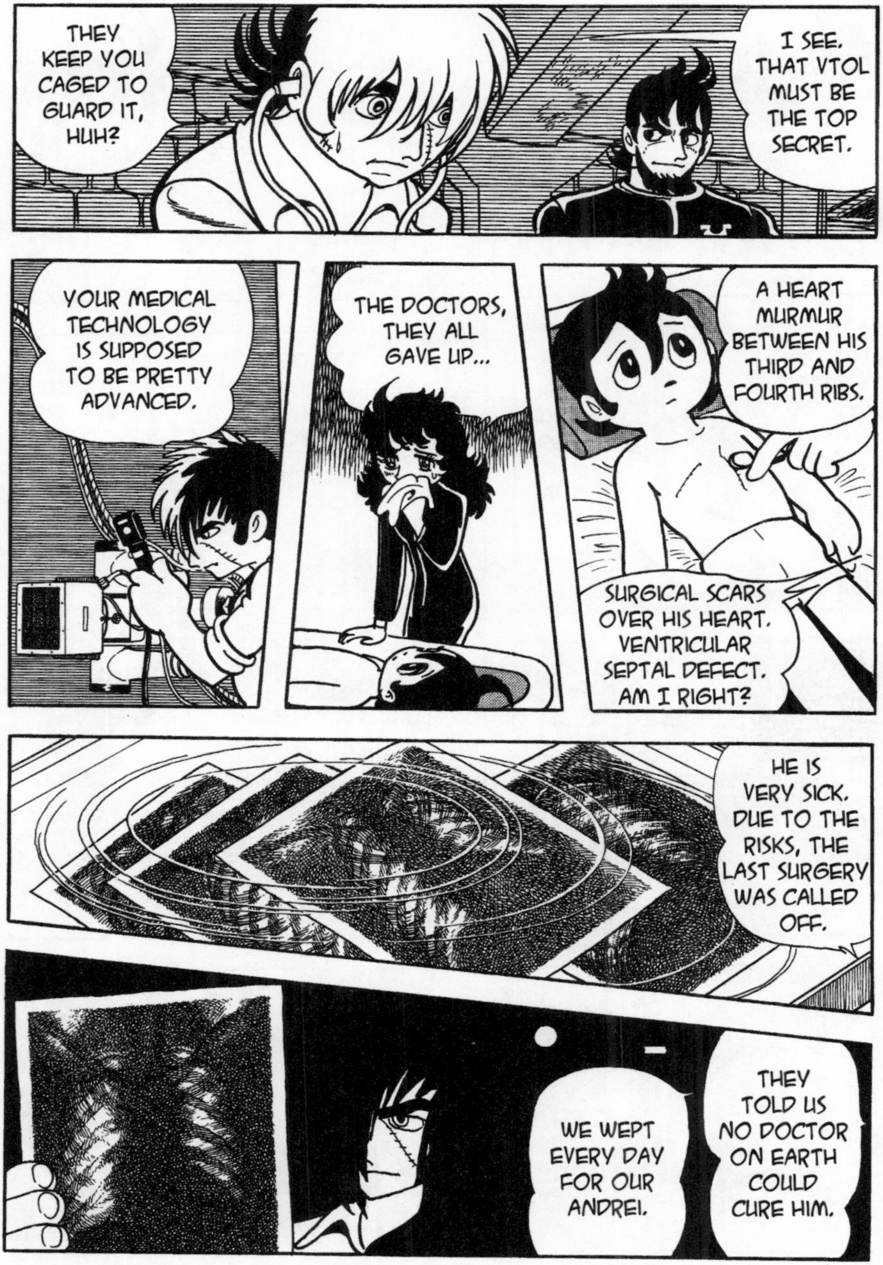
I SEE. THAT VTOL MUST BE THE TOP SECRET.
THEY KEEP YOU CAGED TO GUARD IT, HUH?
A HEART MURMUR BETWEEN HIS THIRD AND FOURTH RIBS.
SURGICAL SCARS OVER HIS HEART. VENTRICULAR SEPTAL DEFECT. AM I RIGHT?
THE DOCTORS, THEY ALL GAVE UP...
YOUR MEDICAL TECHNOLOGY IS SUPPOSED TO BE PRETTY ADVANCED.
HE IS VERY SICK. DUE TO THE RISKS, THE LAST SURGERY WAS CALLED OFF.
THEY TOLD US NO DOCTOR ON EARTH COULD CURE HIM.
WE WEPT EVERY DAY FOR OUR ANDREI.

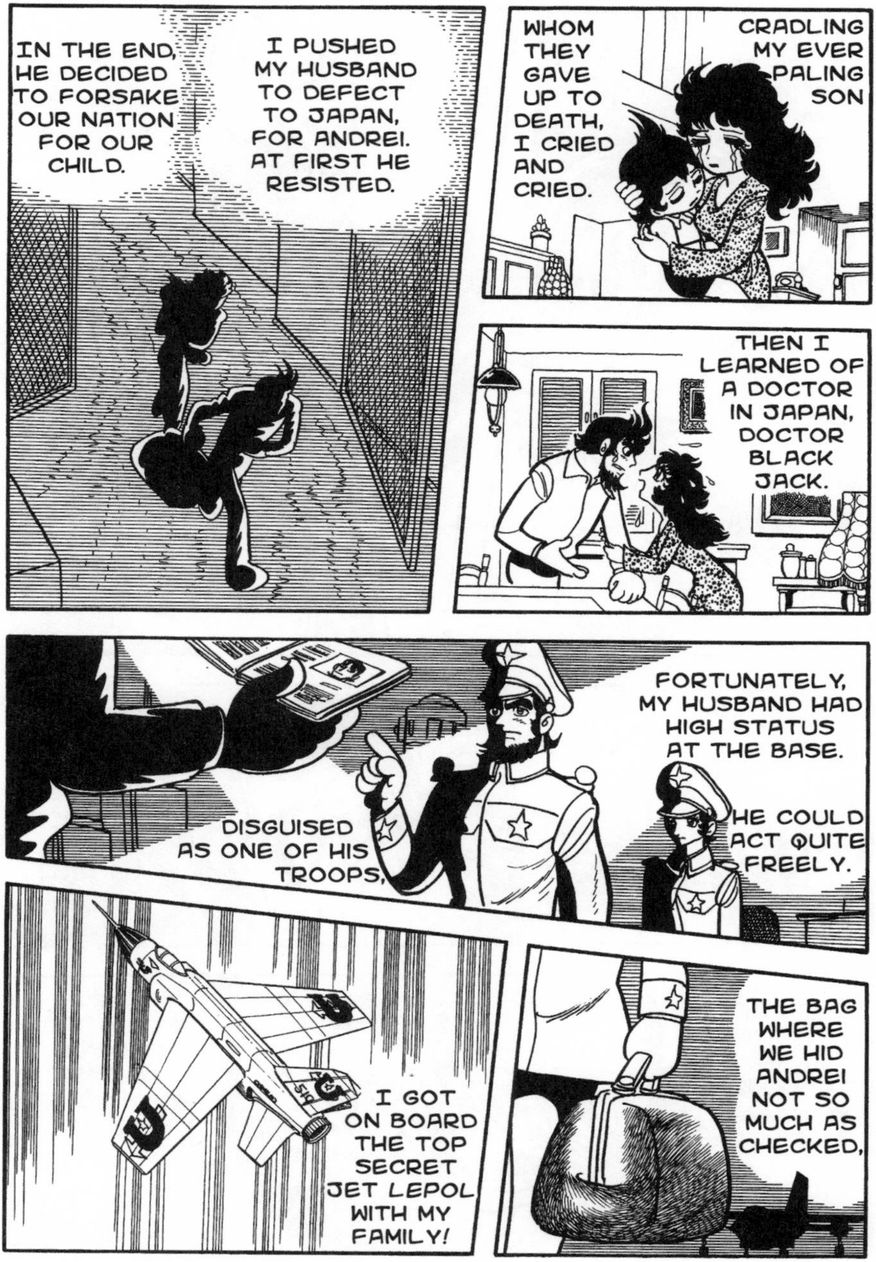
CRADLING MY EVER PALING SON
WHOM THEY GAVE UP TO DEATH, I CRIED AND CRIED.
THEN I LEARNED OF A DOCTOR IN JAPAN, DOCTOR BLACK JACK.
I PUSHED MY HUSBAND TO DEFECT TO JAPAN, FOR ANDREI. AT FIRST HE RESISTED.
IN THE END, HE DECIDED TO FORSAKE OUR NATION FOR OUR CHILD.
FORTUNATELY, MY HUSBAND HAD HIGH STATUS AT THE BASE.
HE COULD ACT QUITE FREELY.
DISGUISED AS ONE OF HIS TROOPS,
THE BAG WHERE WE HID ANDREI NOT SO MUCH AS CHECKED,
I GOT ON BOARD THE TOP SECRET JET LEPOL WITH MY FAMILY!

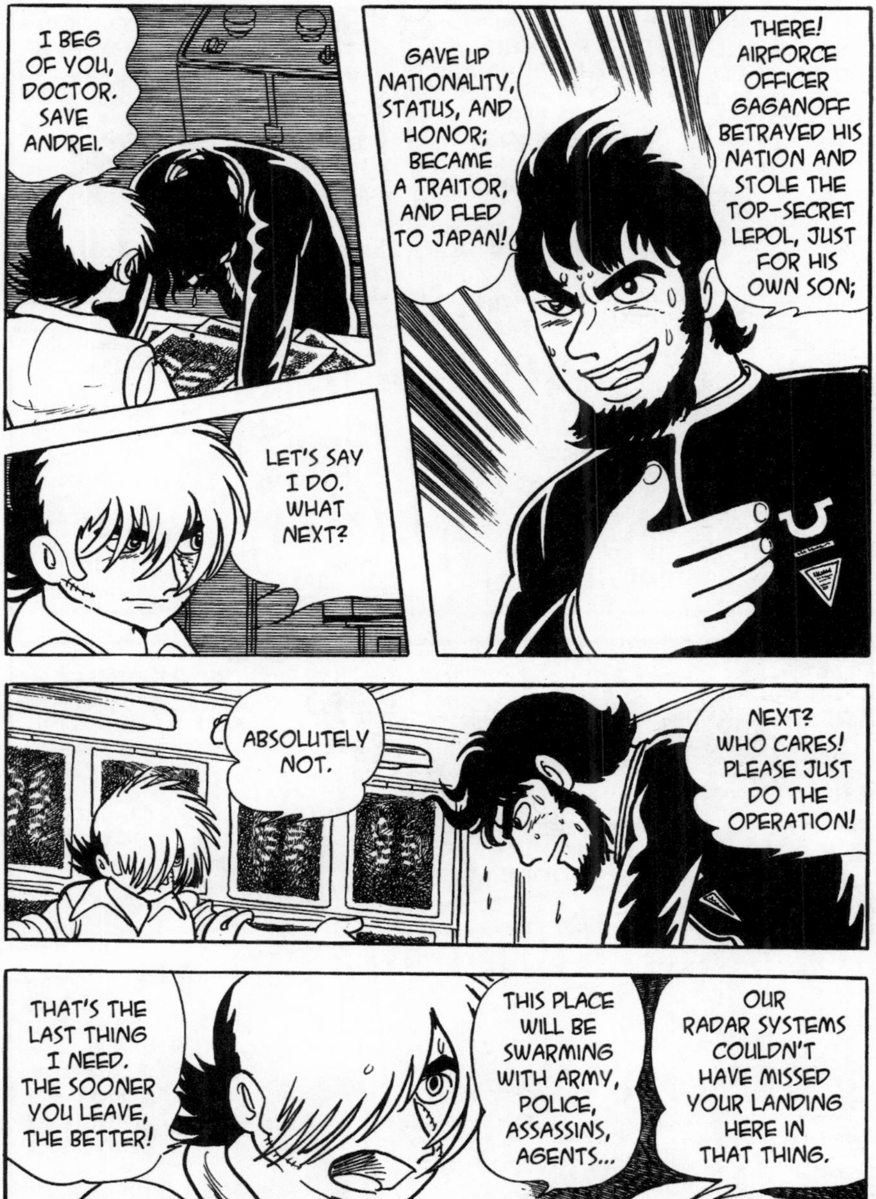
THERE! AIRFORCE OFFICER GAGANOFF BETRAYED HIS NATION AND STOLE THE TOP-SECRET LEPOL, JUST FOR HIS OWN SON;
GAVE UP NATIONALITY, STATUS, AND HONOR; BECAME A TRAITOR, AND FLED TO JAPAN!
I BEG OF YOU, DOCTOR. SAVE ANDREI.
LET'S SAY I DO. WHAT NEXT?
NEXT? WHO CARES! PLEASE JUST DO THE OPERATION!
ABSOLUTELY NOT.
OUR RADAR SYSTEMS COULDN'T HAVE MISSED YOUR LANDING HERE IN THAT THING.
THIS PLACE WILL BE SWARMING WITH ARMY, POLICE, ASSASSINS, AGENTS...
THAT'S THE LAST THING I NEED. THE SOONER YOU LEAVE, THE BETTER!

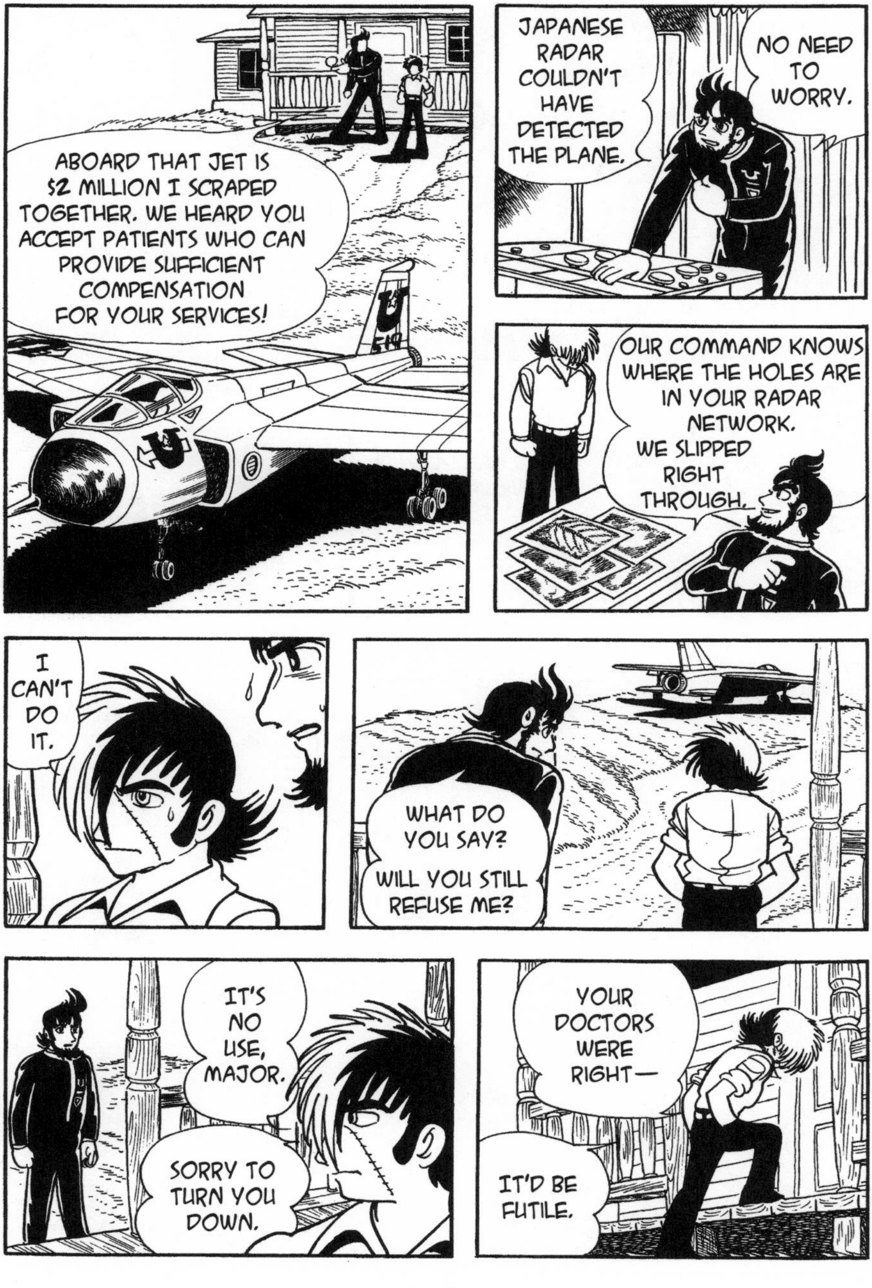
NO NEED TO WORRY.
JAPANESE RADAR COULDN'T HAVE DETECTED THE PLANE.
OUR COMMAND KNOWS WHERE THE HOLES ARE IN YOUR RADAR NETWORK.
WE SLIPPED RIGHT THROUGH.
ABOARD THAT JET IS $2 MILLION I SCRAPED TOGETHER. WE HEARD YOU ACCEPT PATIENTS WHO CAN PROVIDE SUFFICIENT COMPENSATION FOR YOUR SERVICES!
WHAT DO YOU SAY?
WILL YOU STILL REFUSE ME?
I CAN'T DO IT.
YOUR DOCTORS WERE RIGHT—
IT'D BE FUTILE.
IT'S NO USE, MAJOR.
SORRY TO TURN YOU DOWN.

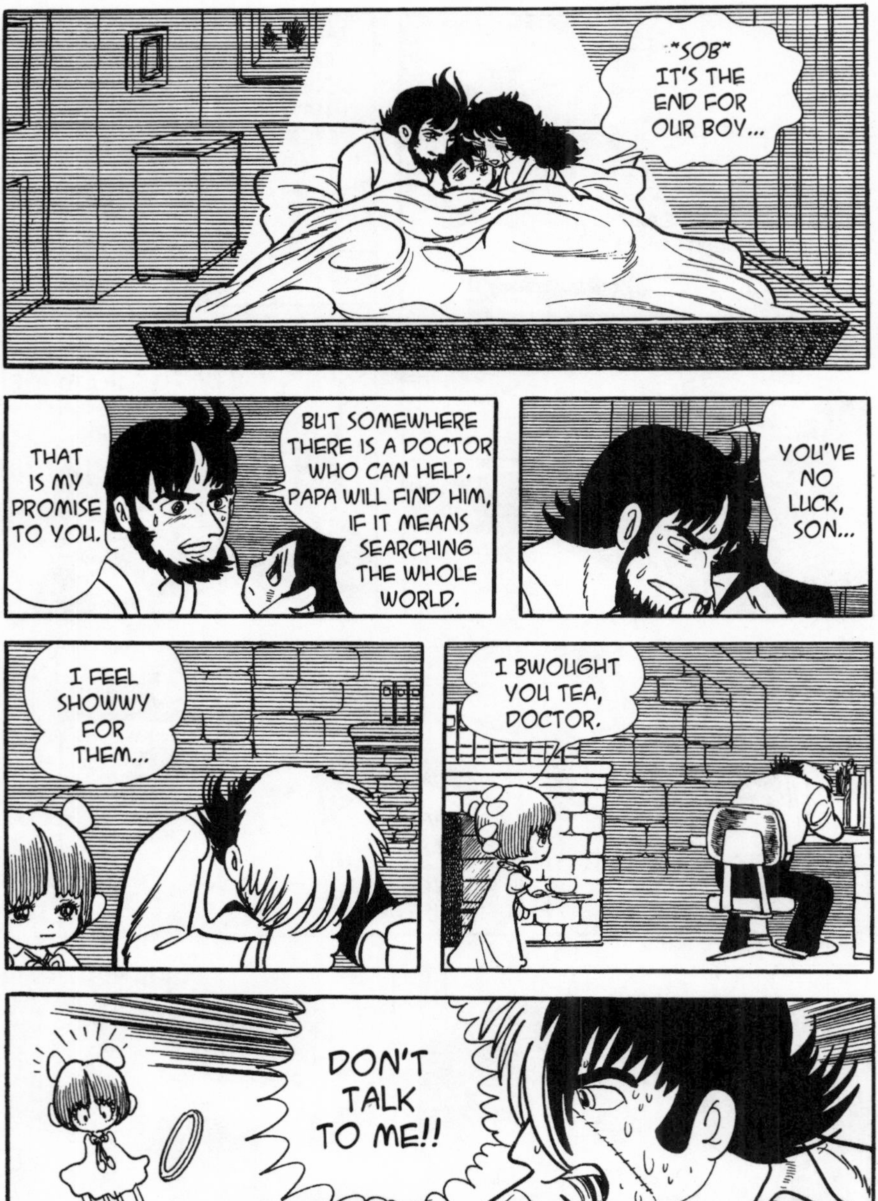
SOB IT'S THE END FOR OUR BOY...
YOU'VE NO LUCK, SON...
BUT SOMEWHERE THERE IS A DOCTOR WHO CAN HELP. PAPA WILL FIND HIM, IF IT MEANS SEARCHING THE WHOLE WORLD.
THAT IS MY PROMISE TO YOU.
I BWOUGHT YOU TEA, DOCTOR.
I FEEL SHOWWY FOR THEM...
DON'T TALK TO ME!!

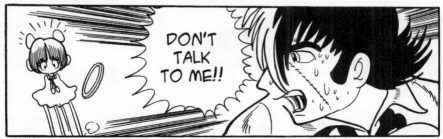

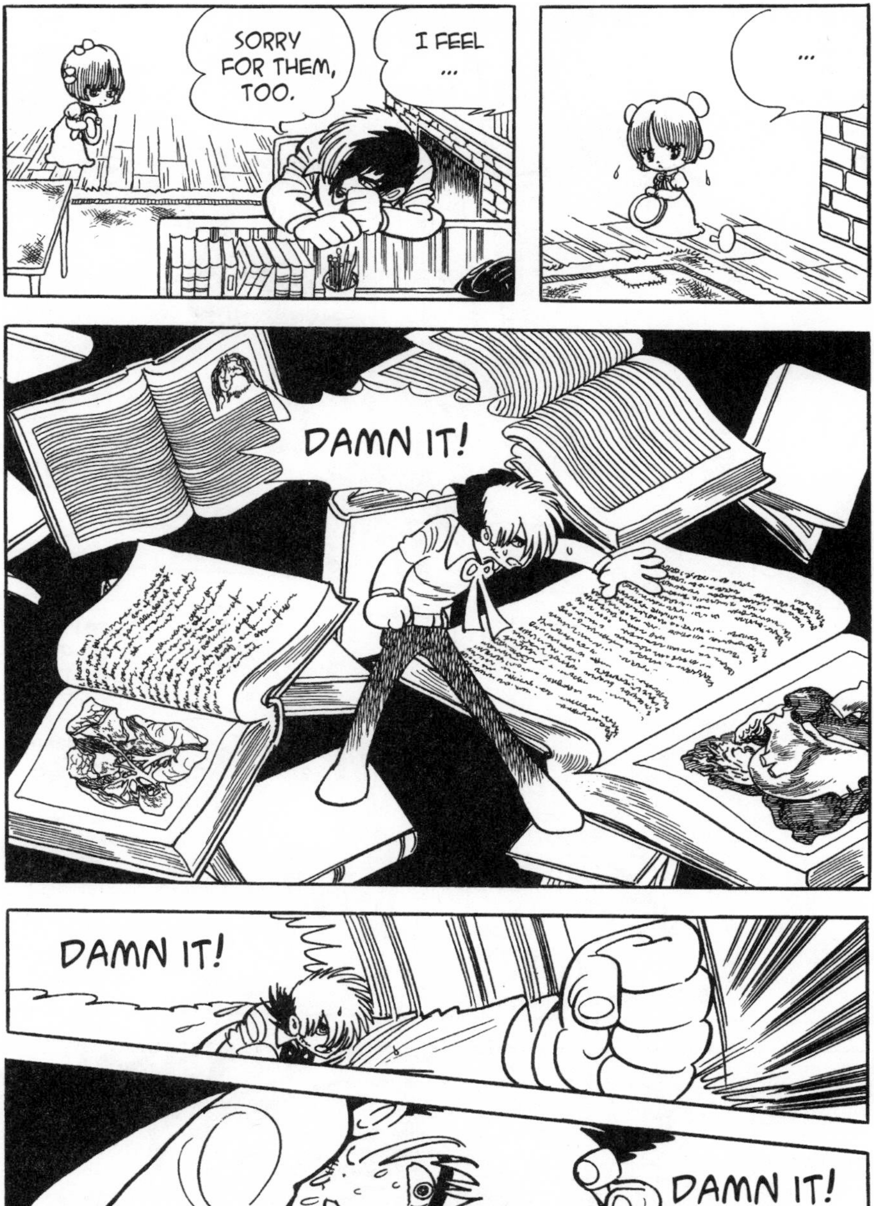
...
I FEEL ...
SORRY FOR THEM, TOO.
DAMN IT!
DAMN IT!
DAMN IT!

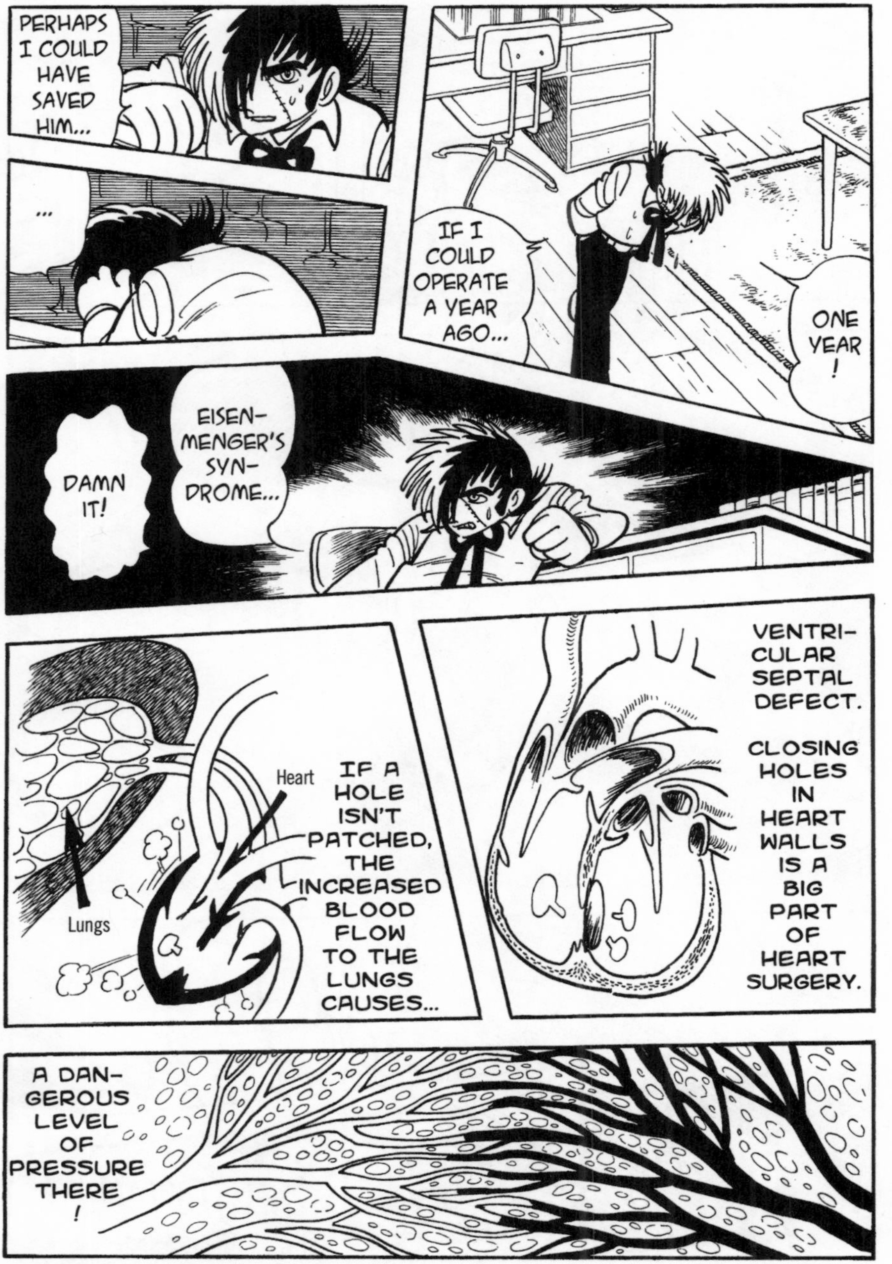
ONE YEAR!
IF I COULD OPERATE A YEAR AGO...
PERHAPS I COULD HAVE SAVED HIM...
...
EISEN-MENGER'S SYN-DROME...
DAMN IT!
VENTRI-CULAR SEPTAL DEFECT.
CLOSING HOLES IN HEART WALLS IS A BIG PART OF HEART SURGERY.
IF A HOLE ISN'T PATCHED, THE INCREASED BLOOD FLOW TO THE LUNGS CAUSES...
Heart
Lungs
A DAN-GEROUS LEVEL OF PRESSURE THERE!

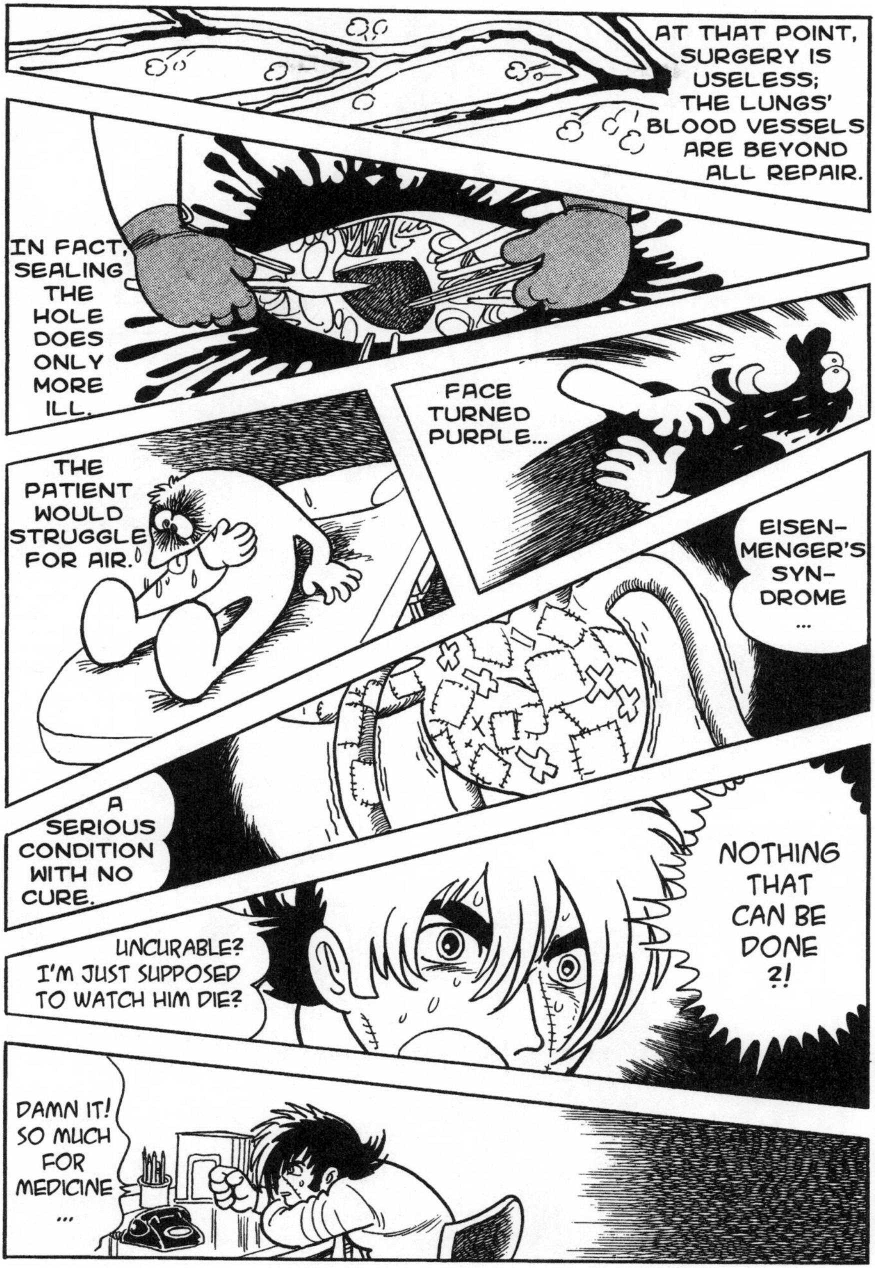
AT THAT POINT, SURGERY IS USELESS; THE LUNGS' BLOOD VESSELS ARE BEYOND ALL REPAIR.
IN FACT, SEALING THE HOLE DOES ONLY MORE ILL.
FACE TURNED PURPLE...
THE PATIENT WOULD STRUGGLE FOR AIR.
EISEN-MENGER'S SYN-DROME ...
A SERIOUS CONDITION WITH NO CURE.
NOTHING THAT CAN BE DONE ?!
UNCURABLE? I'M JUST SUPPOSED TO WATCH HIM DIE?
DAMN IT! SO MUCH FOR MEDICINE ...

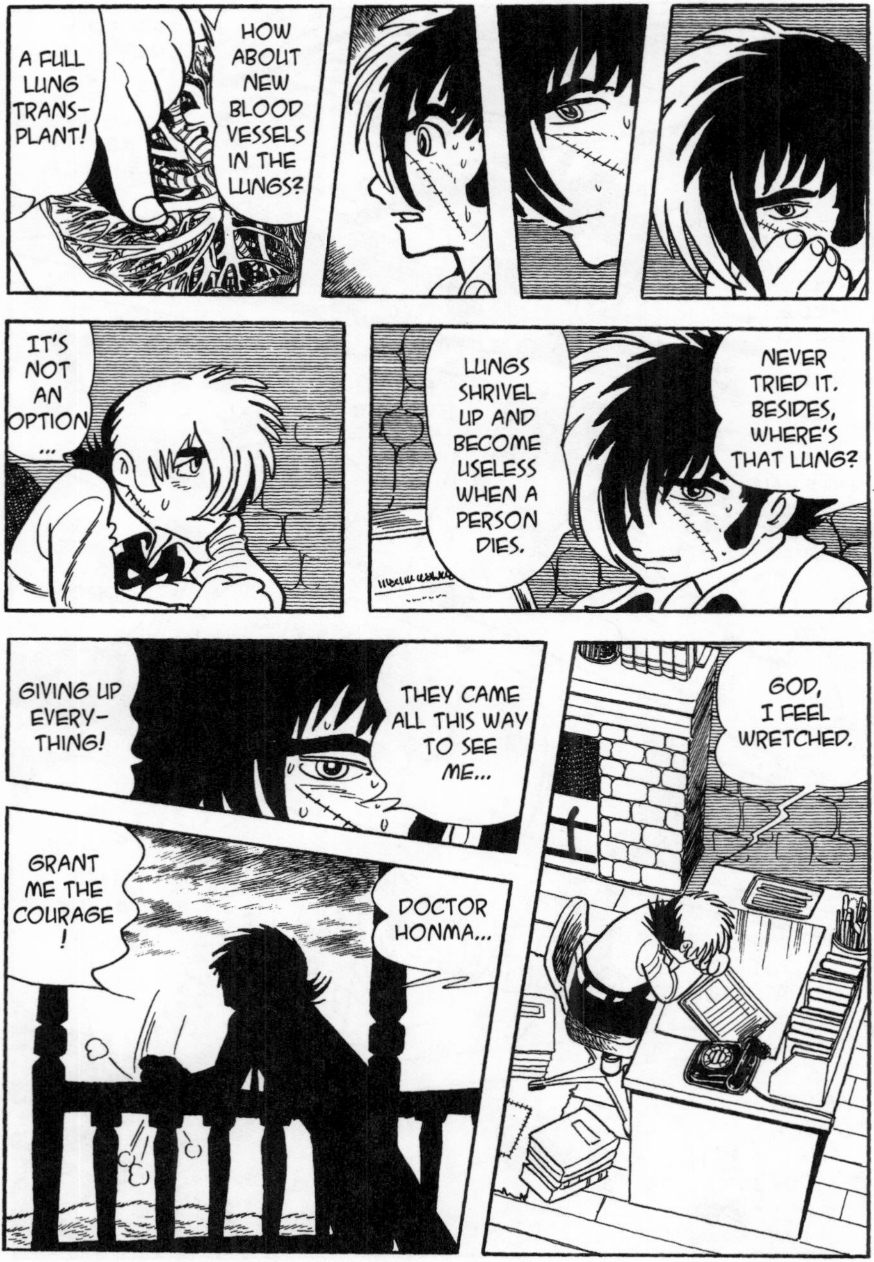
HOW ABOUT NEW BLOOD VESSELS IN THE LUNGS?
A FULL LUNG TRANS-PLANT!
NEVER TRIED IT. BESIDES, WHERE'S THAT LUNG?
LUNGS SHRIVEL UP AND BECOME USELESS WHEN A PERSON DIES.
IT'S NOT AN OPTION ...
GOD, I FEEL WRETCHED.
THEY CAME ALL THIS WAY TO SEE ME...
GIVING UP EVERY-THING!
DOCTOR HONMA...
GRANT ME THE COURAGE !

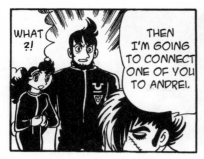

ARE YOU READY TO OFFER YOUR VERY LIVES TO SAVE ANDREI? YOU'D SUFFER ANYTHING FOR YOUR SON?
THAT IS SO!
THEN I'M GOING TO CONNECT ONE OF YOU TO ANDREI.
WHAT ?!
THE BLOOD FROM YOUR LUNGS WILL FLOW DIRECTLY INTO HIS HEART.
I'LL SURGI- CALLY SEAL YOU TO HIM.
IF AND WHEN A HEALTHY SET OF LUNGS BECOMES AVAILABLE, I'LL SEPARATE YOUR BODIES AND PERFORM ON ANDREI. IT WON'T BE SOON.
ARE YOU READY TO SUFFER THIS?
IF IT'LL SAVE HIM !
PUMP
PUMP
PUMP
PUMP

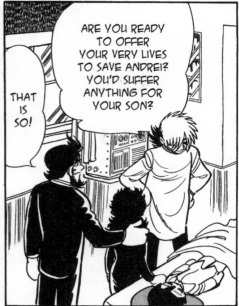

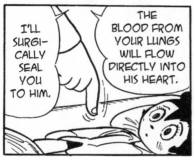

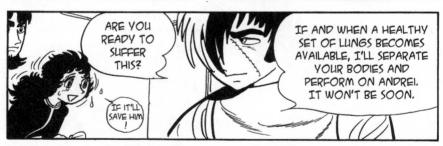

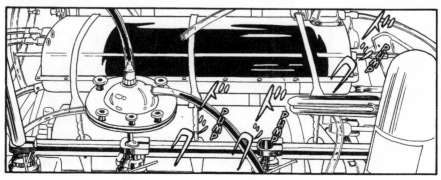

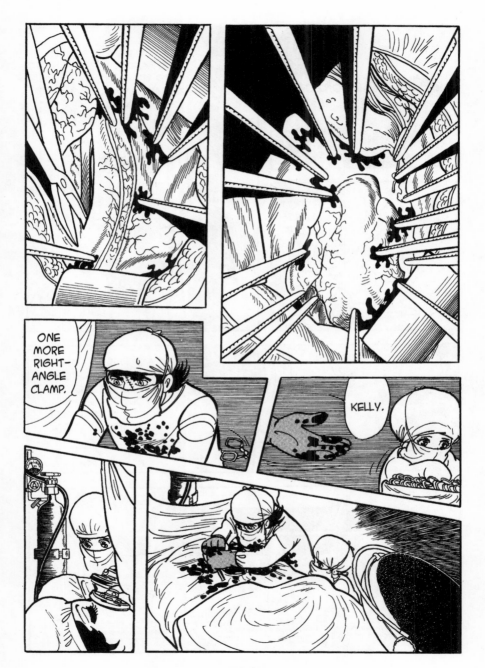

ONE MORE RIGHT-ANGLE CLAMP.

KELLY.

134

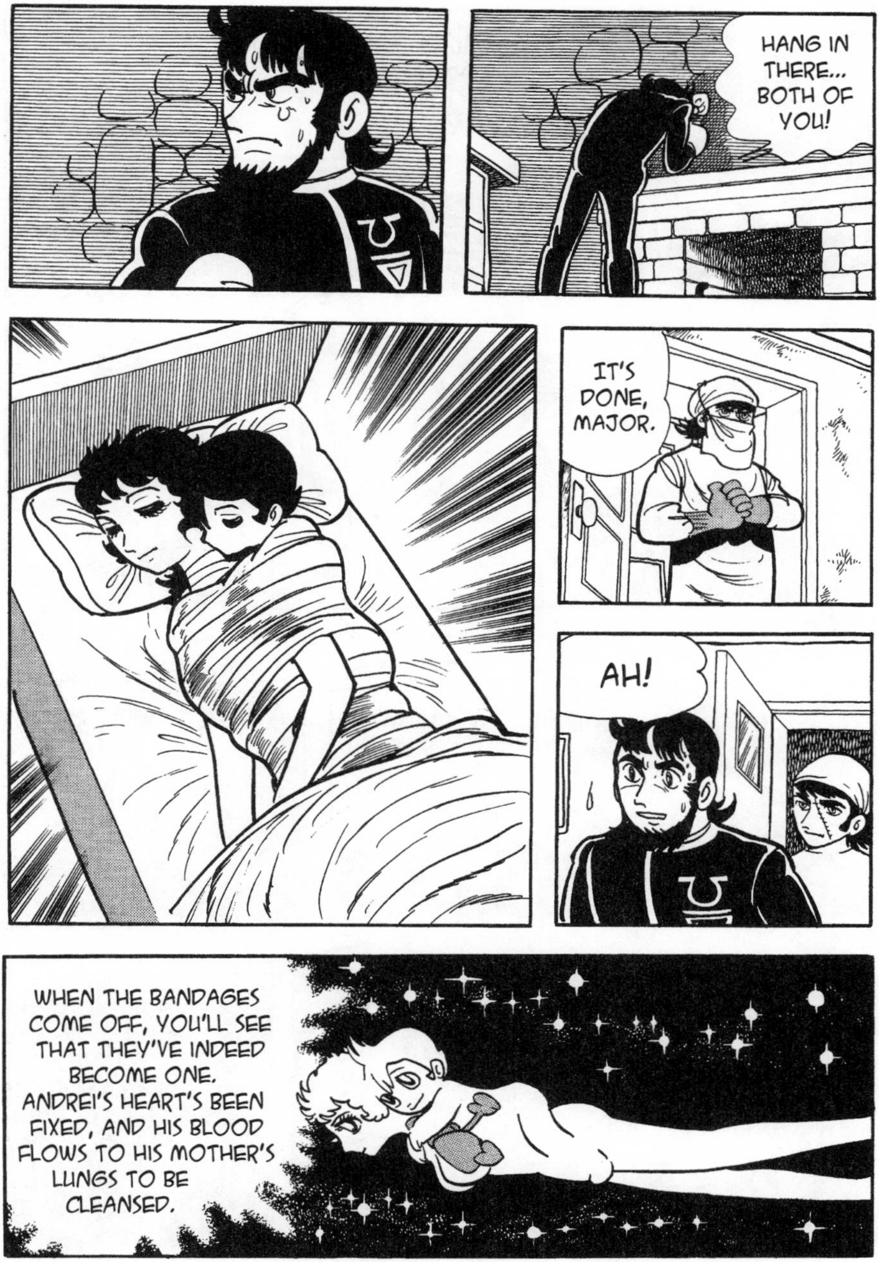
HANG IN THERE... BOTH OF YOU!
IT'S DONE, MAJOR.
AH!
WHEN THE BANDAGES COME OFF, YOU'LL SEE THAT THEY'VE INDEED BECOME ONE. ANDREI'S HEART'S BEEN FIXED, AND HIS BLOOD FLOWS TO HIS MOTHER'S LUNGS TO BE CLEANSED.

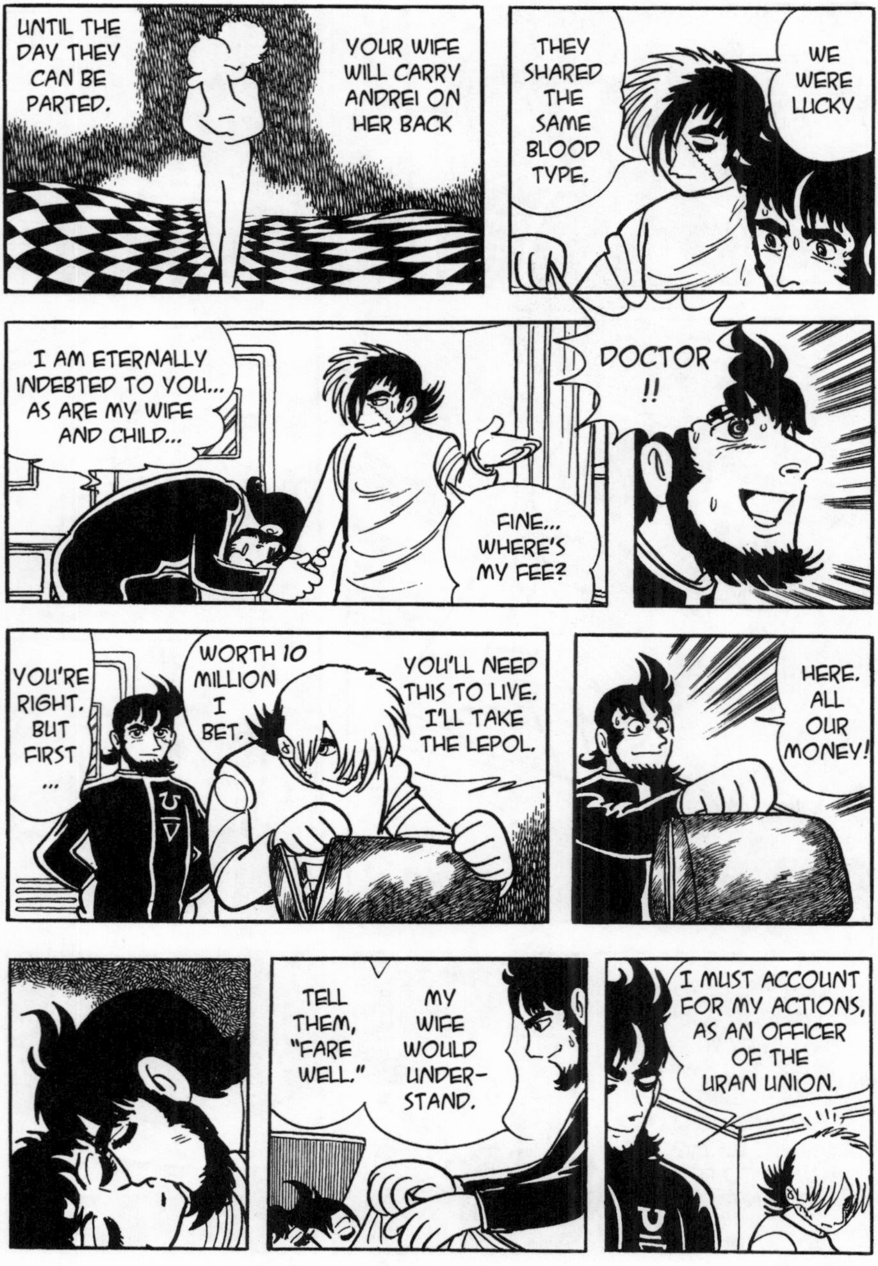
WE WERE LUCKY
THEY SHARED THE SAME BLOOD TYPE.
YOUR WIFE WILL CARRY ANDREI ON HER BACK
UNTIL THE DAY THEY CAN BE PARTED.
DOCTOR !!
I AM ETERNALLY INDEBTED TO YOU... AS ARE MY WIFE AND CHILD...
FINE... WHERE'S MY FEE?
HERE. ALL OUR MONEY!
YOU'LL NEED THIS TO LIVE. I'LL TAKE THE LEPOL.
WORTH 10 MILLION I BET.
YOU'RE RIGHT. BUT FIRST ...
I MUST ACCOUNT FOR MY ACTIONS, AS AN OFFICER OF THE URAN UNION.
MY WIFE WOULD UNDER-STAND.
TELL THEM, "FARE WELL."

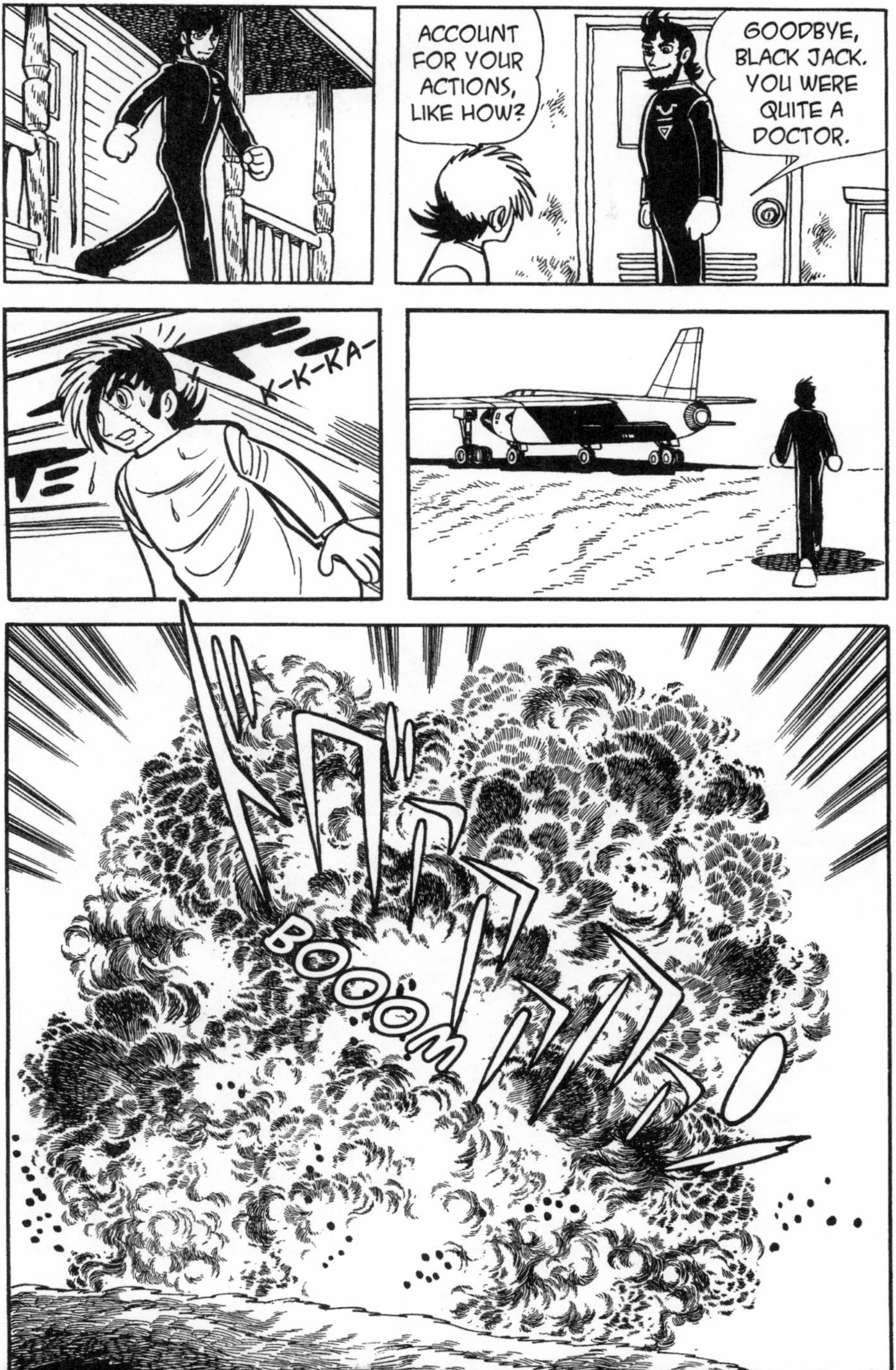
GOODBYE, BLACK JACK. YOU WERE QUITE A DOCTOR.
ACCOUNT FOR YOUR ACTIONS, LIKE HOW?
K-K-KA-
BOOOM

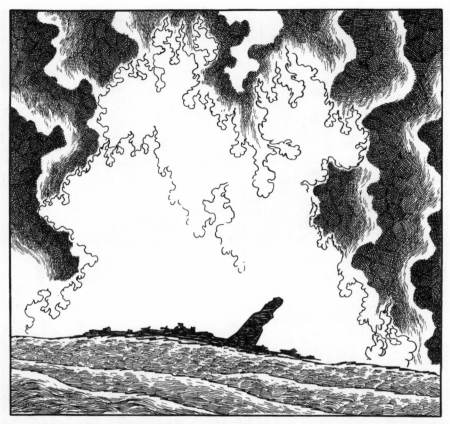

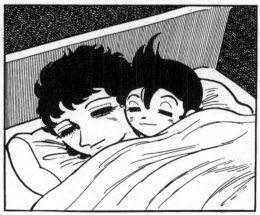

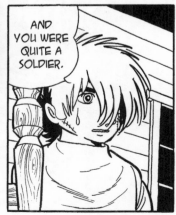

AND YOU WERE QUITE A SOLDIER.

BLACK JACK IN HOSPITAL

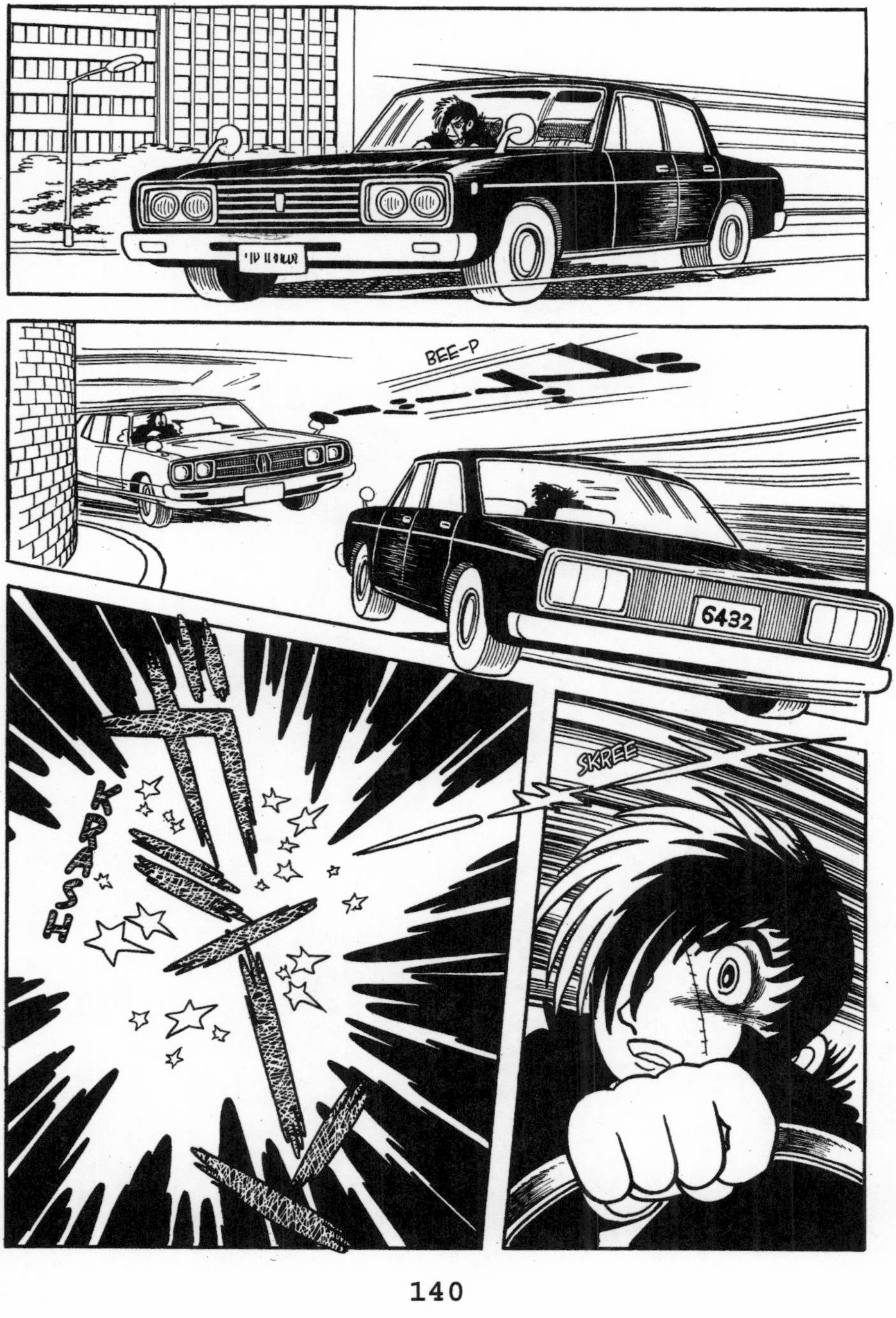
BEE-P
6432
SKREE
KRASH

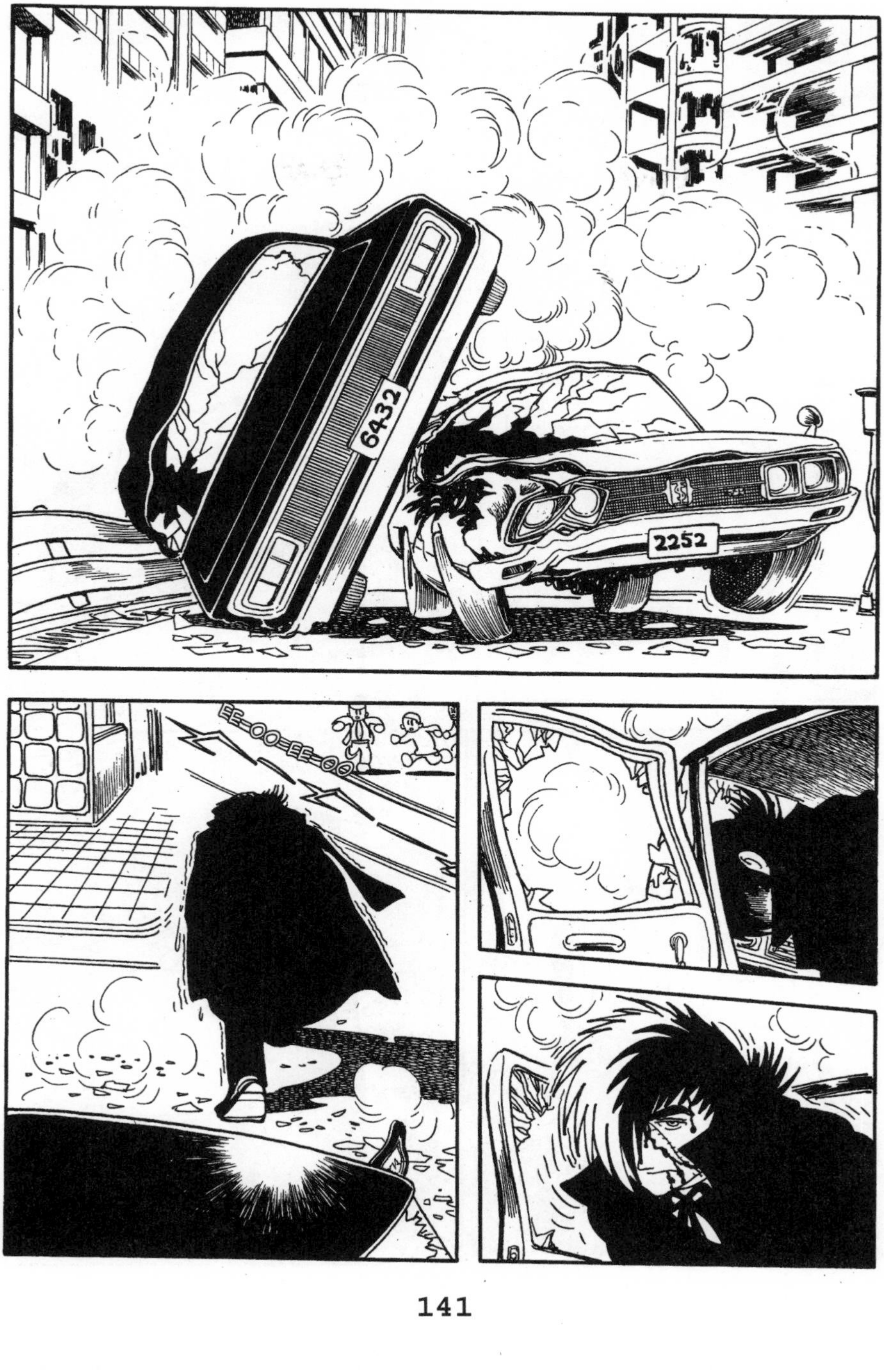
6432
2252
EE-OO-EE-OO

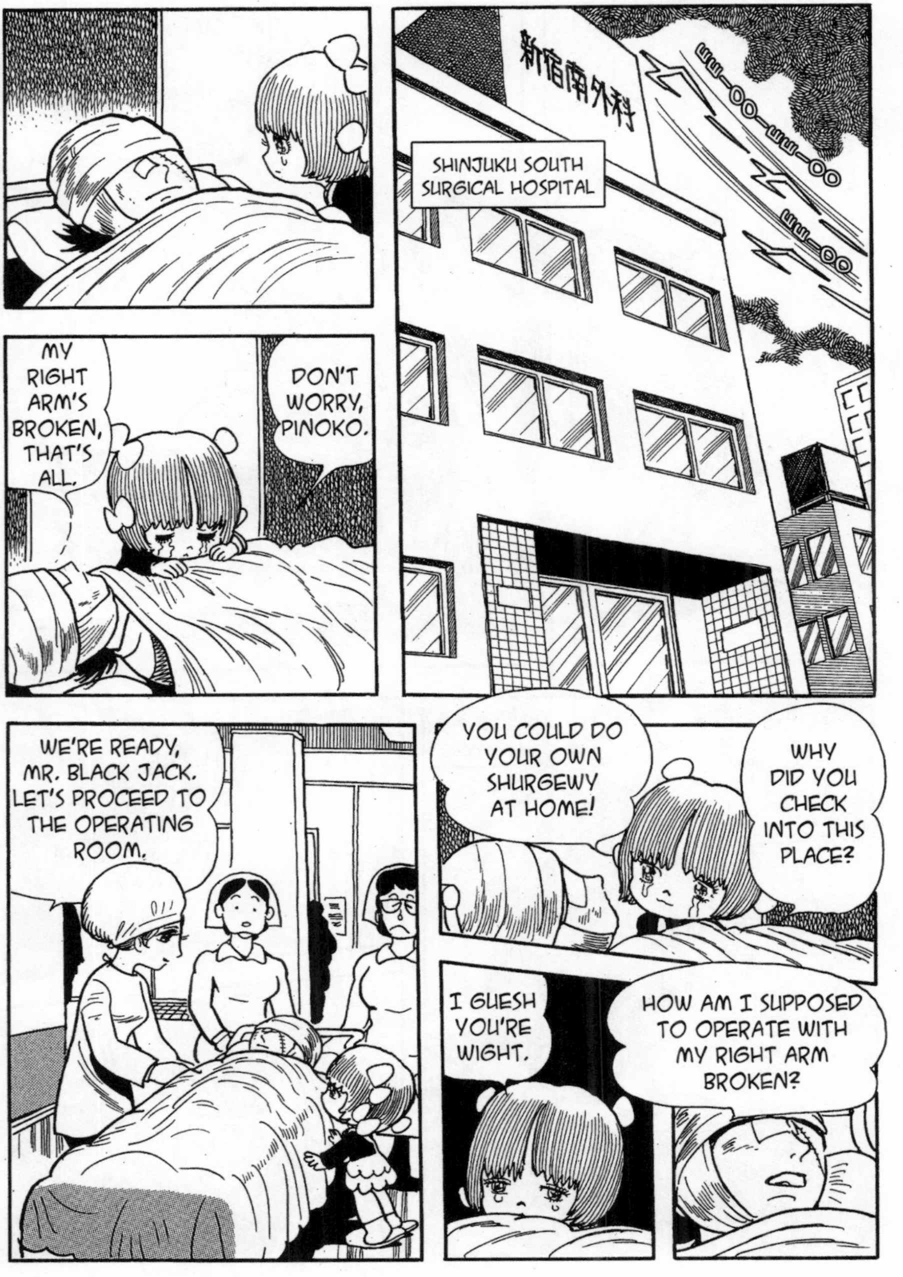

新宿南外科
SHINJUKU SOUTH SURGICAL HOSPITAL
EEE—OO—EEE—OO
EEE—OO
DON'T WORRY, PINOKO.
MY RIGHT ARM'S BROKEN, THAT'S ALL.
WHY DID YOU CHECK INTO THIS PLACE?
YOU COULD DO YOUR OWN SHURGEWY AT HOME!
HOW AM I SUPPOSED TO OPERATE WITH MY RIGHT ARM BROKEN?
I GUESH YOU'RE WIGHT.
WE'RE READY, MR. BLACK JACK. LET'S PROCEED TO THE OPERATING ROOM.

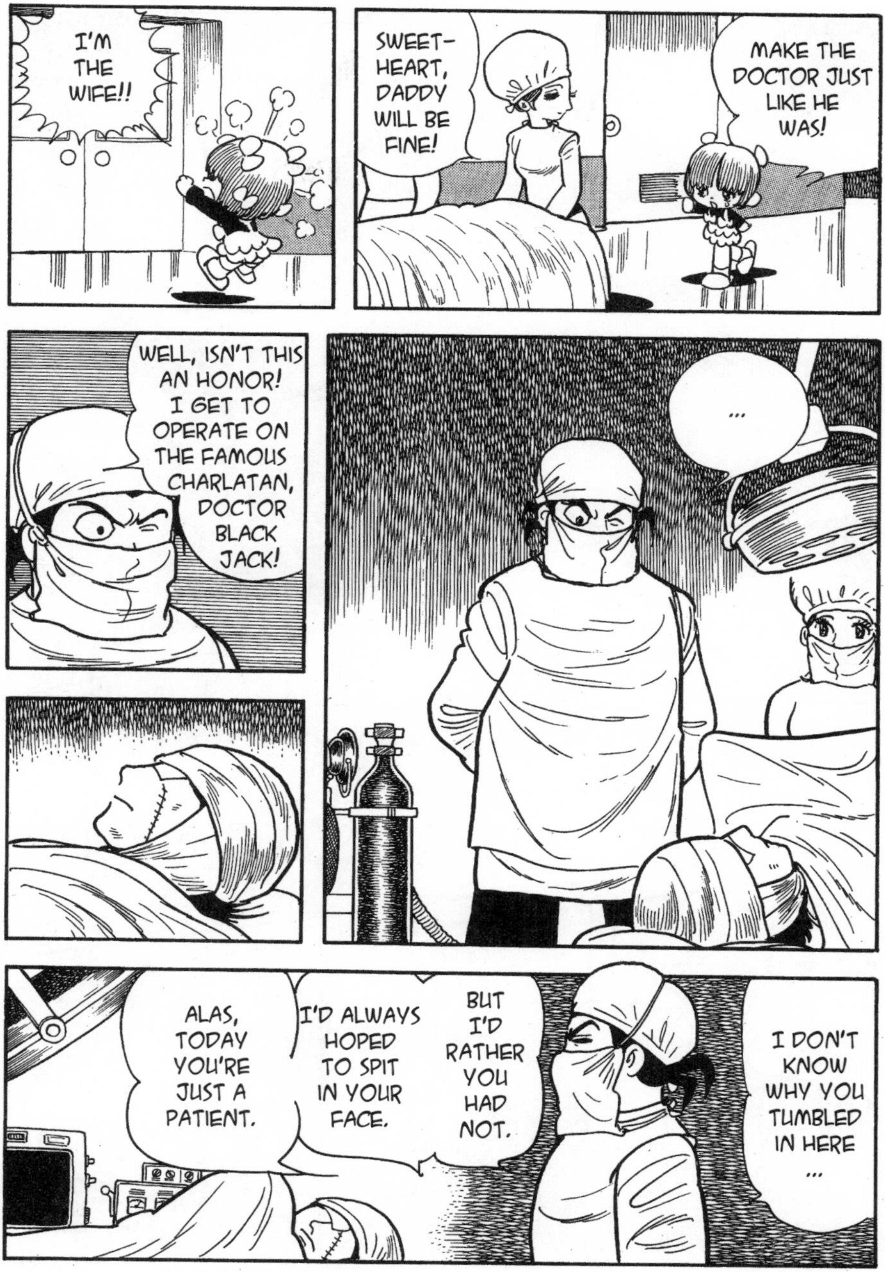
MAKE THE DOCTOR JUST LIKE HE WAS!
SWEET-HEART, DADDY WILL BE FINE!
I'M THE WIFE!!
...
WELL, ISN'T THIS AN HONOR! I GET TO OPERATE ON THE FAMOUS CHARLATAN, DOCTOR BLACK JACK!
I DON'T KNOW WHY YOU TUMBLED IN HERE ...
BUT I'D RATHER YOU HAD NOT.
I'D ALWAYS HOPED TO SPIT IN YOUR FACE.
ALAS, TODAY YOU'RE JUST A PATIENT.

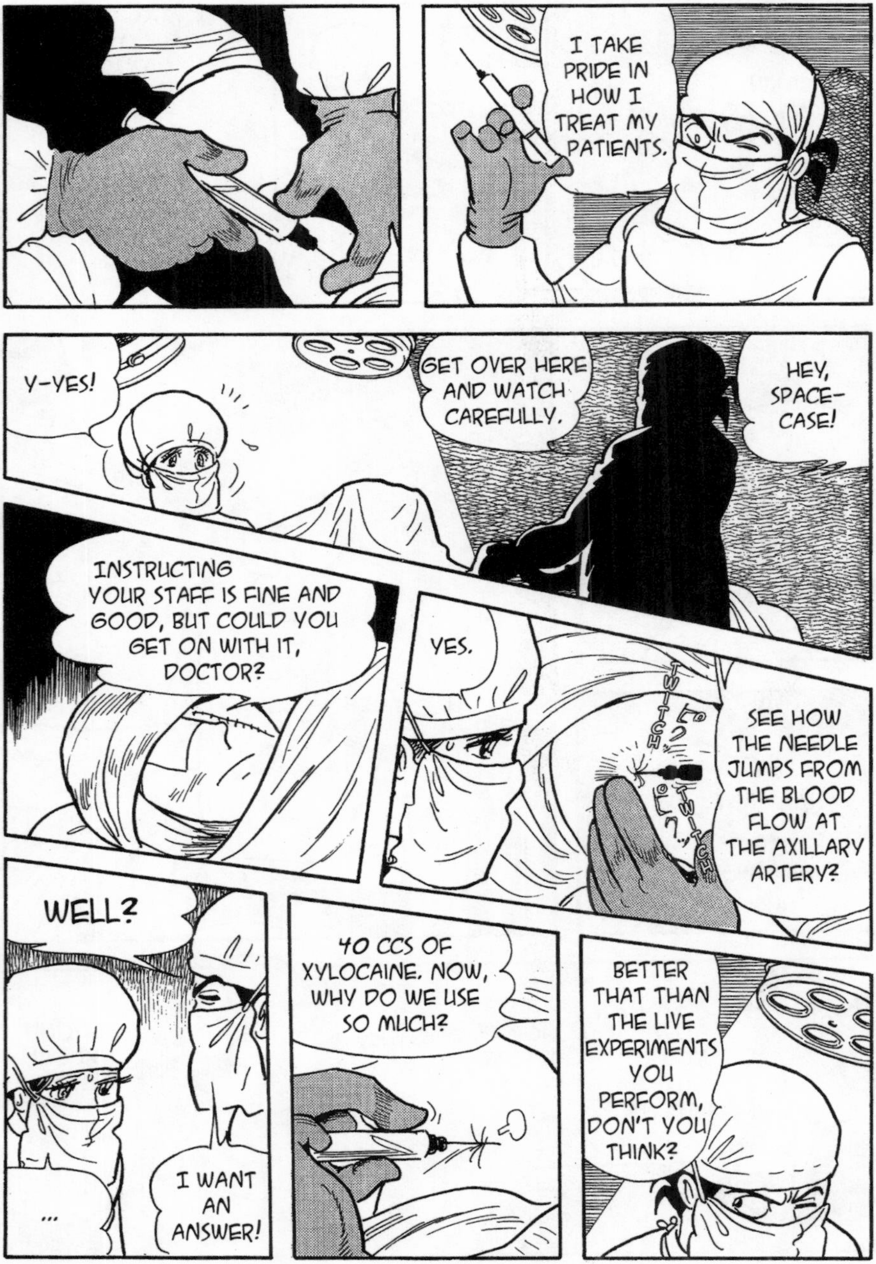
I TAKE PRIDE IN HOW I TREAT MY PATIENTS.
HEY, SPACE-CASE!
GET OVER HERE AND WATCH CAREFULLY.
Y-YES!
SEE HOW THE NEEDLE JUMPS FROM THE BLOOD FLOW AT THE AXILLARY ARTERY?
TWITCH
TWITCH
YES.
INSTRUCTING YOUR STAFF IS FINE AND GOOD, BUT COULD YOU GET ON WITH IT, DOCTOR?
BETTER THAT THAN THE LIVE EXPERIMENTS YOU PERFORM, DON'T YOU THINK?
40 CCS OF XYLOCAINE. NOW, WHY DO WE USE SO MUCH?
WELL?
I WANT AN ANSWER!
...

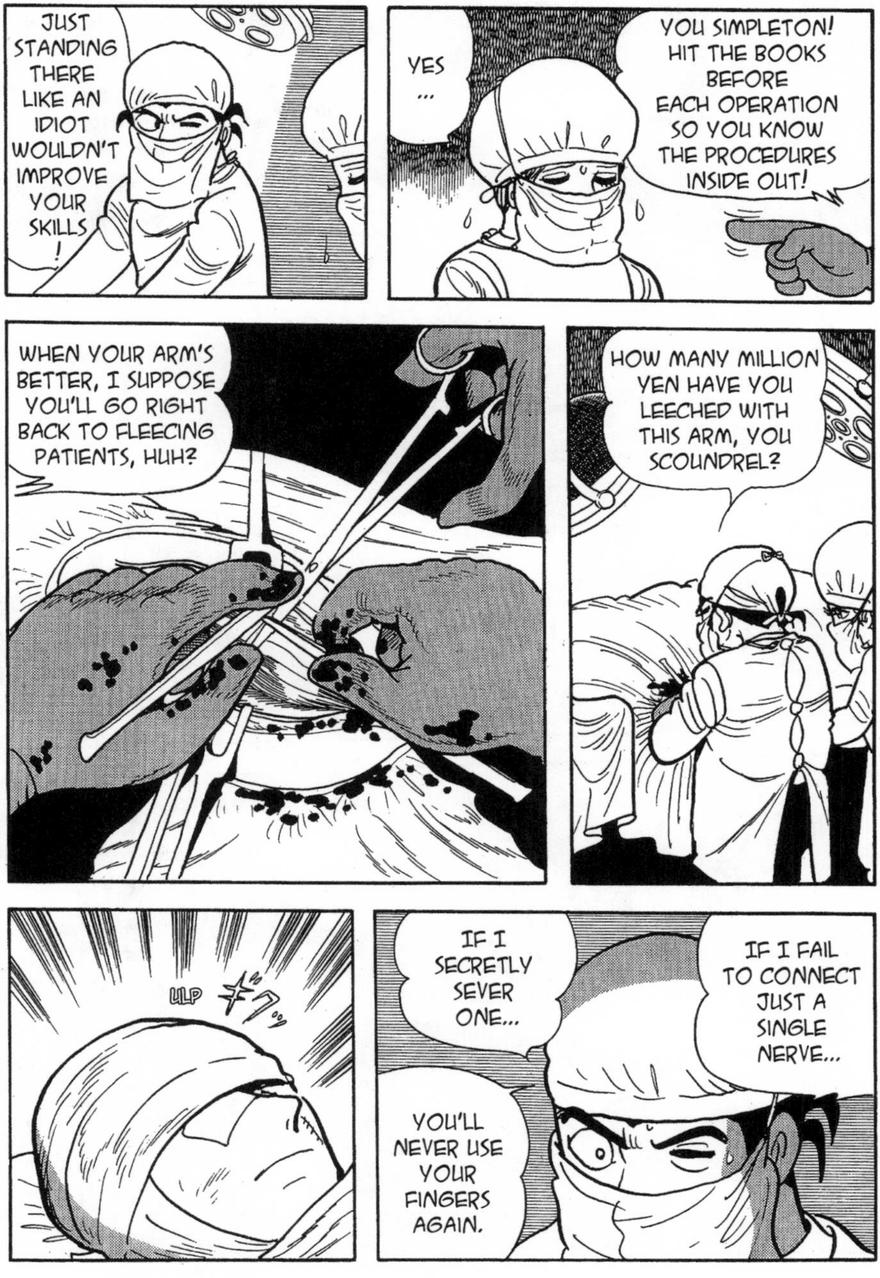
YOU SIMPLETON! HIT THE BOOKS BEFORE EACH OPERATION SO YOU KNOW THE PROCEDURES INSIDE OUT!
YES ...
JUST STANDING THERE LIKE AN IDIOT WOULDN'T IMPROVE YOUR SKILLS !
HOW MANY MILLION YEN HAVE YOU LEECHED WITH THIS ARM, YOU SCOUNDREL?
WHEN YOUR ARM'S BETTER, I SUPPOSE YOU'LL GO RIGHT BACK TO FLEECING PATIENTS, HUH?
IF I FAIL TO CONNECT JUST A SINGLE NERVE...
IF I SECRETLY SEVER ONE...
YOU'LL NEVER USE YOUR FINGERS AGAIN.
ULP

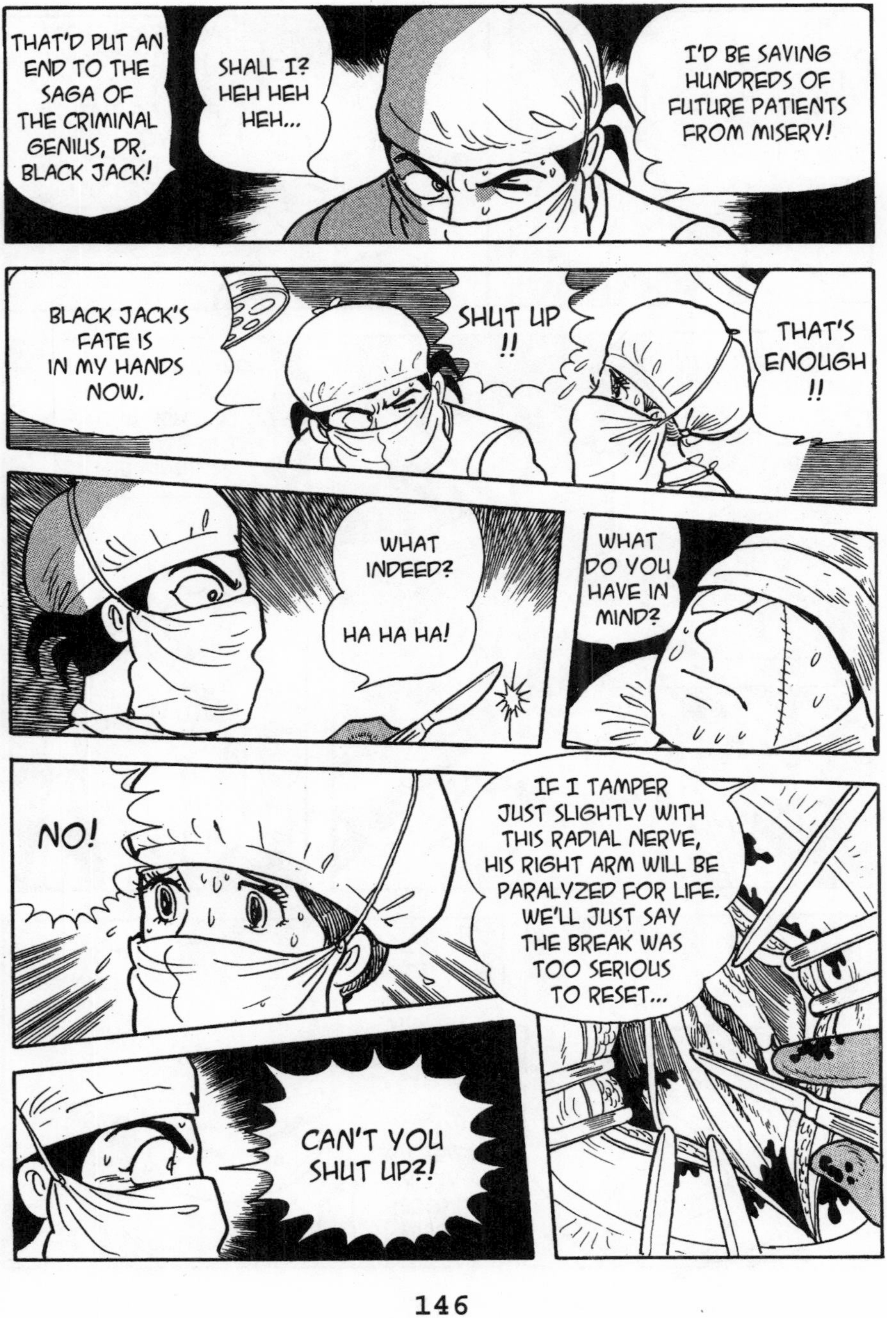
I'D BE SAVING HUNDREDS OF FUTURE PATIENTS FROM MISERY!
SHALL I? HEH HEH HEH...
THAT'D PUT AN END TO THE SAGA OF THE CRIMINAL GENIUS, DR. BLACK JACK!
THAT'S ENOUGH !!
SHUT UP !!
BLACK JACK'S FATE IS IN MY HANDS NOW.
WHAT DO YOU HAVE IN MIND?
WHAT INDEED?
HA HA HA!
IF I TAMPER JUST SLIGHTLY WITH THIS RADIAL NERVE, HIS RIGHT ARM WILL BE PARALYZED FOR LIFE. WE'LL JUST SAY THE BREAK WAS TOO SERIOUS TO RESET...
NO!
CAN'T YOU SHUT UP?!

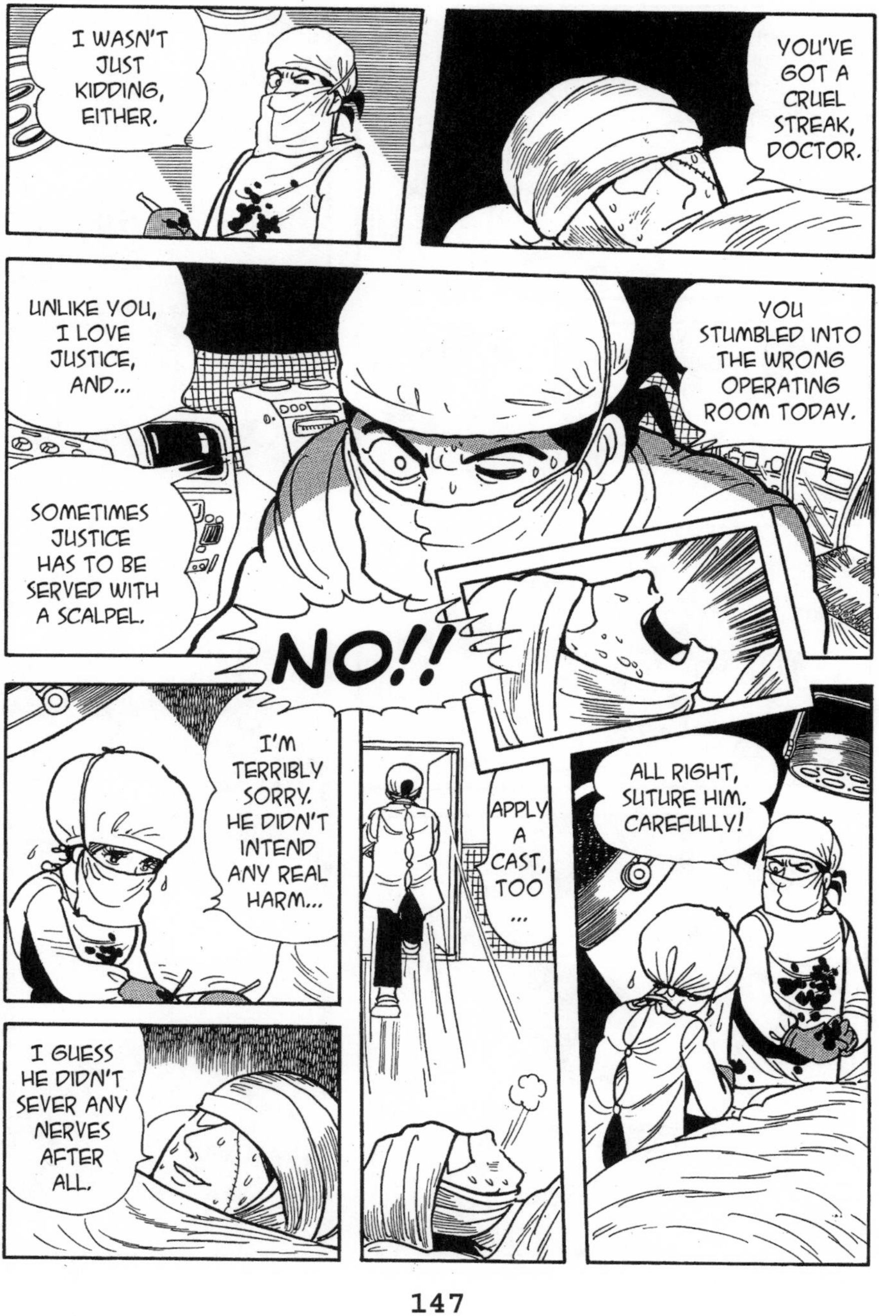
YOU'VE GOT A CRUEL STREAK, DOCTOR.
I WASN'T JUST KIDDING, EITHER.
YOU STUMBLED INTO THE WRONG OPERATING ROOM TODAY.
UNLIKE YOU, I LOVE JUSTICE, AND...
SOMETIMES JUSTICE HAS TO BE SERVED WITH A SCALPEL.
NO!!
ALL RIGHT, SUTURE HIM. CAREFULLY!
APPLY A CAST, TOO ...
I'M TERRIBLY SORRY. HE DIDN'T INTEND ANY REAL HARM...
I GUESS HE DIDN'T SEVER ANY NERVES AFTER ALL.

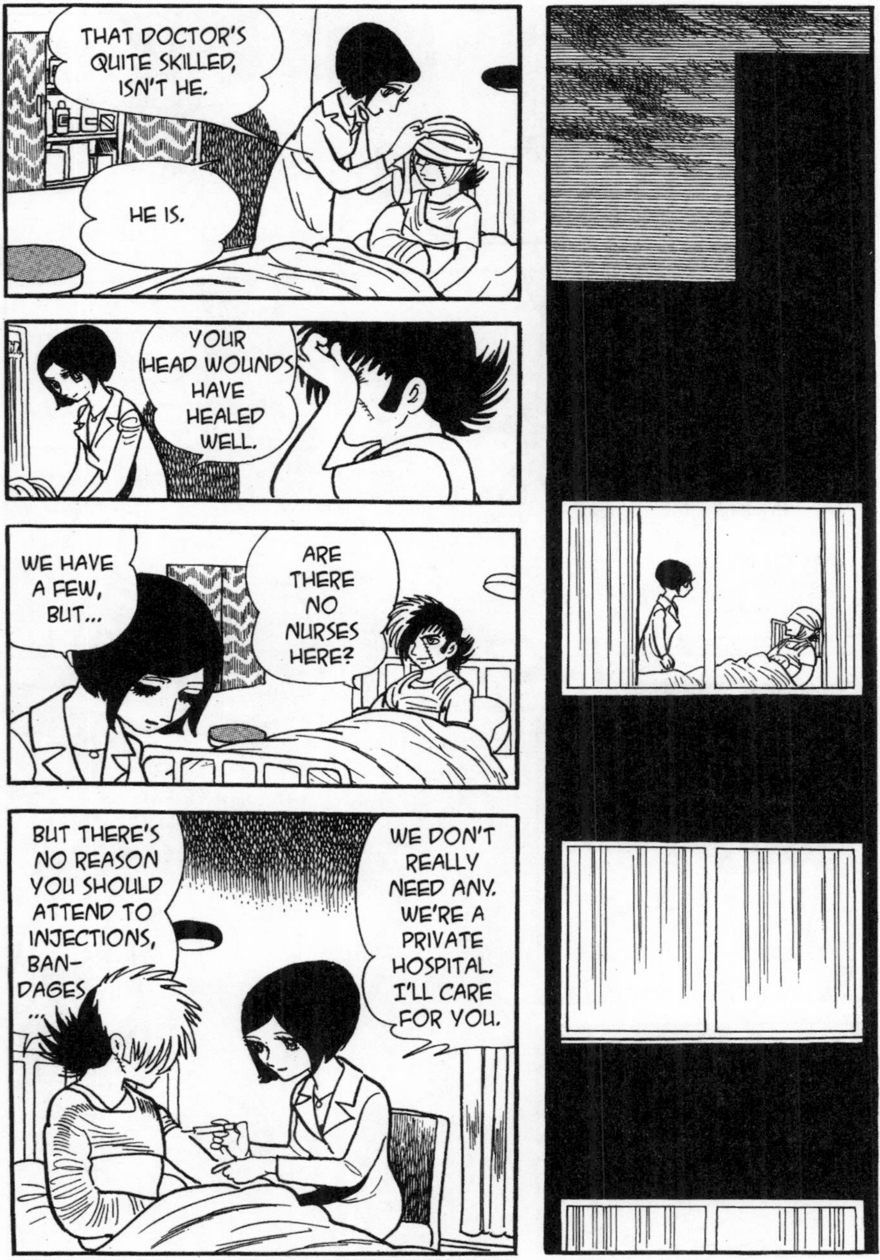
THAT DOCTOR'S QUITE SKILLED, ISN'T HE.
HE IS.
YOUR HEAD WOUNDS HAVE HEALED WELL.
ARE THERE NO NURSES HERE?
WE HAVE A FEW, BUT...
WE DON'T REALLY NEED ANY. WE'RE A PRIVATE HOSPITAL. I'LL CARE FOR YOU.
BUT THERE'S NO REASON YOU SHOULD ATTEND TO INJECTIONS, BANDAGES...

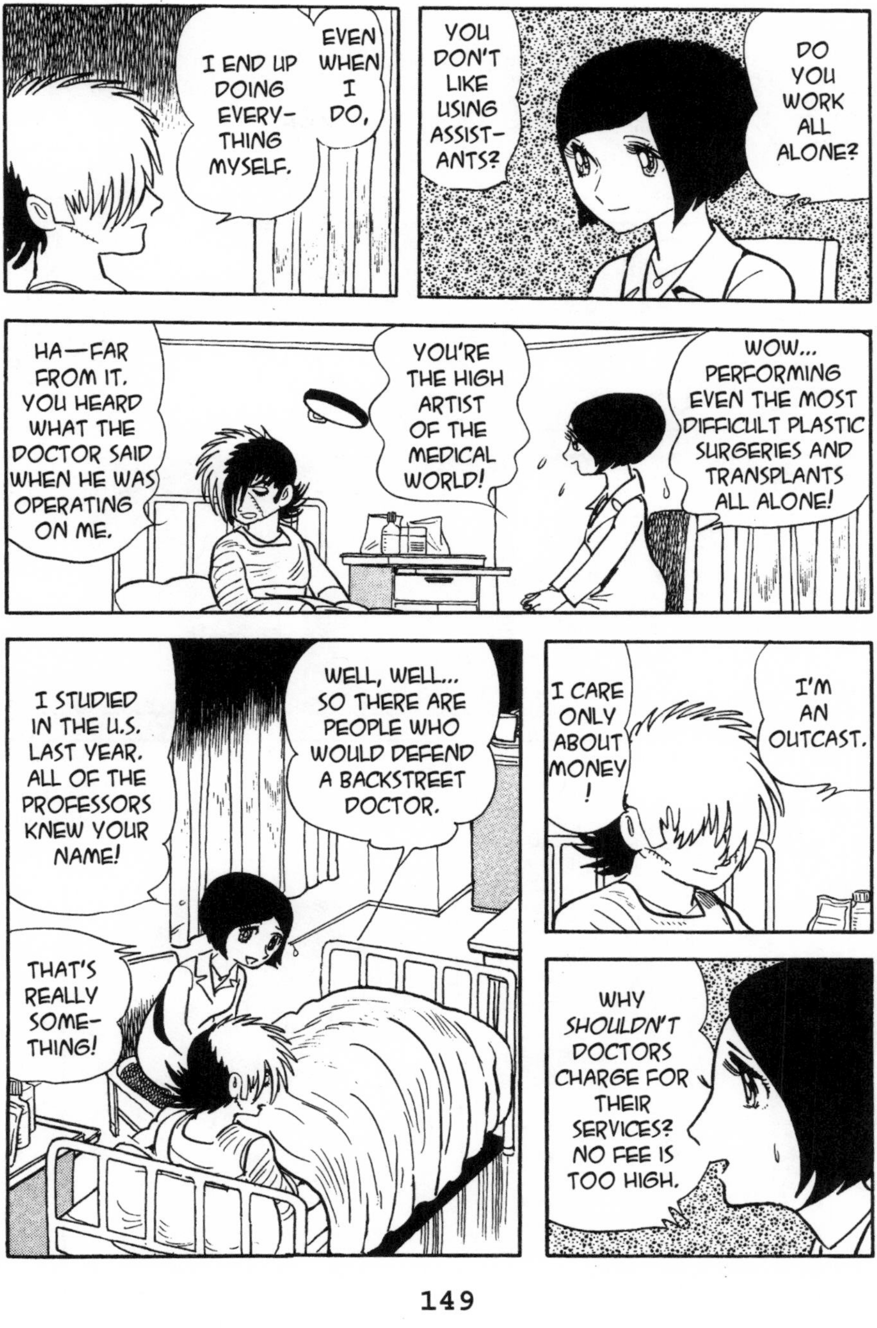
DO YOU WORK ALL ALONE?
YOU DON'T LIKE USING ASSIST-ANTS?
EVEN WHEN I DO,
I END UP DOING EVERY-THING MYSELF.
WOW... PERFORMING EVEN THE MOST DIFFICULT PLASTIC SURGERIES AND TRANSPLANTS ALL ALONE!
YOU'RE THE HIGH ARTIST OF THE MEDICAL WORLD!
HA—FAR FROM IT. YOU HEARD WHAT THE DOCTOR SAID WHEN HE WAS OPERATING ON ME.
I'M AN OUTCAST.
I CARE ONLY ABOUT MONEY!
WHY SHOULDN'T DOCTORS CHARGE FOR THEIR SERVICES? NO FEE IS TOO HIGH.
WELL, WELL... SO THERE ARE PEOPLE WHO WOULD DEFEND A BACKSTREET DOCTOR.
I STUDIED IN THE U.S. LAST YEAR. ALL OF THE PROFESSORS KNEW YOUR NAME!
THAT'S REALLY SOME-THING!

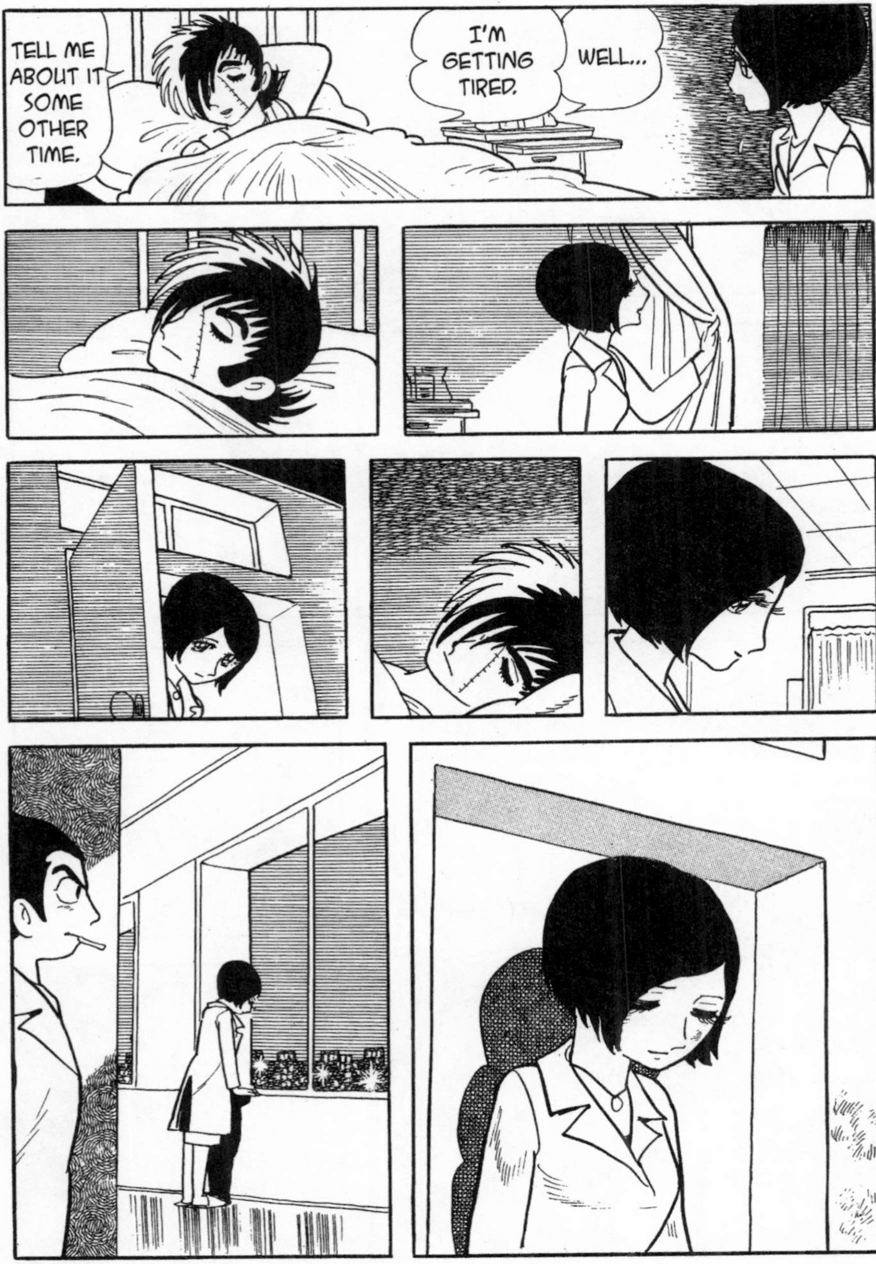
WELL...
I'M GETTING TIRED.
TELL ME ABOUT IT SOME OTHER TIME.

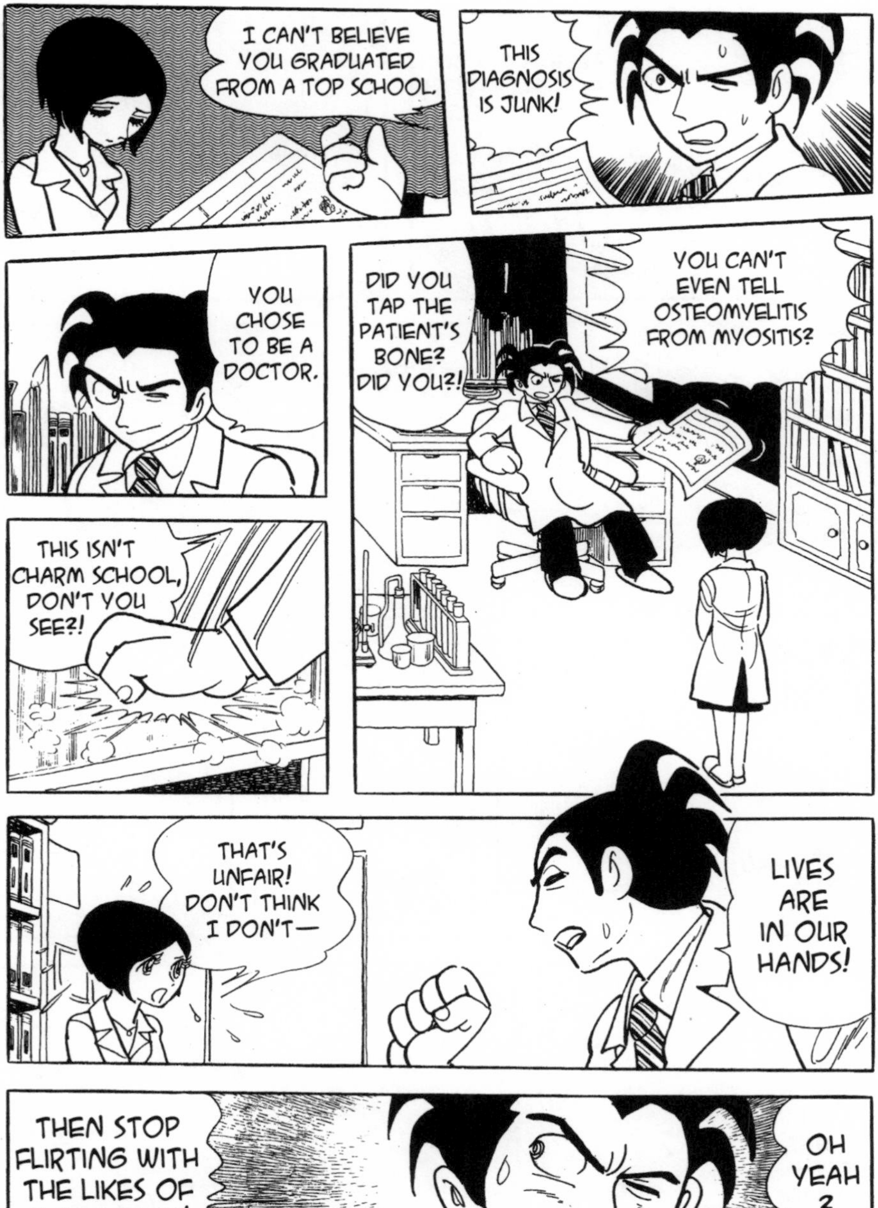
THIS DIAGNOSIS IS JUNK!
I CAN'T BELIEVE YOU GRADUATED FROM A TOP SCHOOL.
YOU CAN'T EVEN TELL OSTEOMYELITIS FROM MYOSITIS?
DID YOU TAP THE PATIENT'S BONE? DID YOU?!
YOU CHOSE TO BE A DOCTOR.
THIS ISN'T CHARM SCHOOL, DON'T YOU SEE?!
LIVES ARE IN OUR HANDS!
THAT'S UNFAIR! DON'T THINK I DON'T—
OH YEAH?
THEN STOP FLIRTING WITH THE LIKES OF BLACK JACK!

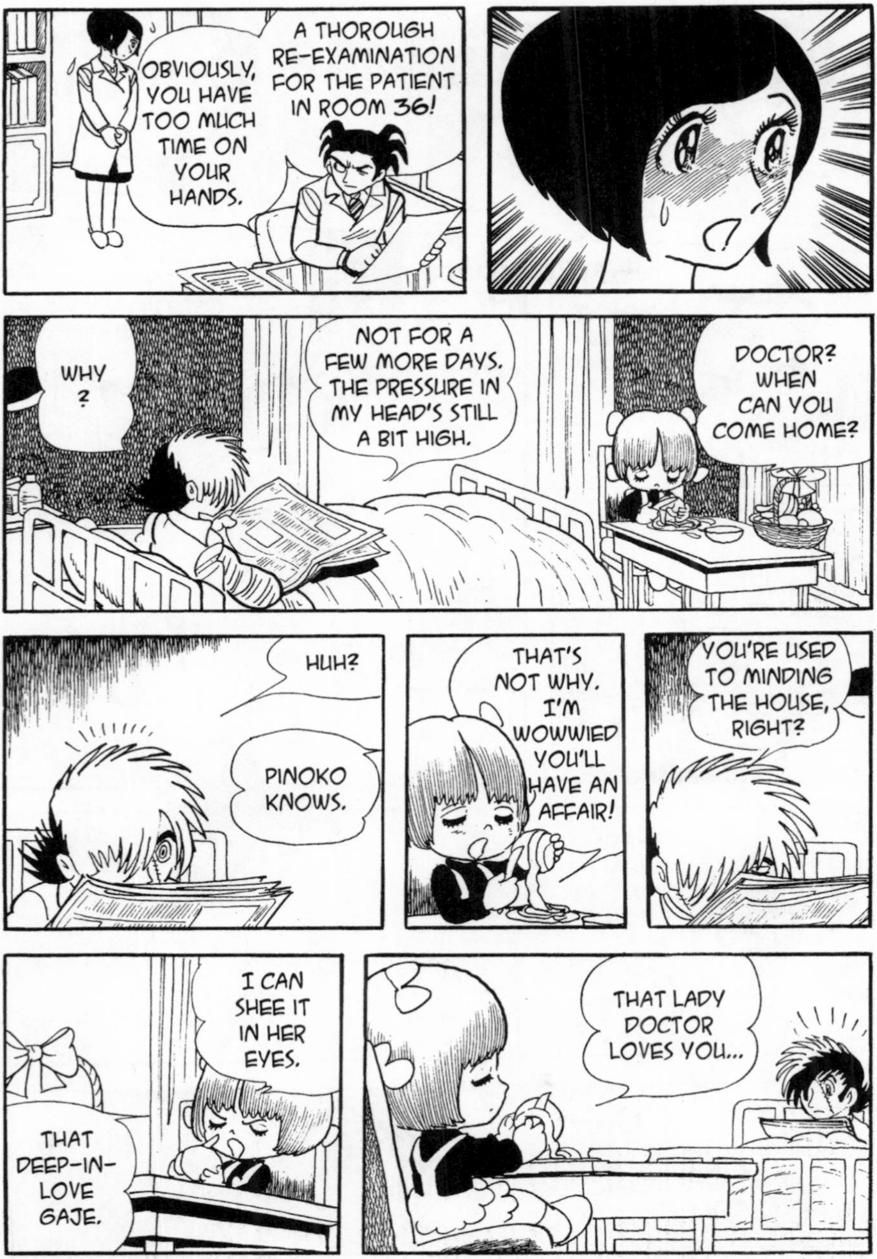
A THOROUGH RE-EXAMINATION FOR THE PATIENT IN ROOM 36!
OBVIOUSLY, YOU HAVE TOO MUCH TIME ON YOUR HANDS.
DOCTOR? WHEN CAN YOU COME HOME?
NOT FOR A FEW MORE DAYS. THE PRESSURE IN MY HEAD'S STILL A BIT HIGH.
WHY ?
YOU'RE USED TO MINDING THE HOUSE, RIGHT?
THAT'S NOT WHY. I'M WOWWIED YOU'LL HAVE AN AFFAIR!
HUH?
PINOKO KNOWS.
THAT LADY DOCTOR LOVES YOU...
I CAN SHEE IT IN HER EYES.
THAT DEEP-IN-LOVE GAJE.

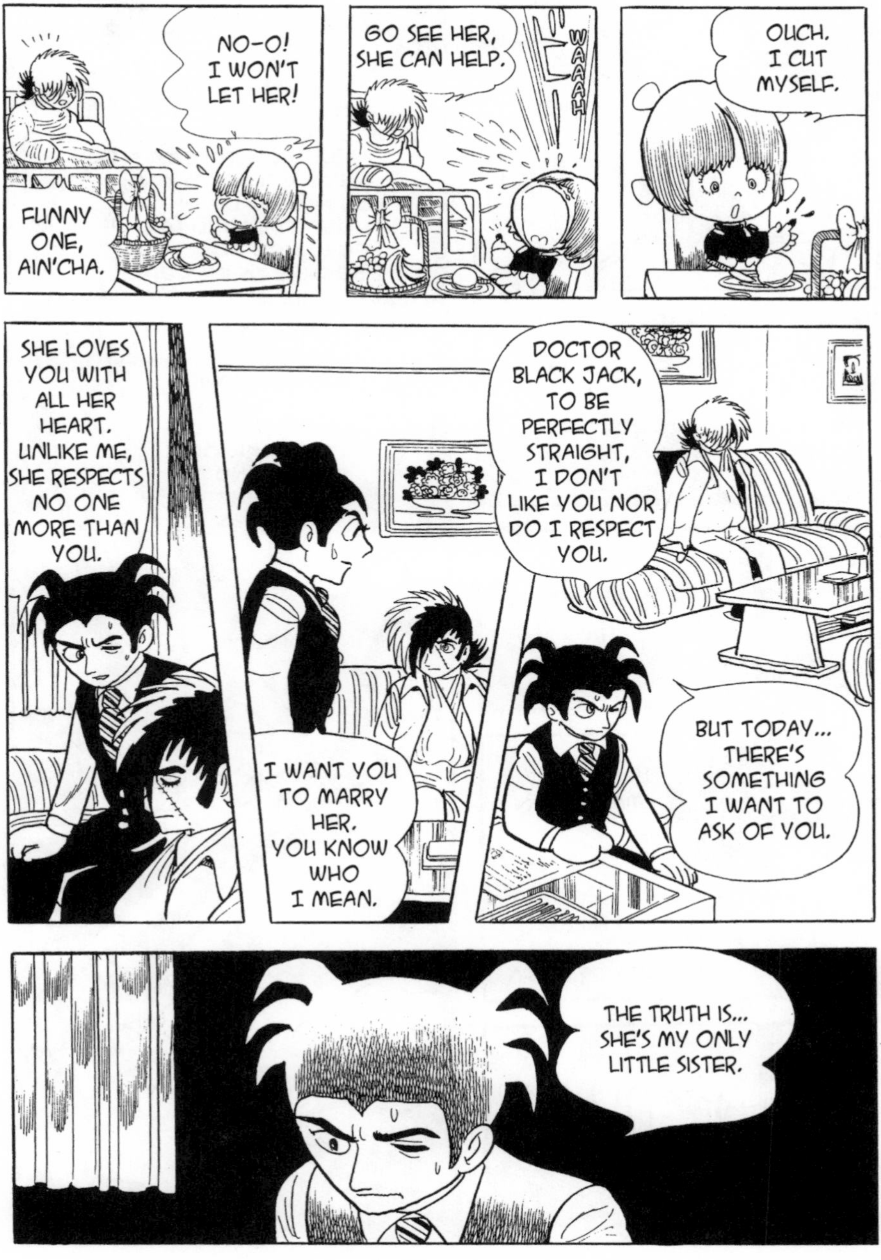
OUCH. I CUT MYSELF.
GO SEE HER, SHE CAN HELP.
WAAAAH
NO-O! I WON'T LET HER!
FUNNY ONE, AIN'CHA.
DOCTOR BLACK JACK, TO BE PERFECTLY STRAIGHT, I DON'T LIKE YOU NOR DO I RESPECT YOU.
BUT TODAY... THERE'S SOMETHING I WANT TO ASK OF YOU.
I WANT YOU TO MARRY HER. YOU KNOW WHO I MEAN.
SHE LOVES YOU WITH ALL HER HEART. UNLIKE ME, SHE RESPECTS NO ONE MORE THAN YOU.
THE TRUTH IS... SHE'S MY ONLY LITTLE SISTER.

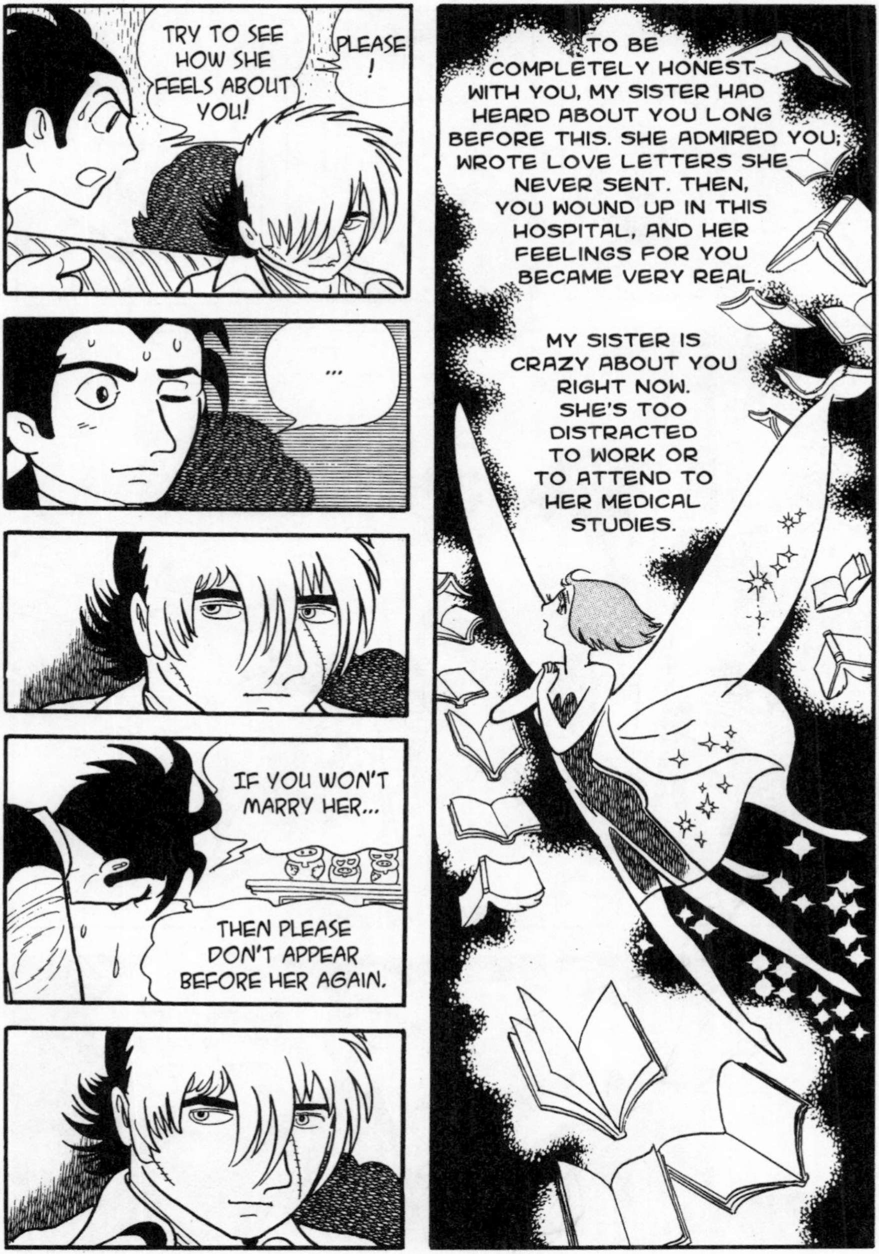
TO BE COMPLETELY HONEST WITH YOU, MY SISTER HAD HEARD ABOUT YOU LONG BEFORE THIS. SHE ADMIRED YOU; WROTE LOVE LETTERS SHE NEVER SENT. THEN, YOU WOUND UP IN THIS HOSPITAL, AND HER FEELINGS FOR YOU BECAME VERY REAL.
MY SISTER IS CRAZY ABOUT YOU RIGHT NOW. SHE'S TOO DISTRACTED TO WORK OR TO ATTEND TO HER MEDICAL STUDIES.
PLEASE!
TRY TO SEE HOW SHE FEELS ABOUT YOU!
...
IF YOU WON'T MARRY HER...
THEN PLEASE DON'T APPEAR BEFORE HER AGAIN.

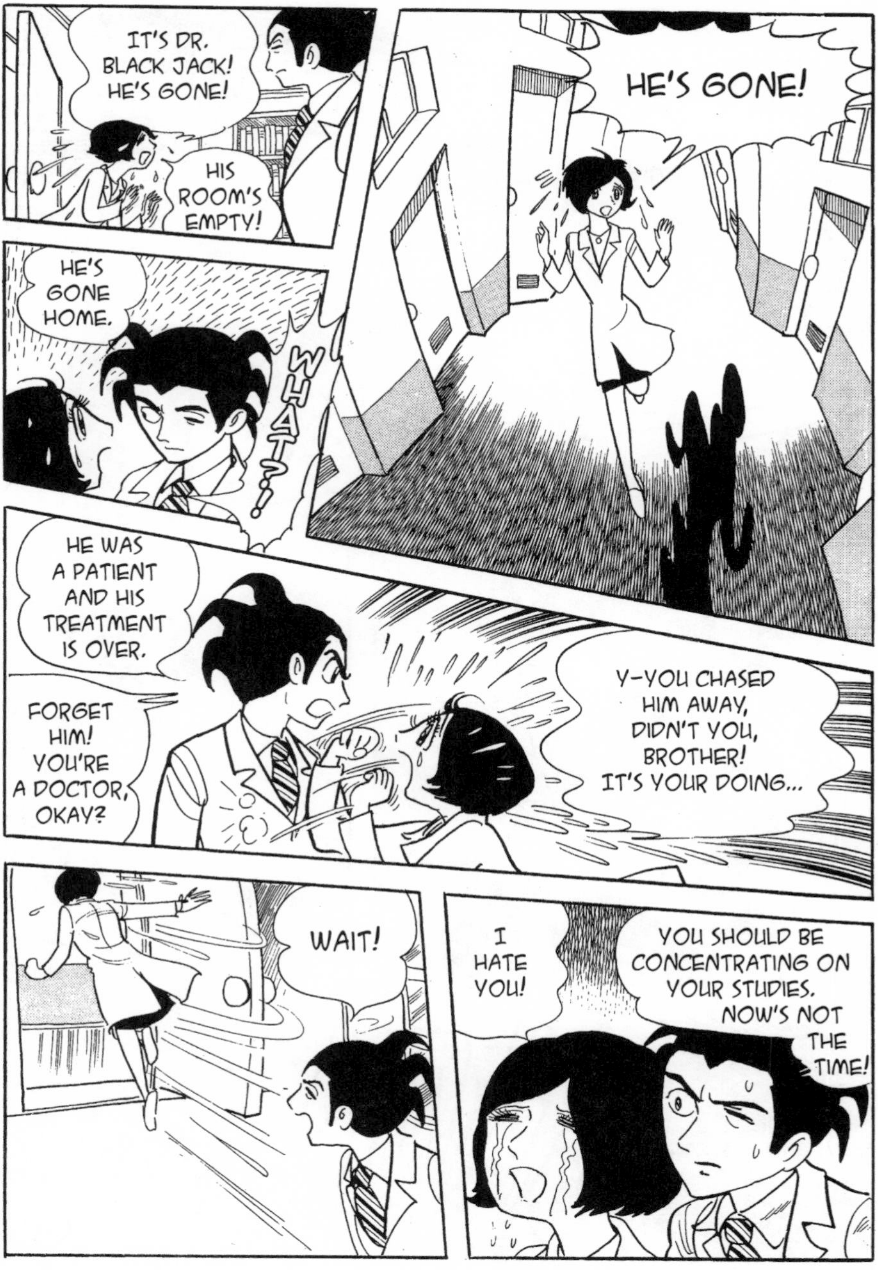
HE'S GONE!
IT'S DR. BLACK JACK! HE'S GONE!
HIS ROOM'S EMPTY!
HE'S GONE HOME.
WHAT?!
HE WAS A PATIENT AND HIS TREATMENT IS OVER.
Y-YOU CHASED HIM AWAY, DIDN'T YOU, BROTHER! IT'S YOUR DOING...
FORGET HIM! YOU'RE A DOCTOR, OKAY?
YOU SHOULD BE CONCENTRATING ON YOUR STUDIES. NOW'S NOT THE TIME!
I HATE YOU!
WAIT!

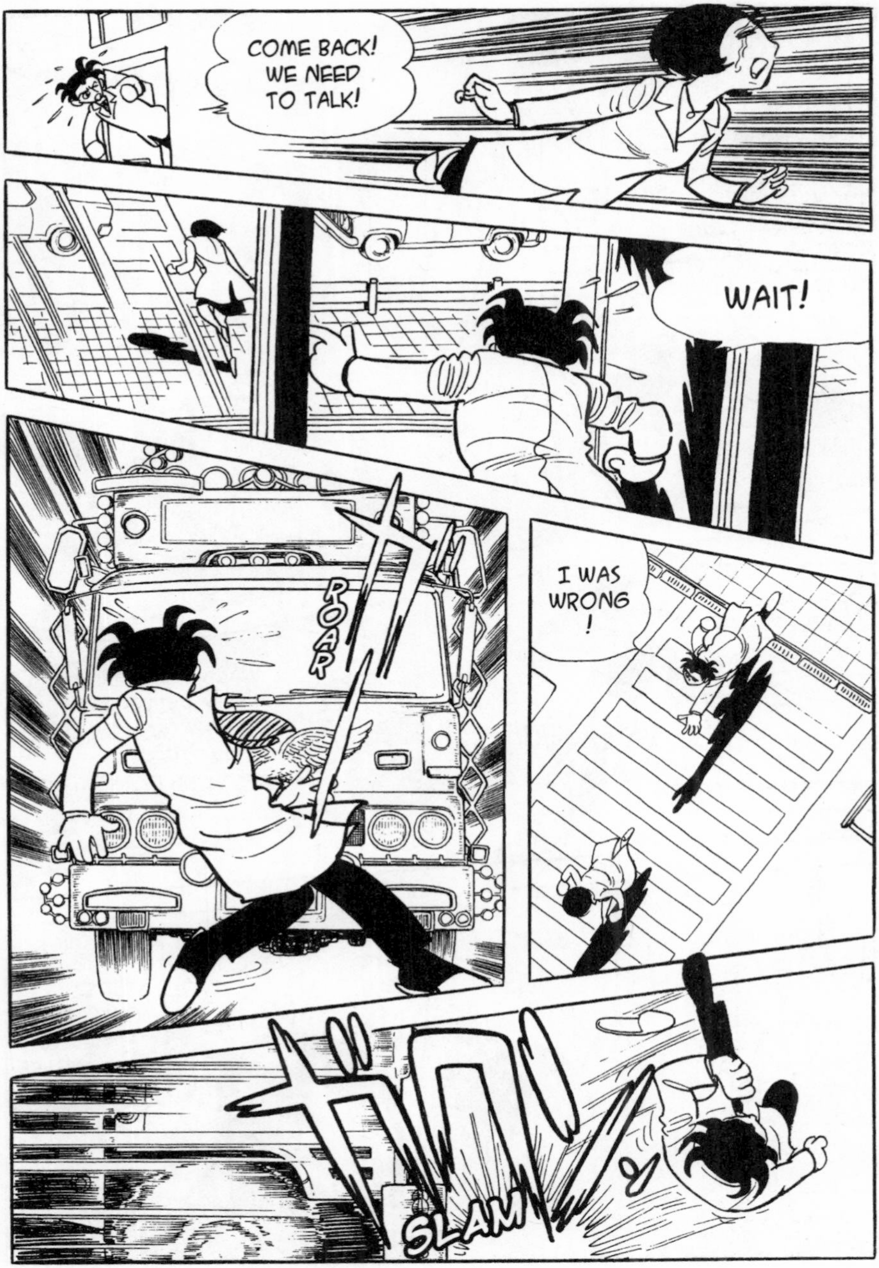
COME BACK! WE NEED TO TALK!
WAIT!
I WAS WRONG!
ROAR
SLAM

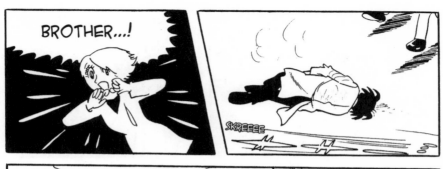

SKREEEE
BROTHER...!
HE WAS HIT?
SOMEONE CALL AN AMBULANCE ...
WAIT, SHE'S A DOCTOR.
BROTHER! C-CAN YOU HEAR ME?
RRRRRING
HELLO?
OH... YOU...
YOUR BROTHER WAS IN AN ACCIDENT? CRITICALLY INJURED?
PLEASE, COME RIGHT AWAY!
UNLESS HE HAS SURGERY NOW, HE WON'T MAKE IT!
HE HAS AN AIR EMBOLISM.
WHAT WOULD YOU HAVE ME DO?
MY RIGHT ARM'S STILL OUT OF COMMISSION.

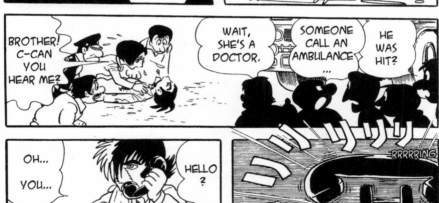

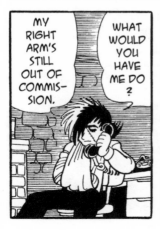

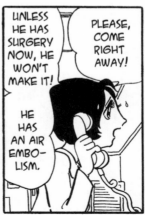

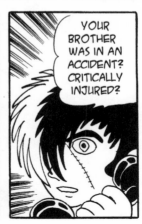

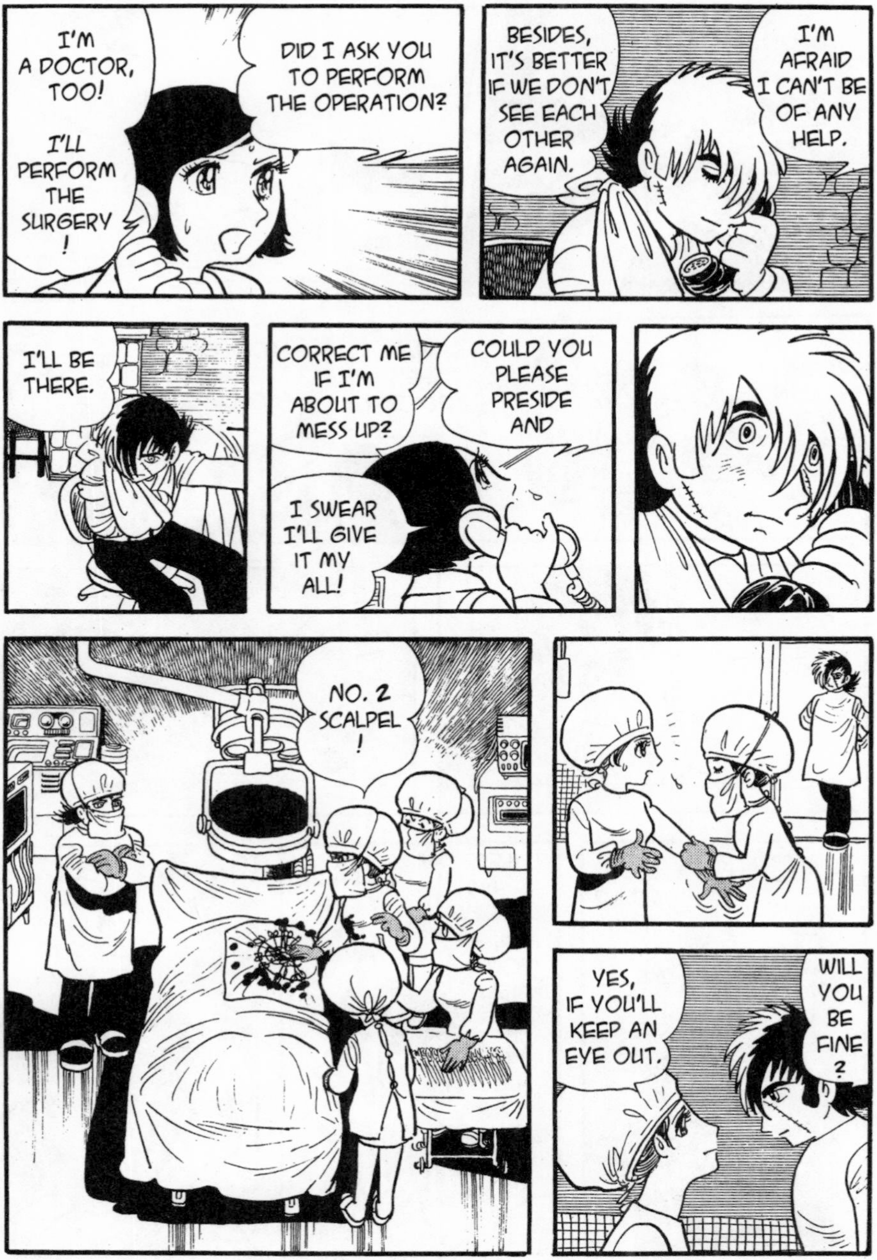
I'M AFRAID I CAN'T BE OF ANY HELP.
BESIDES, IT'S BETTER IF WE DON'T SEE EACH OTHER AGAIN.
DID I ASK YOU TO PERFORM THE OPERATION?
I'M A DOCTOR, TOO!
I'LL PERFORM THE SURGERY!
COULD YOU PLEASE PRESIDE AND
CORRECT ME IF I'M ABOUT TO MESS UP?
I SWEAR I'LL GIVE IT MY ALL!
I'LL BE THERE.
WILL YOU BE FINE?
YES, IF YOU'LL KEEP AN EYE OUT.
NO. 2 SCALPEL!

A WOMAN'S CASE

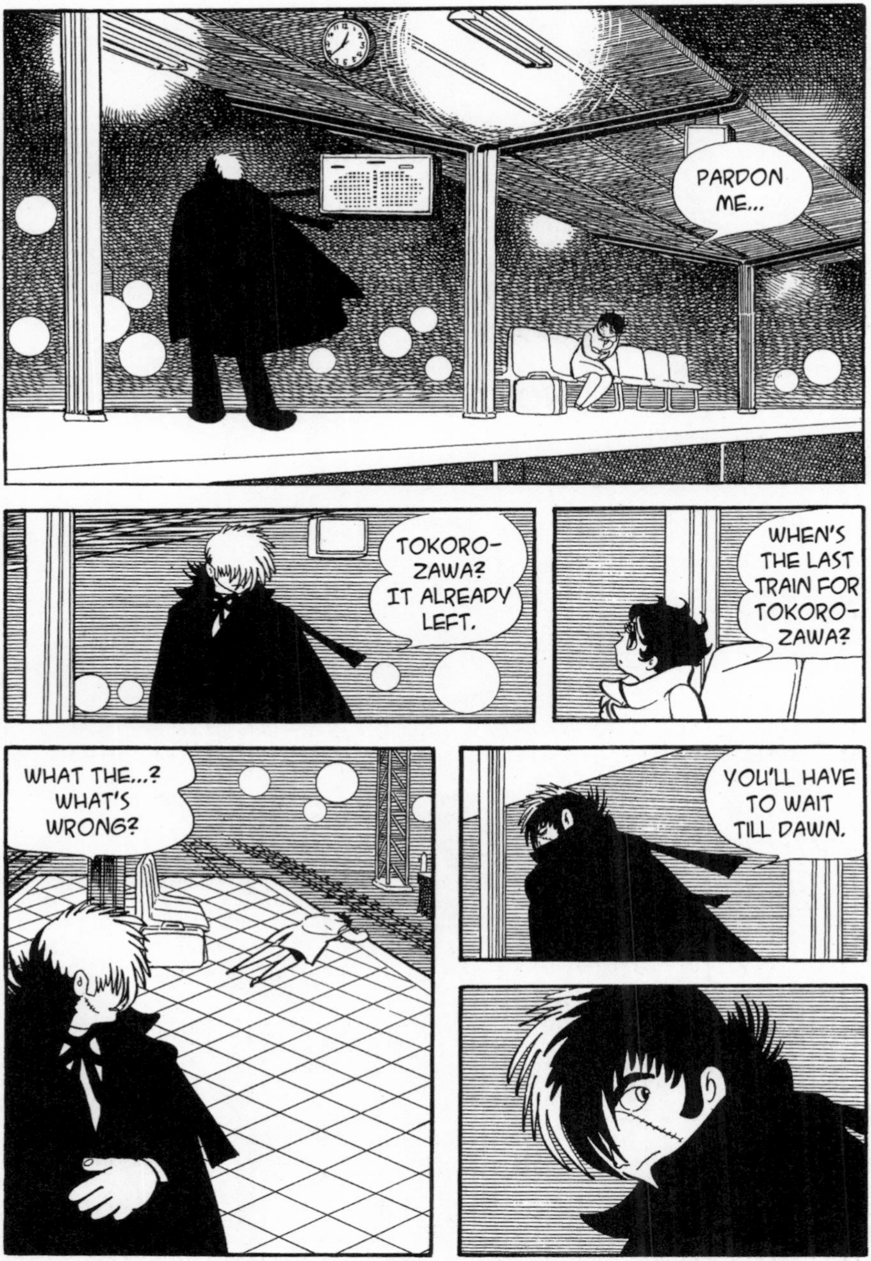
PARDON ME...
WHEN'S THE LAST TRAIN FOR TOKORO-ZAWA?
TOKORO-ZAWA? IT ALREADY LEFT.
YOU'LL HAVE TO WAIT TILL DAWN.
WHAT THE...? WHAT'S WRONG?

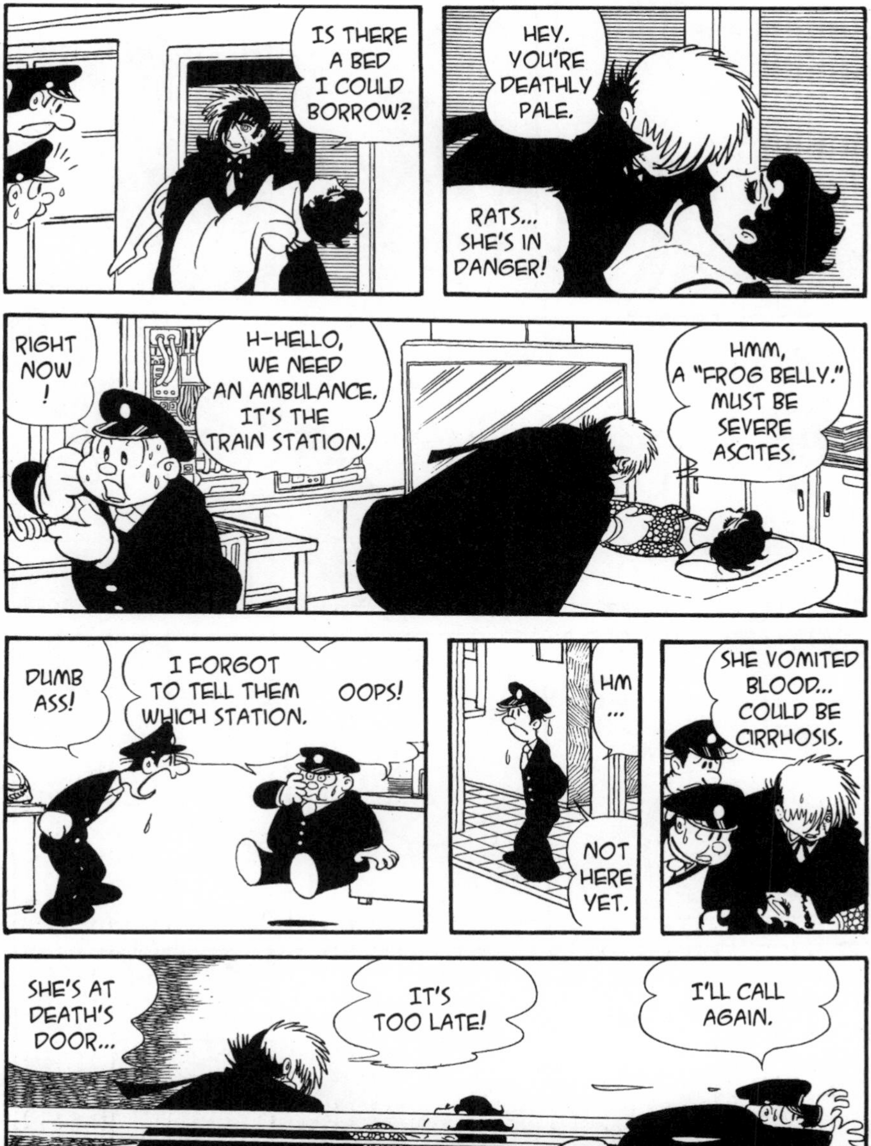
HEY. YOU'RE DEATHLY PALE.
RATS... SHE'S IN DANGER!
IS THERE A BED I COULD BORROW?
HMM, A "FROG BELLY." MUST BE SEVERE ASCITES.
H-HELLO, WE NEED AN AMBULANCE. IT'S THE TRAIN STATION.
RIGHT NOW !
SHE VOMITED BLOOD... COULD BE CIRRHOSIS.
HM ...
NOT HERE YET.
OOPS!
I FORGOT TO TELL THEM WHICH STATION.
DUMB ASS!
I'LL CALL AGAIN.
IT'S TOO LATE!
SHE'S AT DEATH'S DOOR...

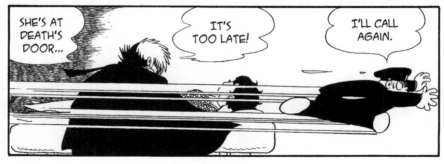

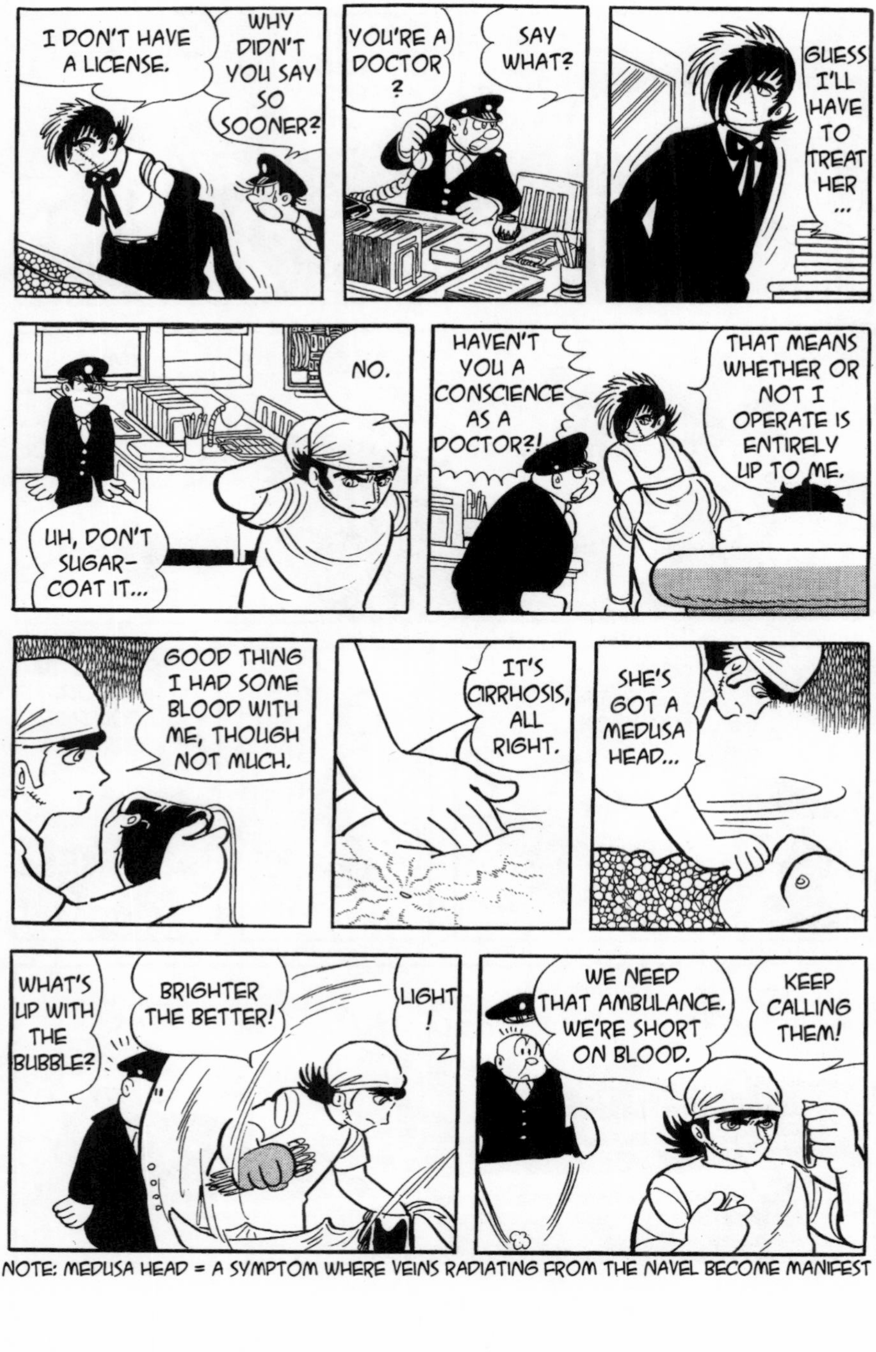
GUESS I'LL HAVE TO TREAT HER ...
SAY WHAT?
YOU'RE A DOCTOR ?
WHY DIDN'T YOU SAY SO SOONER?
I DON'T HAVE A LICENSE.
THAT MEANS WHETHER OR NOT I OPERATE IS ENTIRELY UP TO ME.
HAVEN'T YOU A CONSCIENCE AS A DOCTOR?!
NO.
UH, DON'T SUGAR-COAT IT...
SHE'S GOT A MEDUSA HEAD...
IT'S CIRRHOSIS, ALL RIGHT.
GOOD THING I HAD SOME BLOOD WITH ME, THOUGH NOT MUCH.
KEEP CALLING THEM!
WE NEED THAT AMBULANCE. WE'RE SHORT ON BLOOD.
LIGHT!
BRIGHTER THE BETTER!
WHAT'S UP WITH THE BUBBLE?

NOTE: MEDUSA HEAD = A SYMPTOM WHERE VEINS RADIATING FROM THE NAVEL BECOME MANIFEST

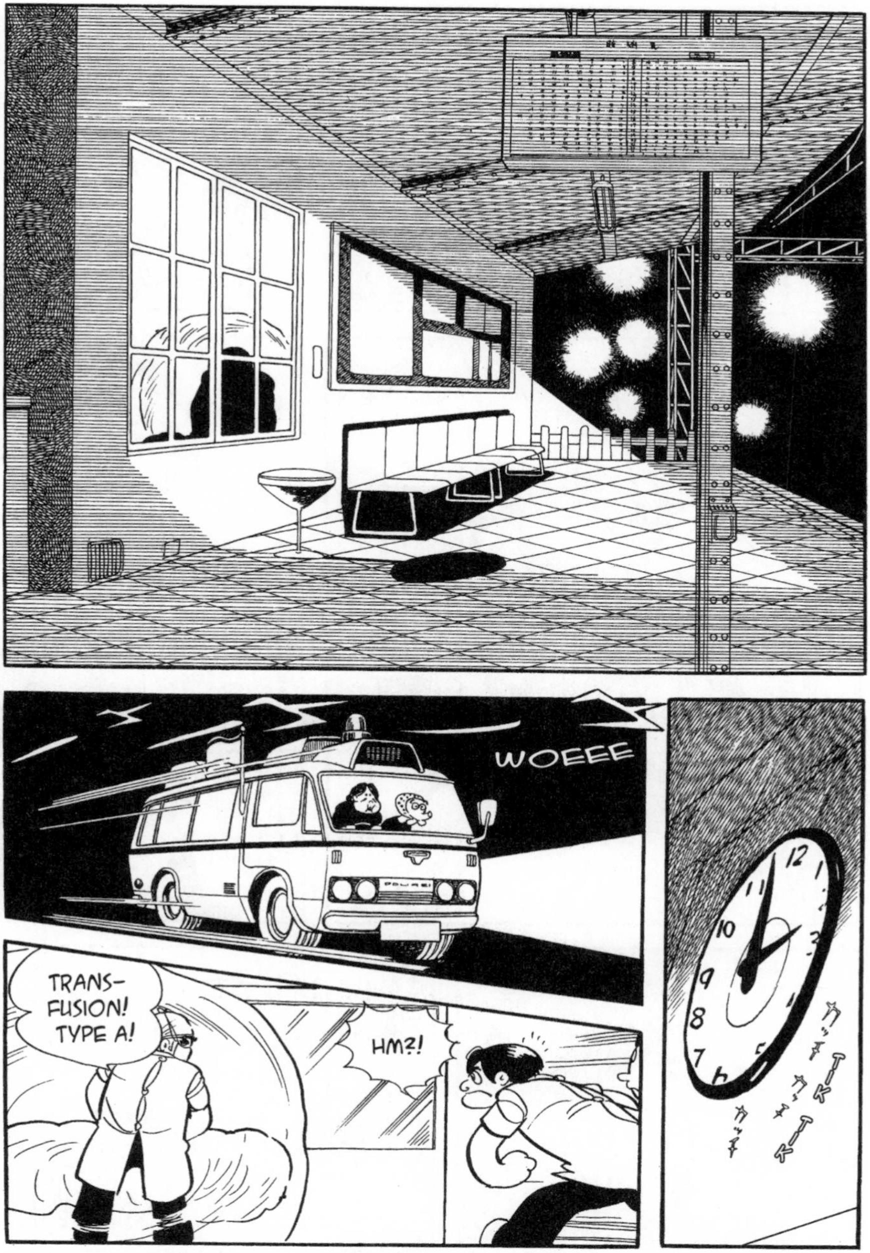
WOEEE
HM?!
TRANS-FUSION! TYPE A!

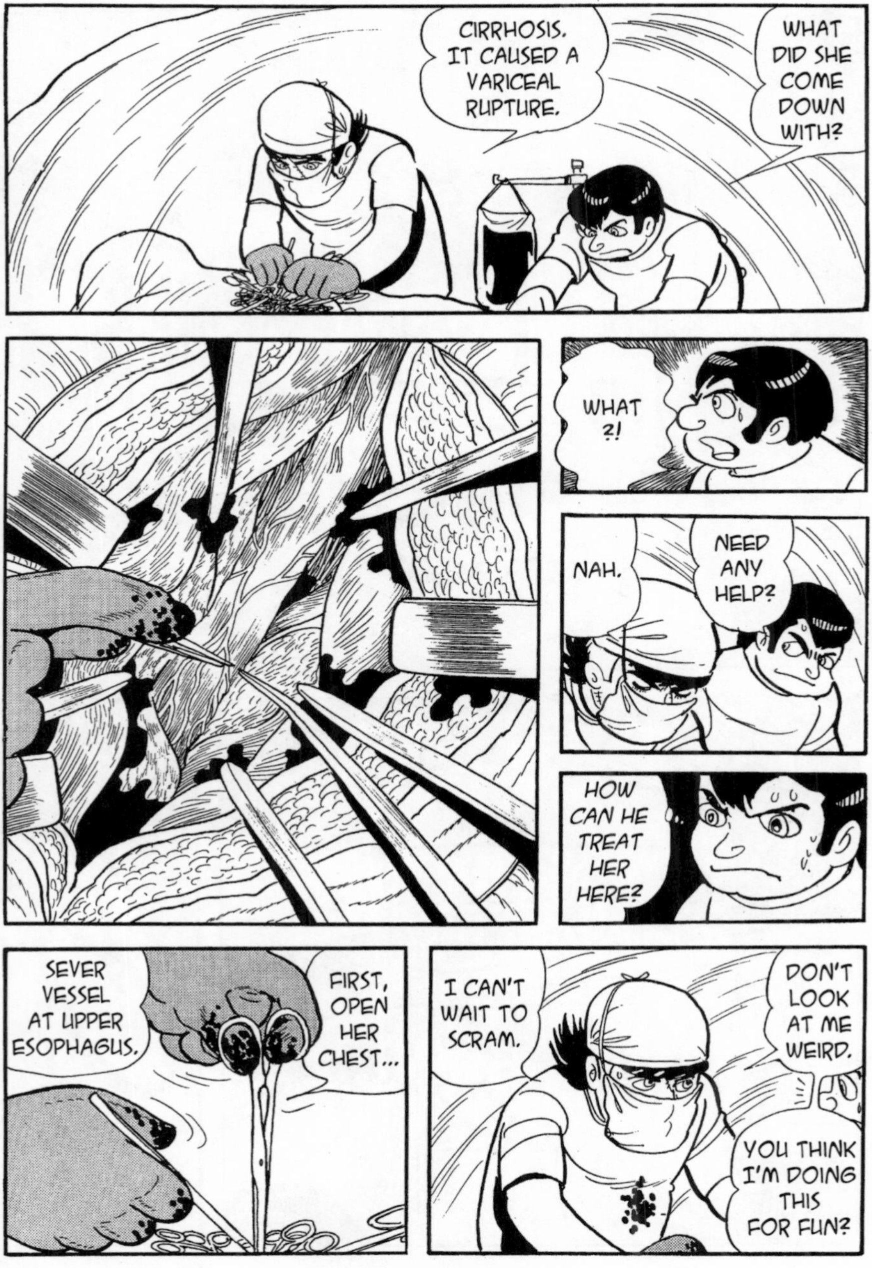
WHAT DID SHE COME DOWN WITH?
CIRRHOSIS. IT CAUSED A VARICEAL RUPTURE.
WHAT ?!
NEED ANY HELP?
NAH.
HOW CAN HE TREAT HER HERE?
DON'T LOOK AT ME WEIRD.
I CAN'T WAIT TO SCRAM.
YOU THINK I'M DOING THIS FOR FUN?
FIRST, OPEN HER CHEST...
SEVER VESSEL AT UPPER ESOPHAGUS.

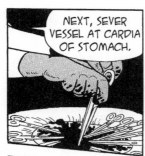

NEXT HER ABDOMEN ...
REMOVE SPLEEN.
WOW ...
HE'S A GOD.
NEXT, SEVER VESSEL AT CARDIA OF STOMACH.
SEVER VAGUS NERVE ADJUSTING STOMACH FLUID.
REFORM PYLORUS OF STOMACH TO AID FOOD PASSAGE.
THAT OUGHT TO DO.
BETTER CLOSE HER UP ...
PLEASE HANDLE IT FROM HERE.
NOW, THAT WAS SURGERY...
I ONLY INTENDED TO GIVE HER FIRST AID.
WHAT A CHUMP I AM !
I GOT CARRIED AWAY...

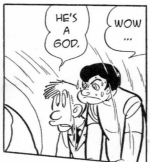

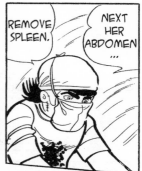

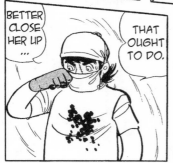

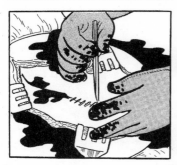

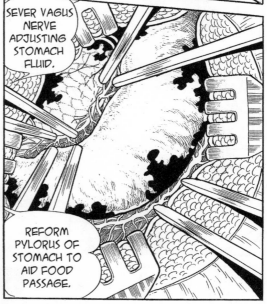

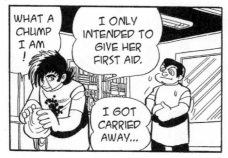

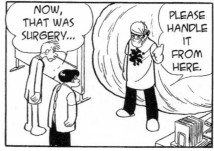

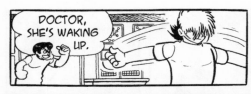

DOCTOR, SHE'S WAKING UP.
THANK YOU.
I'D LIKE TO PAY YOU...
BUT I'M BROKE.
I KNOW THAT.
IF YOU WEREN'T, YOU'D HAVE GONE TO A DOCTOR INSTEAD OF SPENDING THE NIGHT IN PAIN AT A TRAIN STATION.
ONE DAY, DOCTOR, I WILL PAY YOU.
I WILL. I SWEAR TO GOD THAT I'LL PAY YOU.
LOOK, IT'S OKAY.

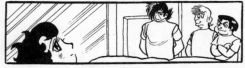

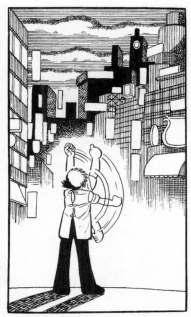

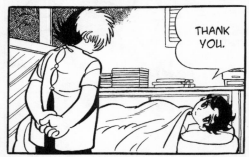

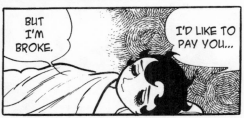

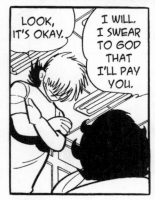

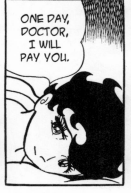

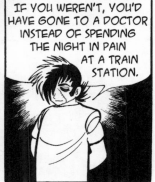

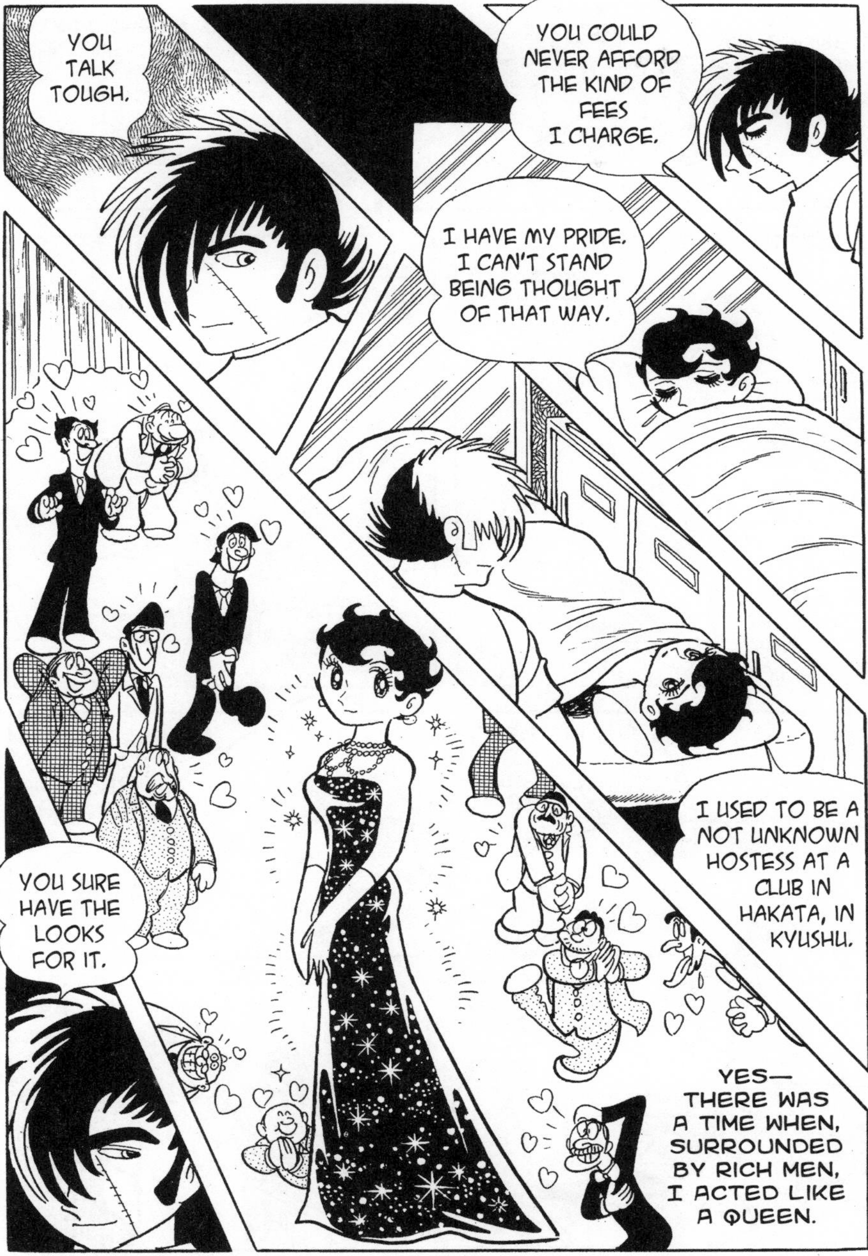
YOU COULD NEVER AFFORD THE KIND OF FEES I CHARGE.
I HAVE MY PRIDE. I CAN'T STAND BEING THOUGHT OF THAT WAY.
YOU TALK TOUGH.
I USED TO BE A NOT UNKNOWN HOSTESS AT A CLUB IN HAKATA, IN KYUSHU.
YOU SURE HAVE THE LOOKS FOR IT.
YES— THERE WAS A TIME WHEN, SURROUNDED BY RICH MEN, I ACTED LIKE A QUEEN.

NOTE: "CLUB" = A HIGH-PRICED BAR LOUNGE WHERE ATTRACTIVE WOMEN, RATHER LIKE THE GEISHA OF OLD, OFFER COMPANIONSHIP BUT ONLY ENTER INTO RELATIONSHIPS AT THEIR OWN DISCRETION

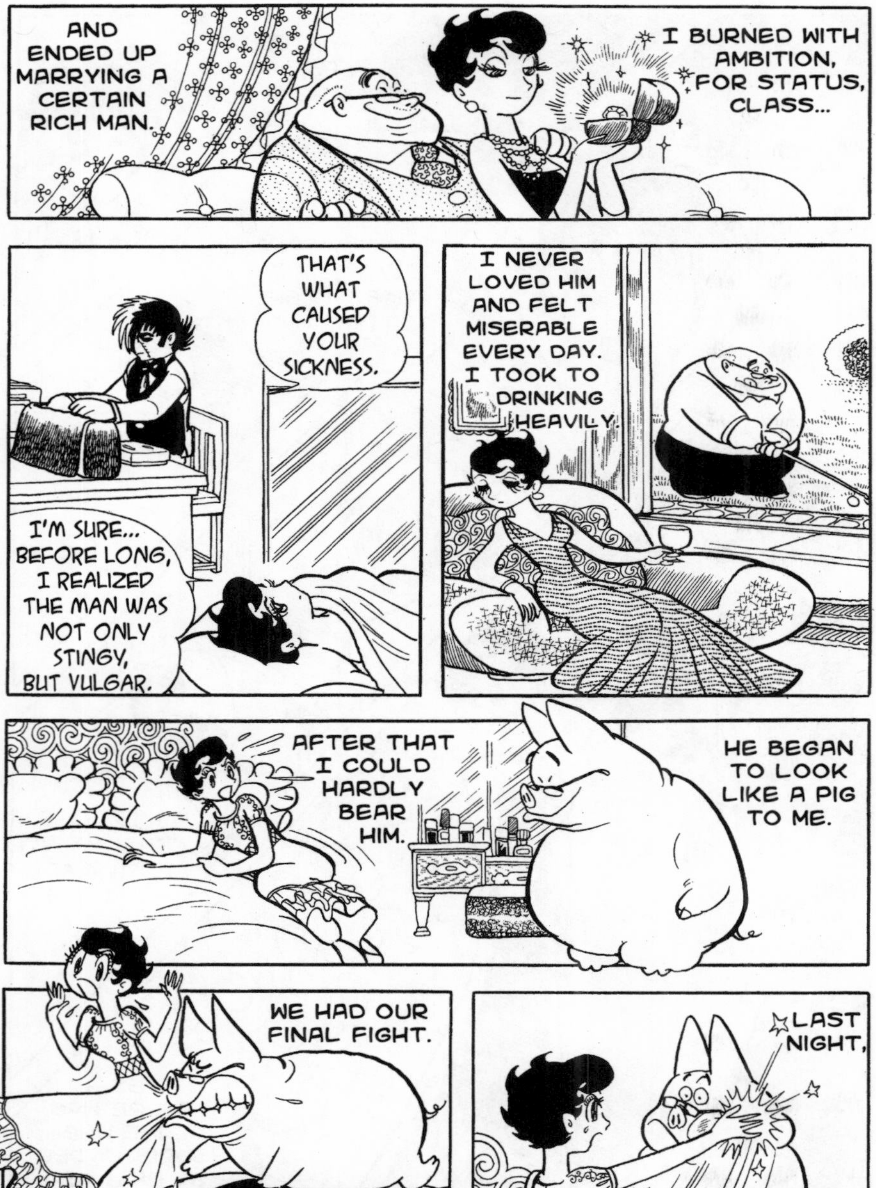
I BURNED WITH AMBITION, FOR STATUS, CLASS...
AND ENDED UP MARRYING A CERTAIN RICH MAN.
I NEVER LOVED HIM AND FELT MISERABLE EVERY DAY. I TOOK TO DRINKING HEAVILY.
THAT'S WHAT CAUSED YOUR SICKNESS.
I'M SURE... BEFORE LONG, I REALIZED THE MAN WAS NOT ONLY STINGY, BUT VULGAR.
HE BEGAN TO LOOK LIKE A PIG TO ME.
AFTER THAT I COULD HARDLY BEAR HIM.
LAST NIGHT,
WE HAD OUR FINAL FIGHT.

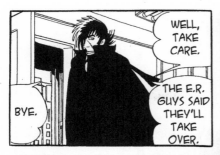

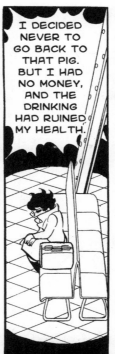

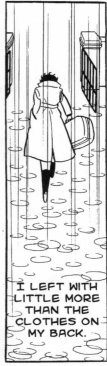

I LEFT WITH LITTLE MORE THAN THE CLOTHES ON MY BACK.
I DECIDED NEVER TO GO BACK TO THAT PIG. BUT I HAD NO MONEY, AND THE DRINKING HAD RUINED MY HEALTH.
WELL, TAKE CARE.
THE E.R. GUYS SAID THEY'LL TAKE OVER.
BYE.
DOCTOR...
AT LEAST TELL ME HOW MUCH I OWE YOU.
LET'S SEE... YOU COULD TREAT ME TO A BOWL OF RAMEN NOODLES.
I'D RATHER YOU DIDN'T JOKE AROUND ABOUT THIS. I'M ASKING IN EARNEST.
LOOK, MY FEES ARE WELL BEYOND YOUR CURRENT MEANS.
JUST BUY ME SOME RAMEN ONE OF THESE DAYS.
DOCTOR!
I'M IN YOUR DEBT...

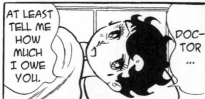

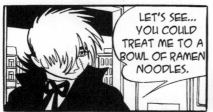

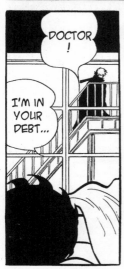

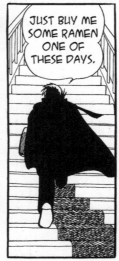

NOTE: "RAMEN," OR NOODLE SOUP, IS AN INEXPENSIVE TREAT COMMON AROUND TRAIN STATIONS.

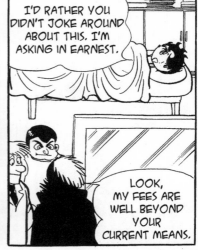

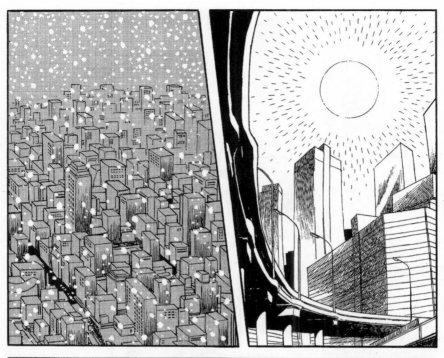

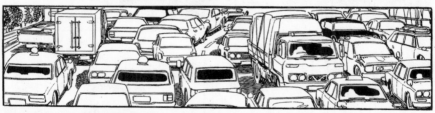

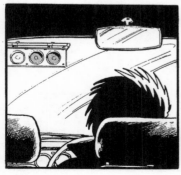

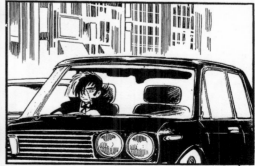

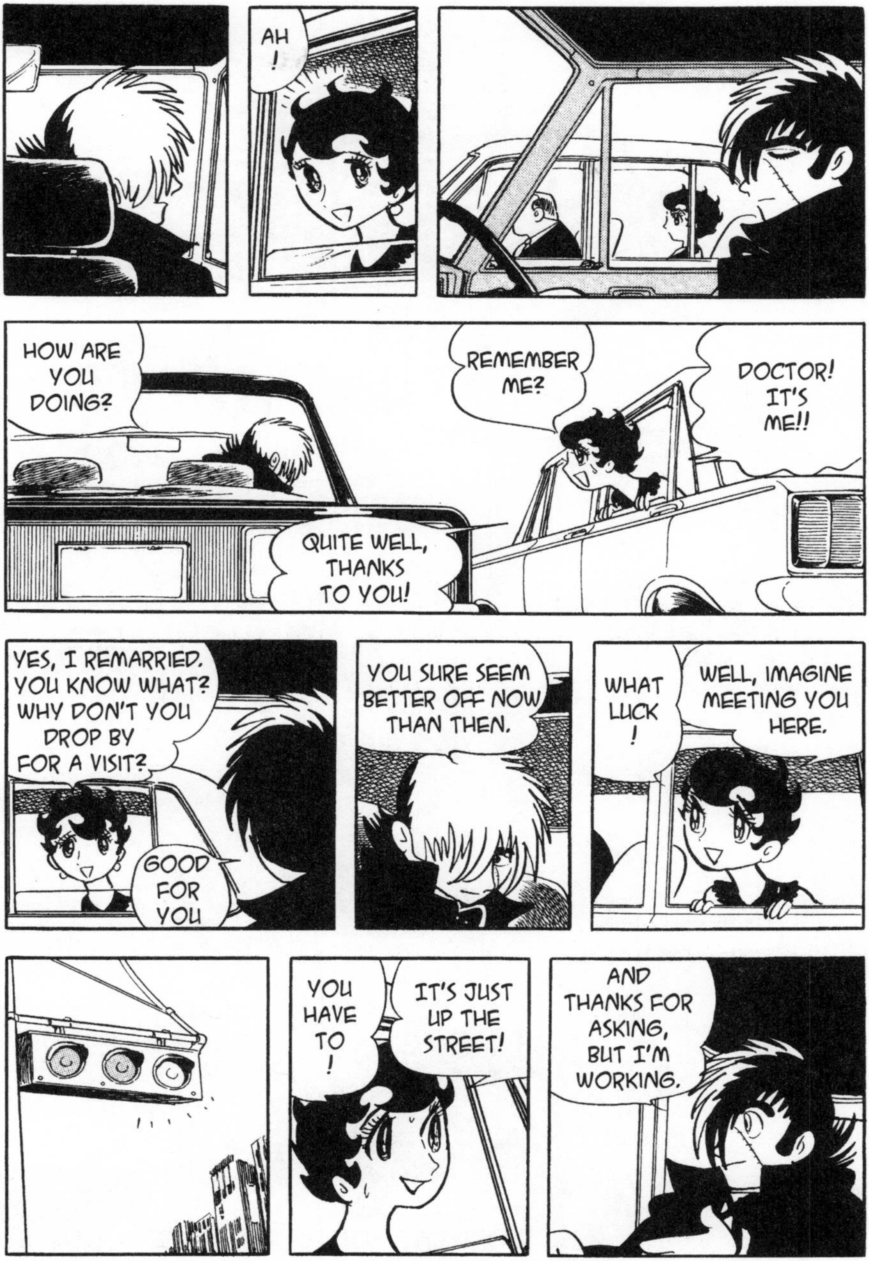
AH!
DOCTOR! IT'S ME!!
REMEMBER ME?
HOW ARE YOU DOING?
QUITE WELL, THANKS TO YOU!
WELL, IMAGINE MEETING YOU HERE.
WHAT LUCK!
YOU SURE SEEM BETTER OFF NOW THAN THEN.
YES, I REMARRIED. YOU KNOW WHAT? WHY DON'T YOU DROP BY FOR A VISIT?
GOOD FOR YOU
AND THANKS FOR ASKING, BUT I'M WORKING.
IT'S JUST UP THE STREET!
YOU HAVE TO!

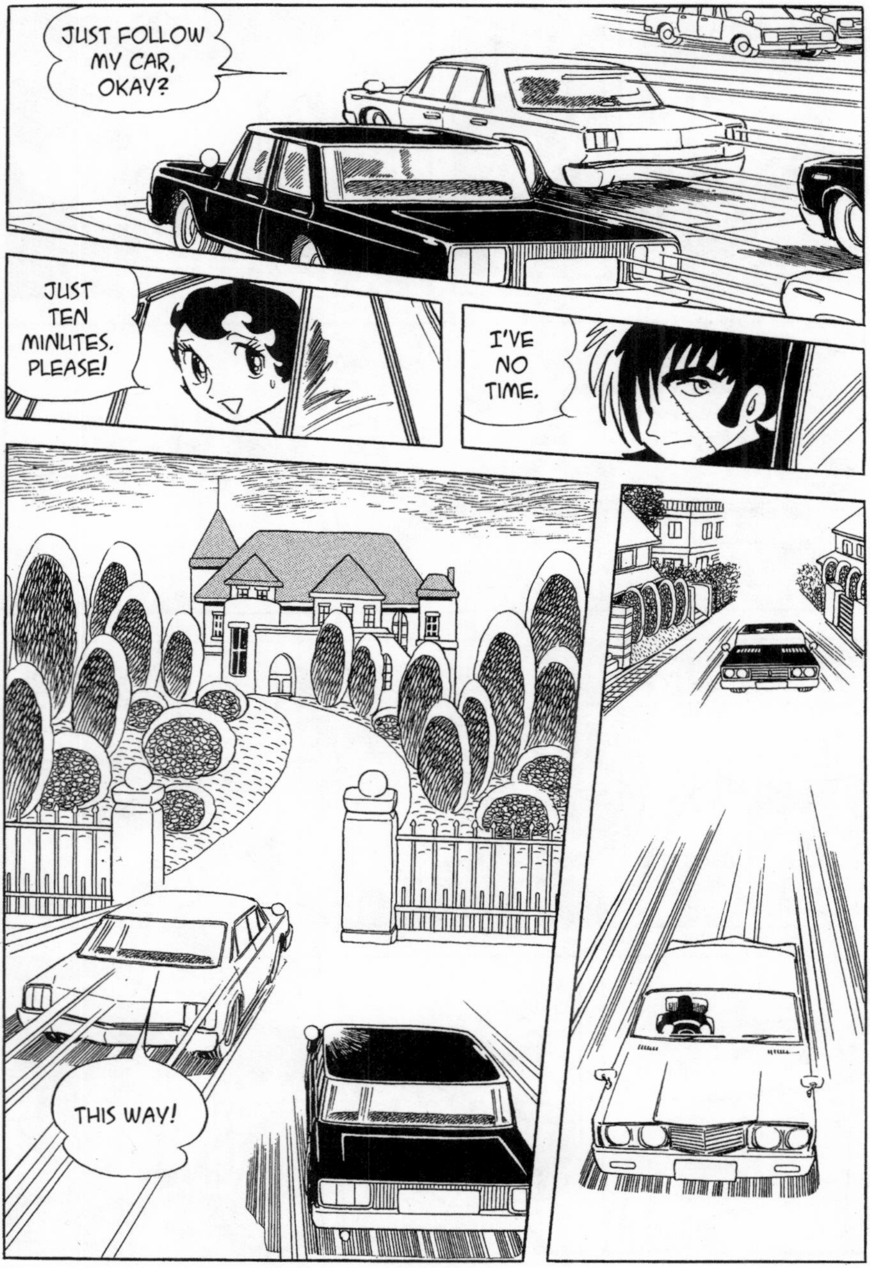
JUST FOLLOW MY CAR, OKAY?
I'VE NO TIME.
JUST TEN MINUTES. PLEASE!
THIS WAY!

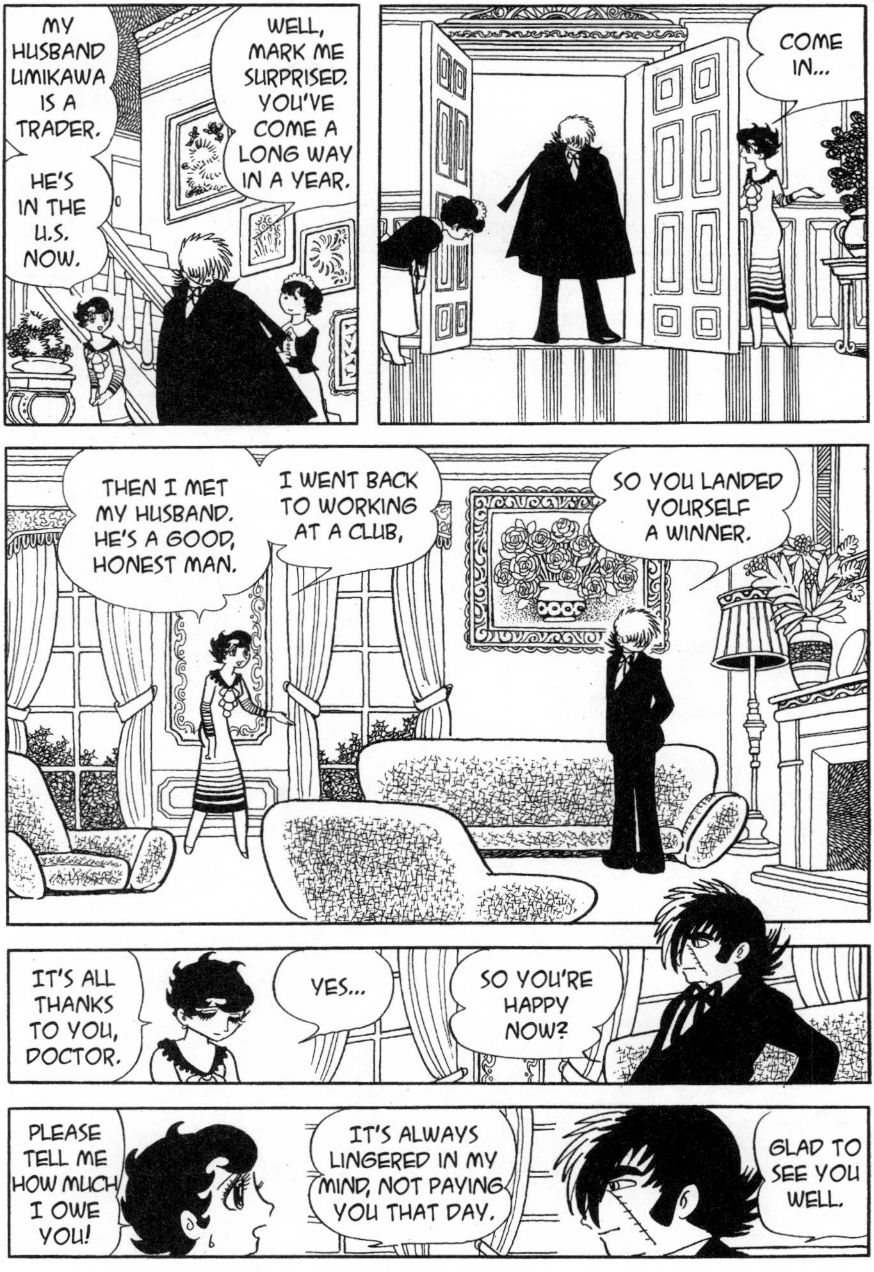
COME IN...
WELL, MARK ME SURPRISED. YOU'VE COME A LONG WAY IN A YEAR.
MY HUSBAND UMIKAWA IS A TRADER.
HE'S IN THE U.S. NOW.
SO YOU LANDED YOURSELF A WINNER.
I WENT BACK TO WORKING AT A CLUB,
THEN I MET MY HUSBAND. HE'S A GOOD, HONEST MAN.
SO YOU'RE HAPPY NOW?
YES...
IT'S ALL THANKS TO YOU, DOCTOR.
GLAD TO SEE YOU WELL.
IT'S ALWAYS LINGERED IN MY MIND, NOT PAYING YOU THAT DAY.
PLEASE TELL ME HOW MUCH I OWE YOU!

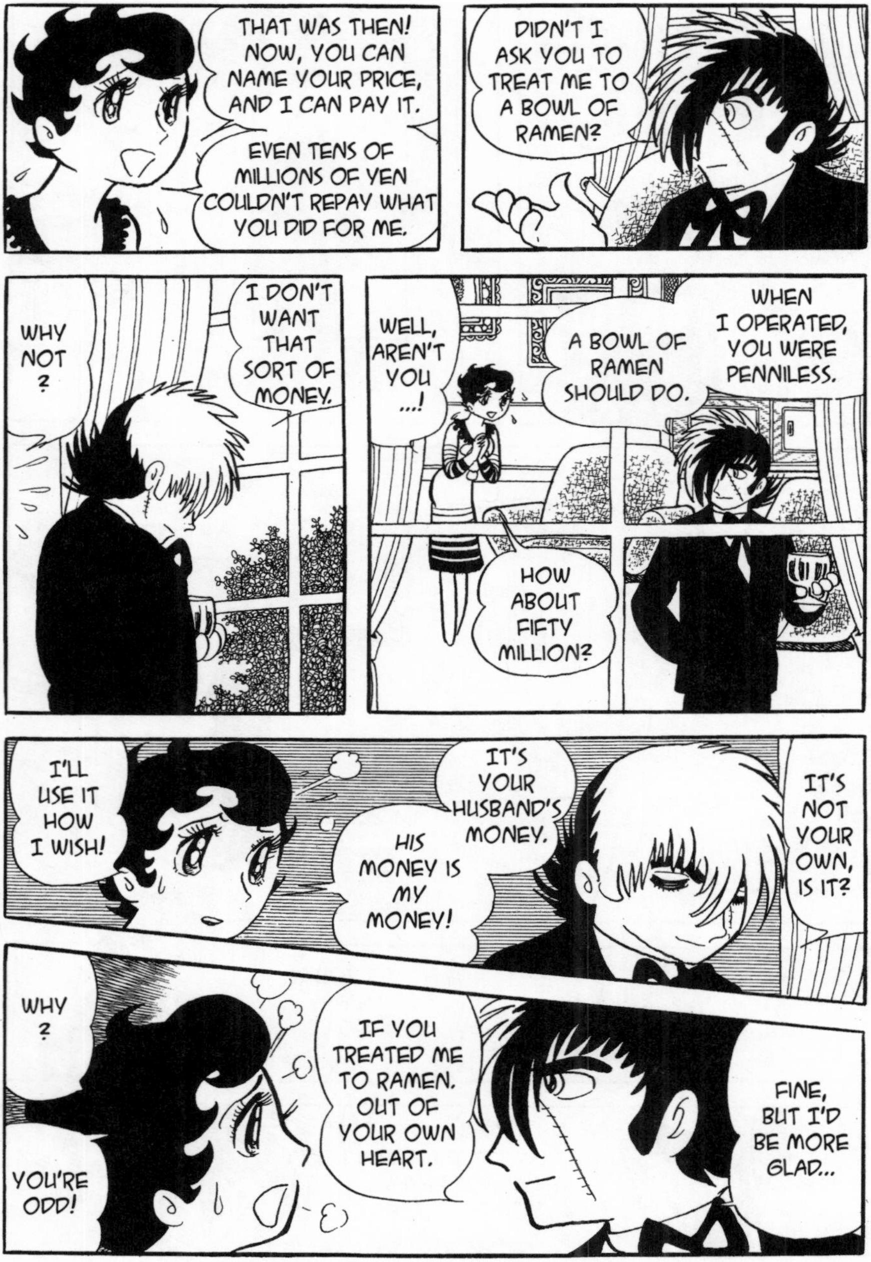
DIDN'T I ASK YOU TO TREAT ME TO A BOWL OF RAMEN?
THAT WAS THEN! NOW, YOU CAN NAME YOUR PRICE, AND I CAN PAY IT.
EVEN TENS OF MILLIONS OF YEN COULDN'T REPAY WHAT YOU DID FOR ME.
WHEN I OPERATED, YOU WERE PENNILESS.
A BOWL OF RAMEN SHOULD DO.
WELL, AREN'T YOU ...!
HOW ABOUT FIFTY MILLION?
I DON'T WANT THAT SORT OF MONEY.
WHY NOT?
IT'S NOT YOUR OWN, IS IT?
IT'S YOUR HUSBAND'S MONEY.
HIS MONEY IS MY MONEY!
I'LL USE IT HOW I WISH!
FINE, BUT I'D BE MORE GLAD...
IF YOU TREATED ME TO RAMEN. OUT OF YOUR OWN HEART.
WHY?
YOU'RE ODD!

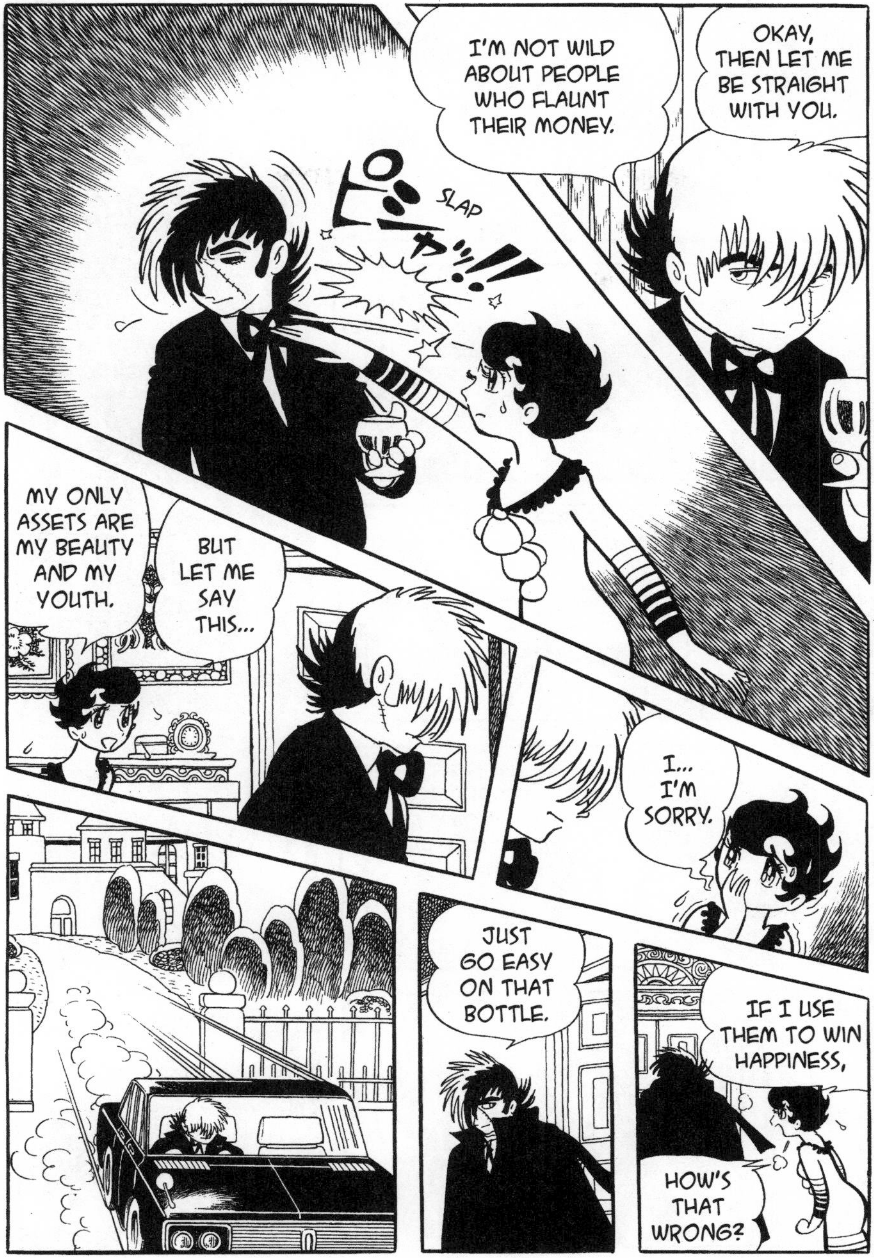
OKAY, THEN LET ME BE STRAIGHT WITH YOU.
I'M NOT WILD ABOUT PEOPLE WHO FLAUNT THEIR MONEY.
SLAP
I... I'M SORRY.
BUT LET ME SAY THIS...
MY ONLY ASSETS ARE MY BEAUTY AND MY YOUTH.
IF I USE THEM TO WIN HAPPINESS,
HOW'S THAT WRONG?
JUST GO EASY ON THAT BOTTLE.

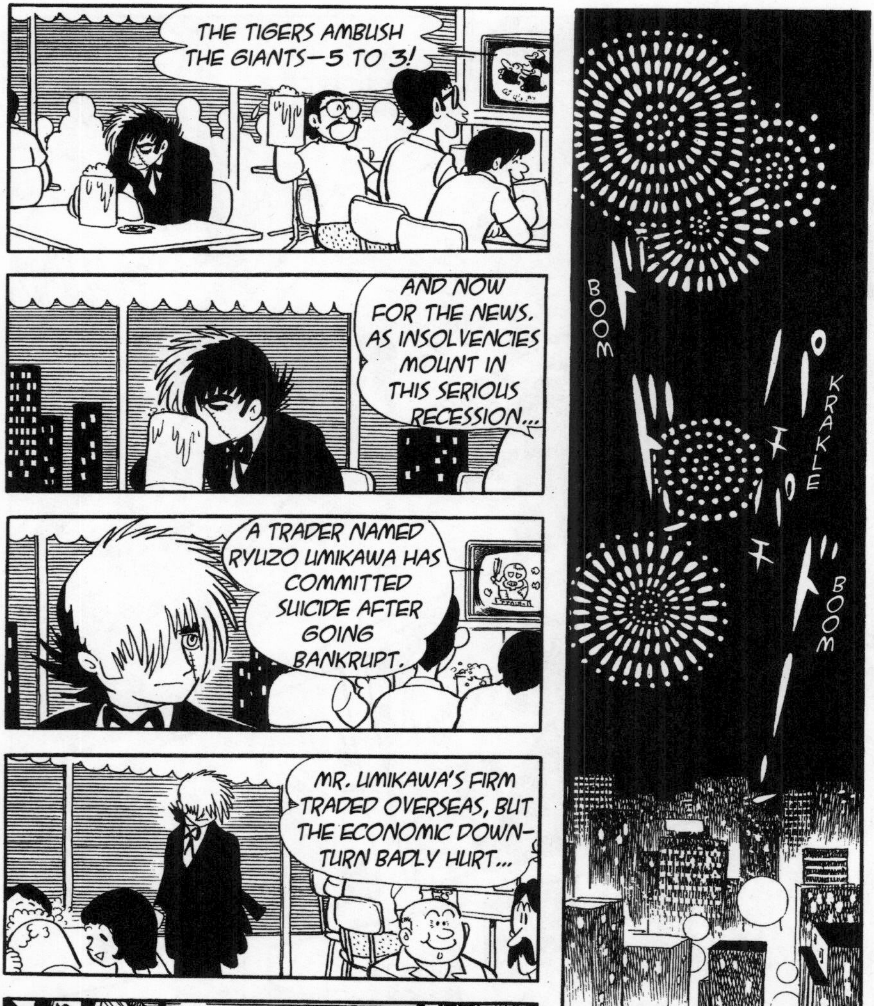
BOOM
KRAKLE
BOOM
THE TIGERS AMBUSH THE GIANTS—5 TO 3!
AND NOW FOR THE NEWS. AS INSOLVENCIES MOUNT IN THIS SERIOUS RECESSION...
A TRADER NAMED RYUZO UMIKAWA HAS COMMITTED SUICIDE AFTER GOING BANKRUPT.
MR. UMIKAWA'S FIRM TRADED OVERSEAS, BUT THE ECONOMIC DOWN-TURN BADLY HURT...

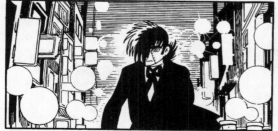

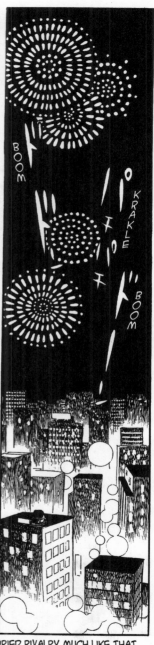

NOTE: "TIGERS" AND "GIANTS" = BASEBALL TEAMS WITH A STORIED RIVALRY MUCH LIKE THAT BETWEEN THE RED SOX AND THE YANKEES

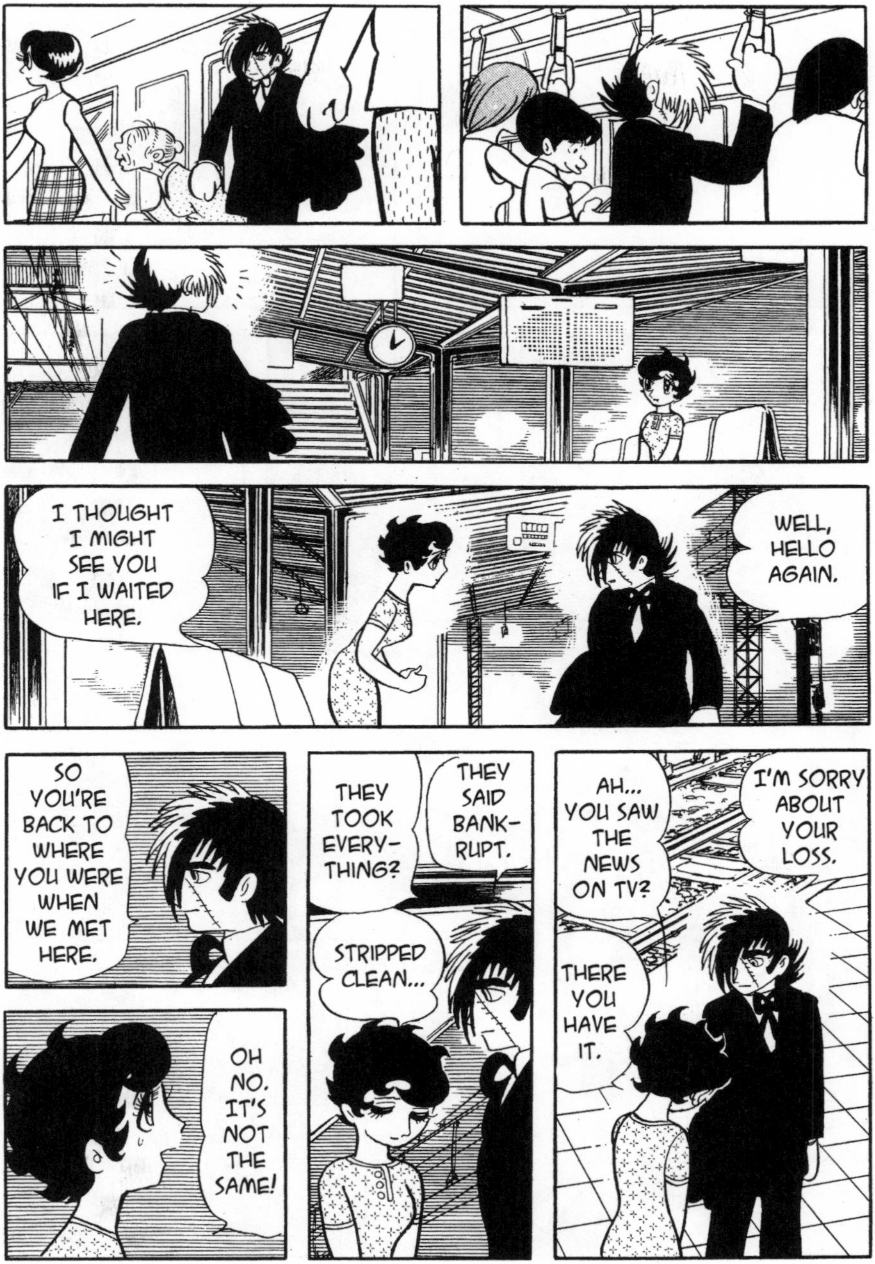
WELL, HELLO AGAIN.
I THOUGHT I MIGHT SEE YOU IF I WAITED HERE.
I'M SORRY ABOUT YOUR LOSS.
AH... YOU SAW THE NEWS ON TV?
THERE YOU HAVE IT.
THEY SAID BANK-RUPT.
THEY TOOK EVERY-THING?
STRIPPED CLEAN...
SO YOU'RE BACK TO WHERE YOU WERE WHEN WE MET HERE.
OH NO. IT'S NOT THE SAME!

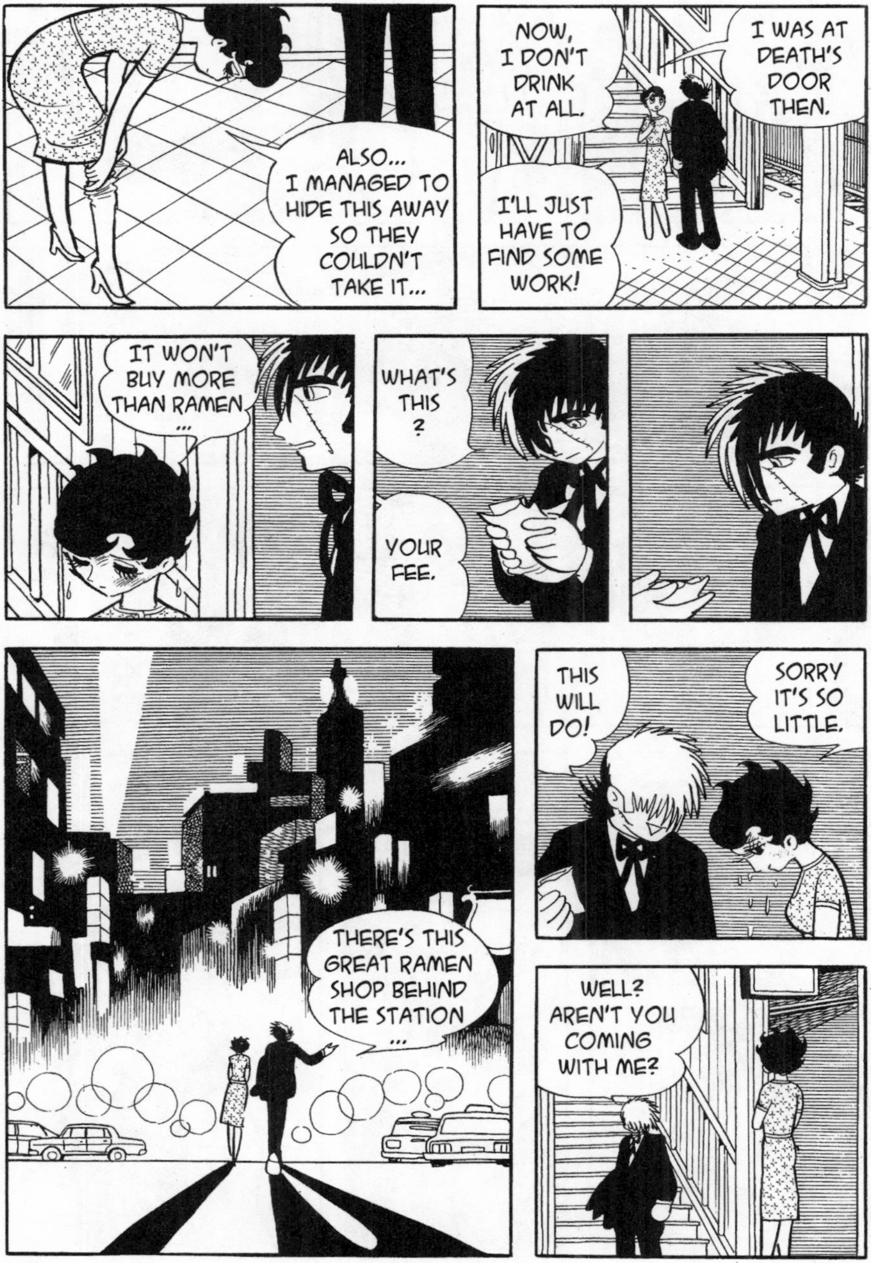
I WAS AT DEATH'S DOOR THEN.
NOW, I DON'T DRINK AT ALL.
I'LL JUST HAVE TO FIND SOME WORK!
ALSO... I MANAGED TO HIDE THIS AWAY SO THEY COULDN'T TAKE IT...
WHAT'S THIS ?
YOUR FEE.
IT WON'T BUY MORE THAN RAMEN ...
SORRY IT'S SO LITTLE.
THIS WILL DO!
WELL? AREN'T YOU COMING WITH ME?
THERE'S THIS GREAT RAMEN SHOP BEHIND THE STATION ...

TWO DARK DOCTORS

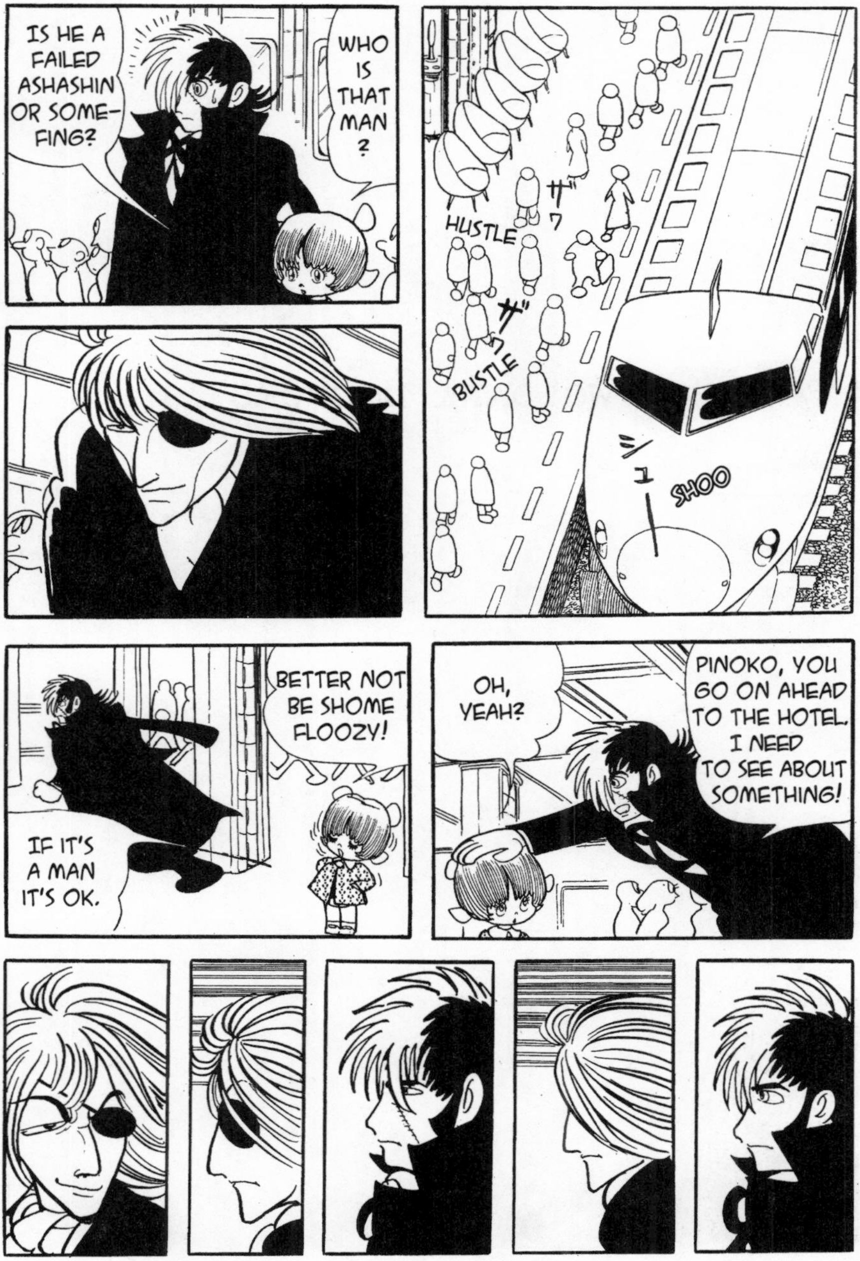
ザワ
HUSTLE
ザワ
BUSTLE
シュー
SHOO
WHO IS THAT MAN?
IS HE A FAILED ASHASHIN OR SOME-FING?
PINOKO, YOU GO ON AHEAD TO THE HOTEL. I NEED TO SEE ABOUT SOMETHING!
OH, YEAH?
BETTER NOT BE SHOME FLOOZY!
IF IT'S A MAN IT'S OK.

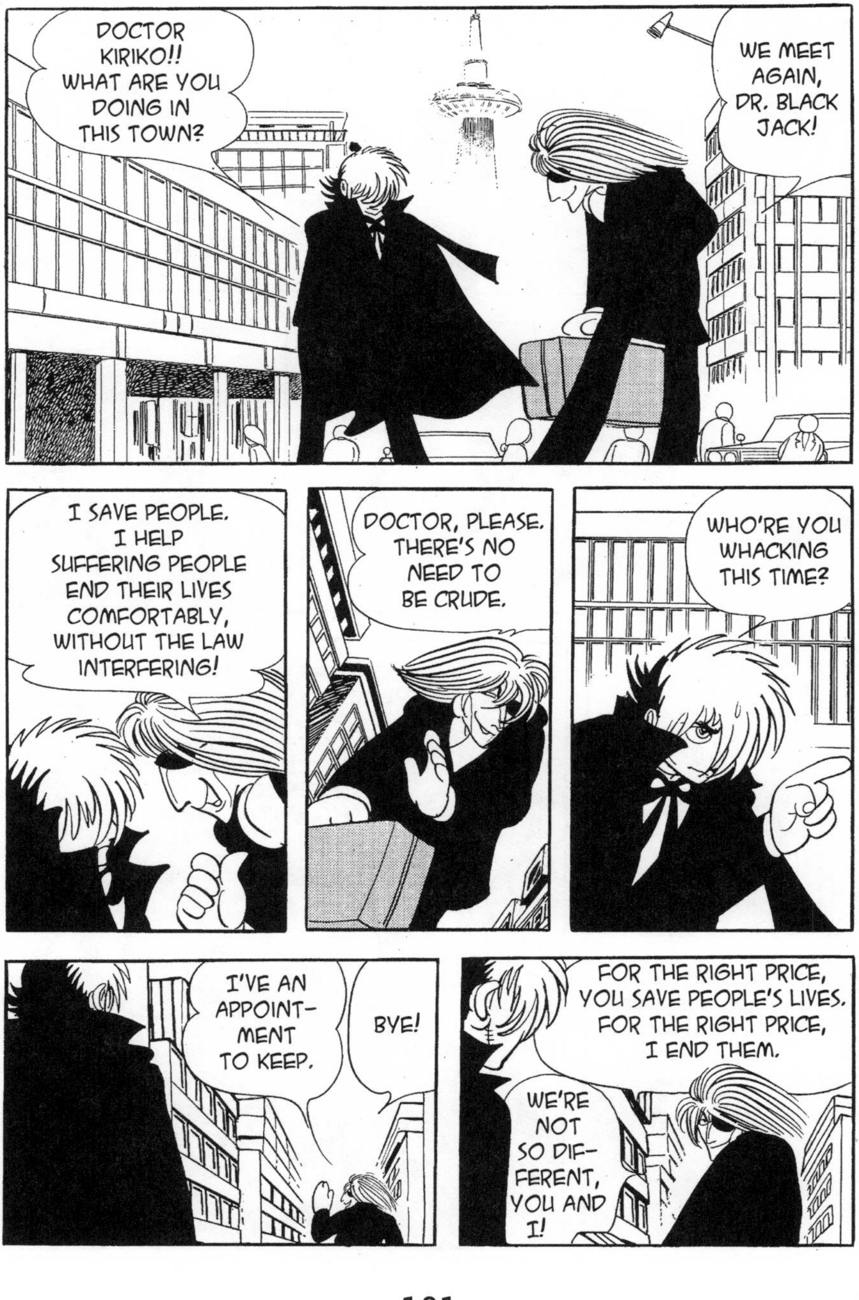
WE MEET AGAIN, DR. BLACK JACK!
DOCTOR KIRIKO!! WHAT ARE YOU DOING IN THIS TOWN?
WHO'RE YOU WHACKING THIS TIME?
DOCTOR, PLEASE. THERE'S NO NEED TO BE CRUDE.
I SAVE PEOPLE. I HELP SUFFERING PEOPLE END THEIR LIVES COMFORTABLY, WITHOUT THE LAW INTERFERING!
FOR THE RIGHT PRICE, YOU SAVE PEOPLE'S LIVES. FOR THE RIGHT PRICE, I END THEM.
WE'RE NOT SO DIF-FERENT, YOU AND I!
BYE!
I'VE AN APPOINT-MENT TO KEEP.

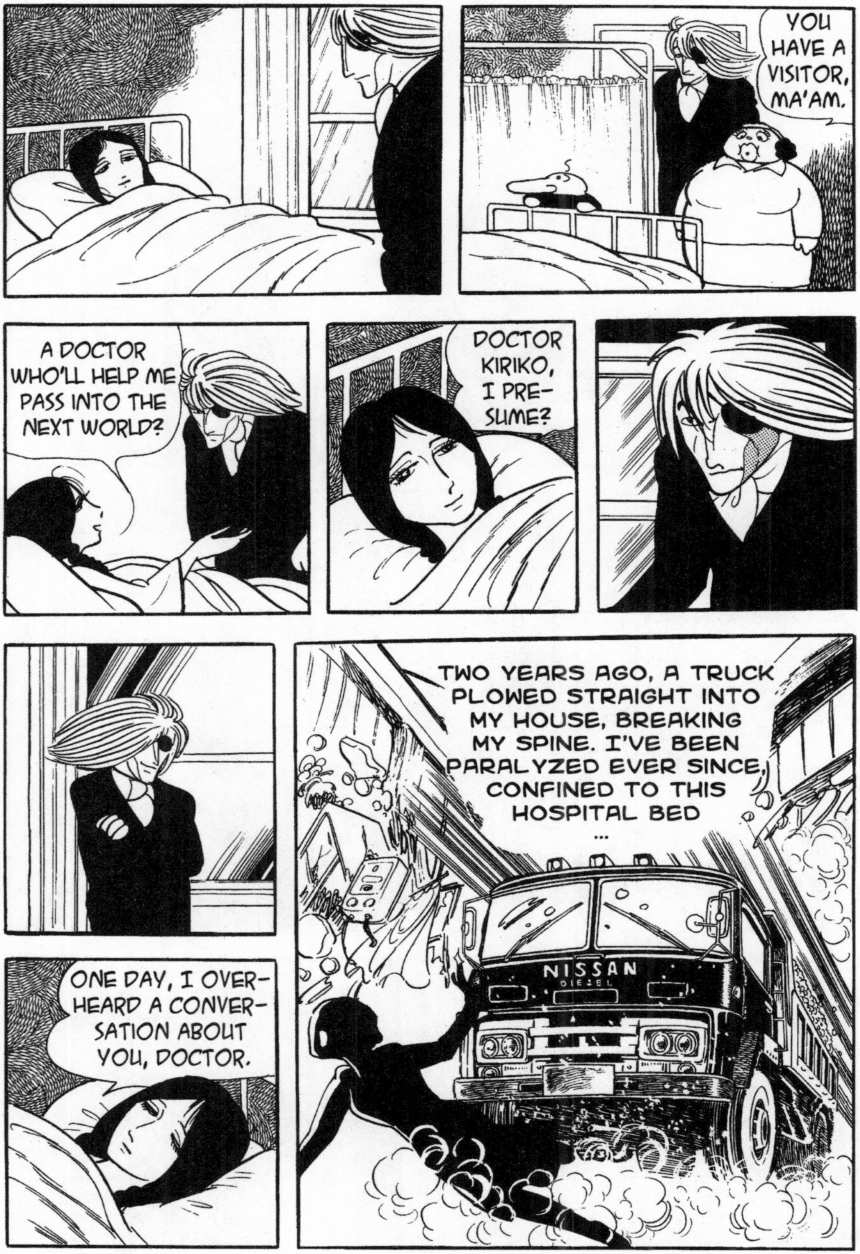
YOU HAVE A VISITOR, MA'AM.
DOCTOR KIRIKO, I PRE-SUME?
A DOCTOR WHO'LL HELP ME PASS INTO THE NEXT WORLD?
TWO YEARS AGO, A TRUCK PLOWED STRAIGHT INTO MY HOUSE, BREAKING MY SPINE. I'VE BEEN PARALYZED EVER SINCE, CONFINED TO THIS HOSPITAL BED ...
NISSAN
DIESEL
ONE DAY, I OVER-HEARD A CONVER-SATION ABOUT YOU, DOCTOR.

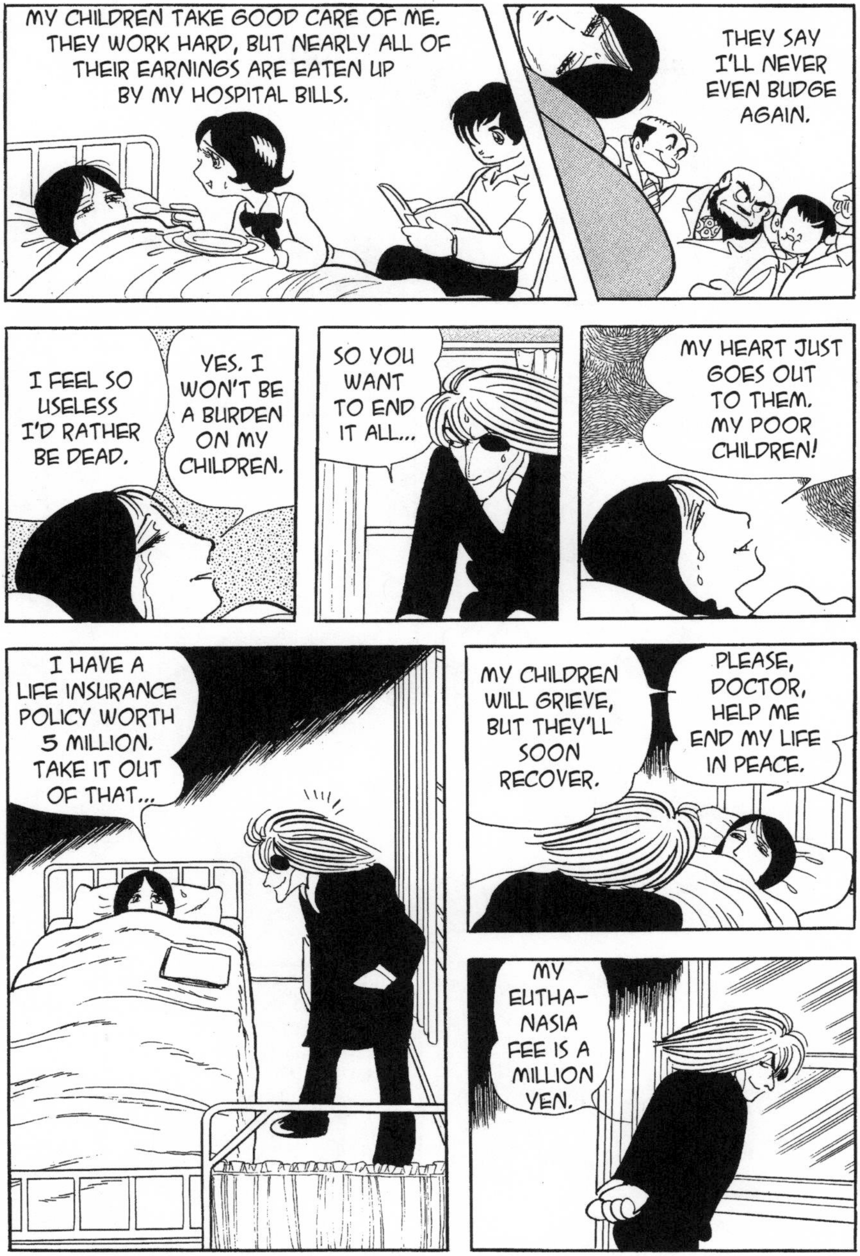
MY CHILDREN TAKE GOOD CARE OF ME. THEY WORK HARD, BUT NEARLY ALL OF THEIR EARNINGS ARE EATEN UP BY MY HOSPITAL BILLS.
THEY SAY I'LL NEVER EVEN BUDGE AGAIN.
I FEEL SO USELESS I'D RATHER BE DEAD.
YES. I WON'T BE A BURDEN ON MY CHILDREN.
SO YOU WANT TO END IT ALL...
MY HEART JUST GOES OUT TO THEM. MY POOR CHILDREN!
I HAVE A LIFE INSURANCE POLICY WORTH 5 MILLION. TAKE IT OUT OF THAT...
MY CHILDREN WILL GRIEVE, BUT THEY'LL SOON RECOVER.
PLEASE, DOCTOR, HELP ME END MY LIFE IN PEACE.
MY EUTHA-NASIA FEE IS A MILLION YEN.

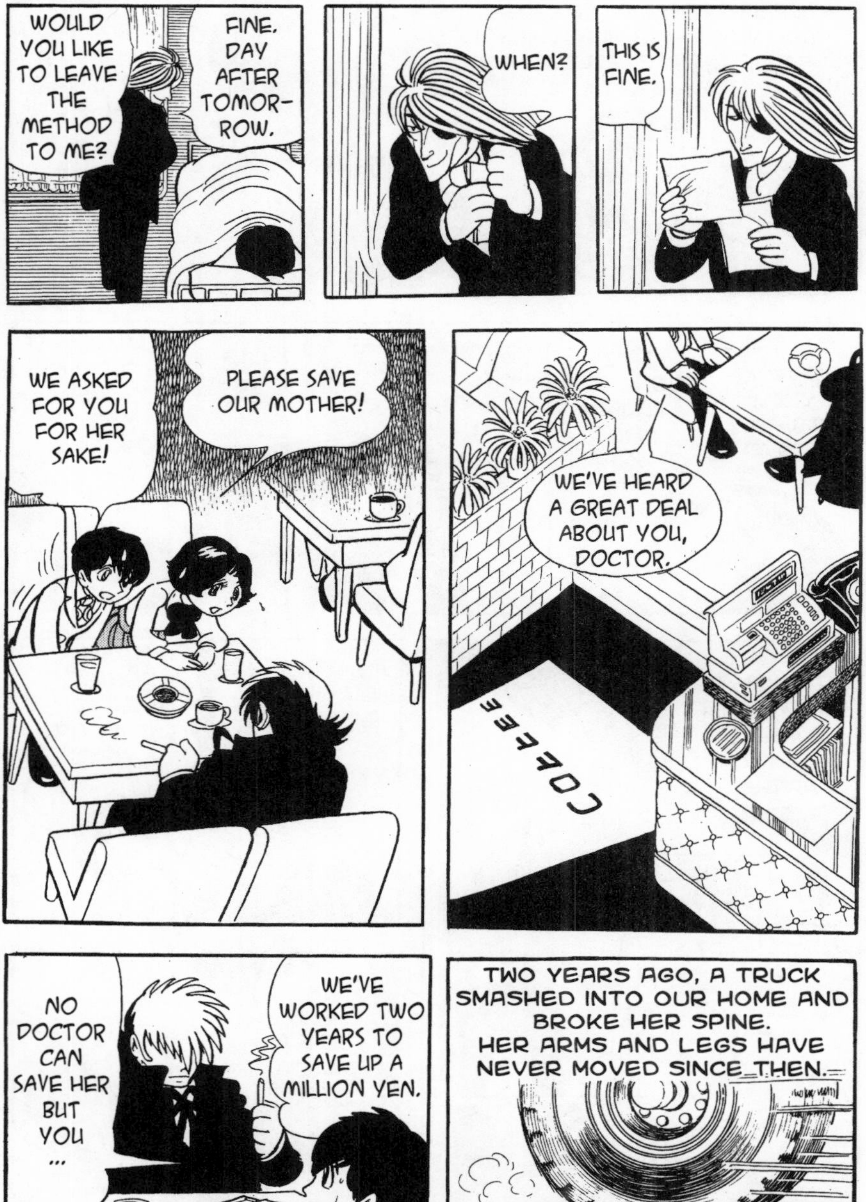
THIS IS FINE.
WHEN?
FINE. DAY AFTER TOMORROW.
WOULD YOU LIKE TO LEAVE THE METHOD TO ME?
WE'VE HEARD A GREAT DEAL ABOUT YOU, DOCTOR.
COFFEE
PLEASE SAVE OUR MOTHER!
WE ASKED FOR YOU FOR HER SAKE!
TWO YEARS AGO, A TRUCK SMASHED INTO OUR HOME AND BROKE HER SPINE. HER ARMS AND LEGS HAVE NEVER MOVED SINCE THEN.
WE'VE WORKED TWO YEARS TO SAVE UP A MILLION YEN.
NO DOCTOR CAN SAVE HER BUT YOU ...

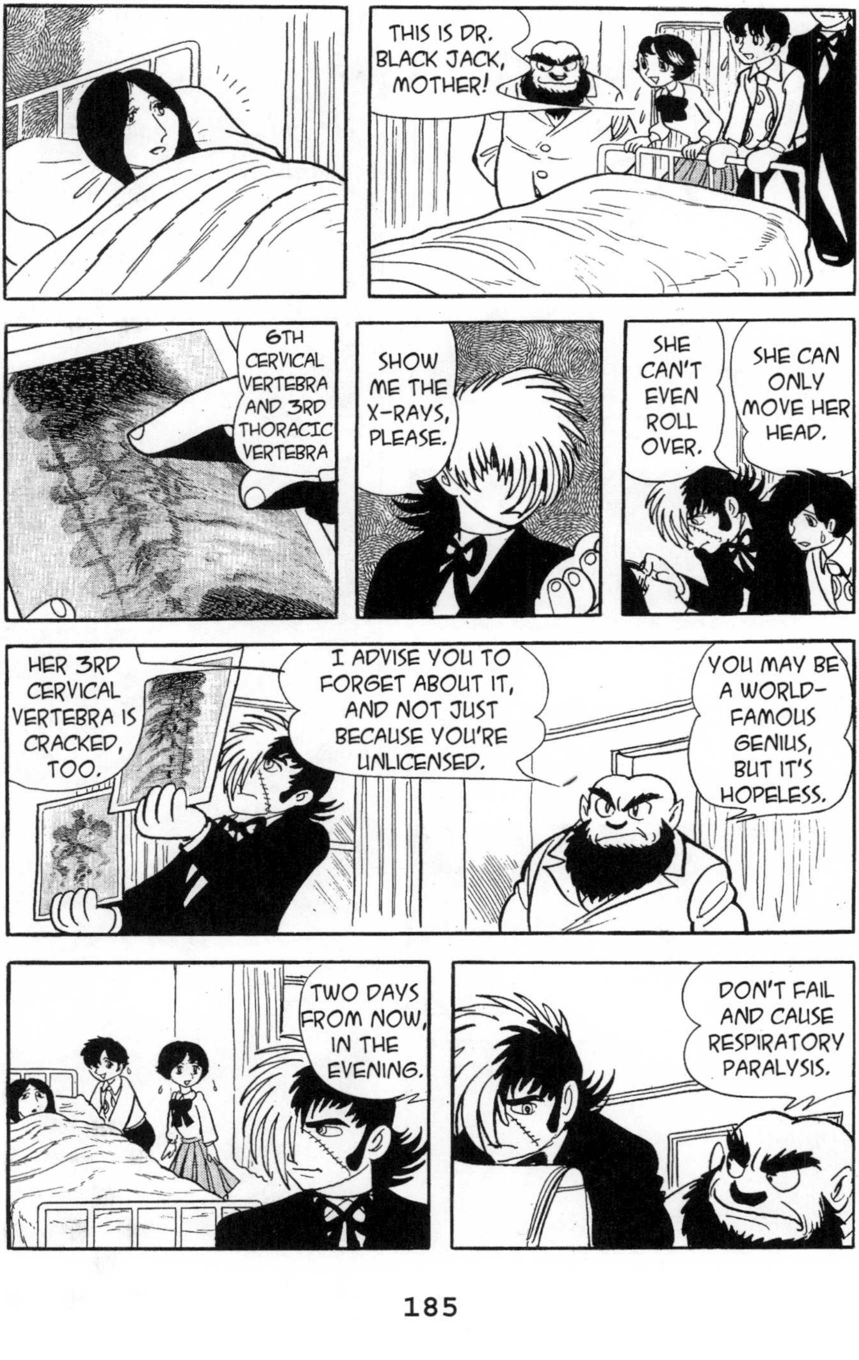
THIS IS DR. BLACK JACK, MOTHER!
SHE CAN ONLY MOVE HER HEAD.
SHE CAN'T EVEN ROLL OVER.
SHOW ME THE X-RAYS, PLEASE.
6TH CERVICAL VERTEBRA AND 3RD THORACIC VERTEBRA
YOU MAY BE A WORLD-FAMOUS GENIUS, BUT IT'S HOPELESS.
I ADVISE YOU TO FORGET ABOUT IT, AND NOT JUST BECAUSE YOU'RE UNLICENSED.
HER 3RD CERVICAL VERTEBRA IS CRACKED, TOO.
DON'T FAIL AND CAUSE RESPIRATORY PARALYSIS.
TWO DAYS FROM NOW, IN THE EVENING.

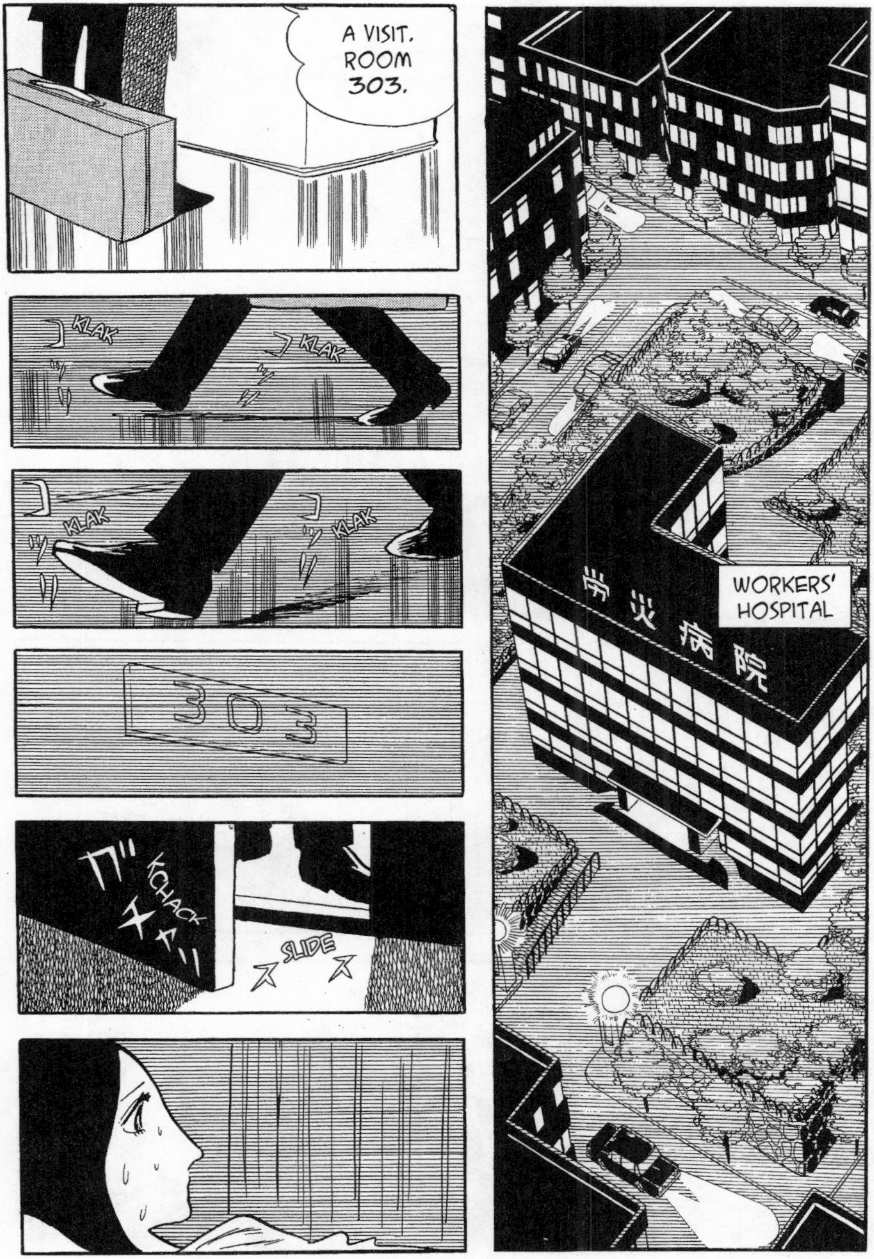

労災病院
WORKERS' HOSPITAL
A VISIT. ROOM 303.
コツ KLAK
コツ KLAK
コツ KLAK
コツ KLAK
303
ガチャッ KCHACK
ス SLIDE ス

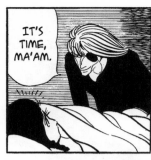

WHO'S THERE?
IT'S TIME, MA'AM.
WHAT'S THAT?
A DEVICE FOR A PEACEFUL DEATH.
I WILL ATTACH ELECTRODES TO THE BACK OF YOUR HEAD AND SEND ULTRA-SONIC WAVES. IT WILL SLOWLY PARALYZE YOUR MEDULLA OBLONGATA.
YOUR RESPIRATORY CENTER WILL CEASE TO FUNCTION. YOU'LL DIE.
BUT FIRST, YOU'LL BEGIN TO FEEL DREAMY. YOU WILL BREATHE YOUR LAST IN THAT STATE...
IT WILL BE SEEN AS A NATURAL DEATH.
NOW IF YOU'RE READY, WE WILL BEGIN.
BEEP
BEEP

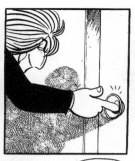

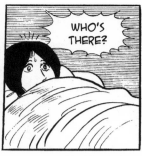

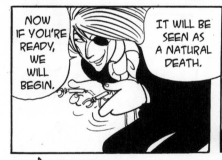

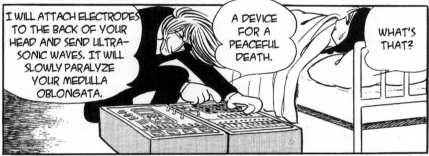

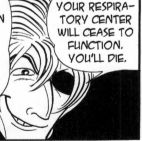

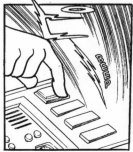

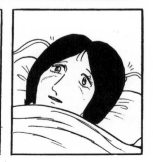

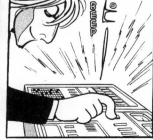

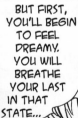

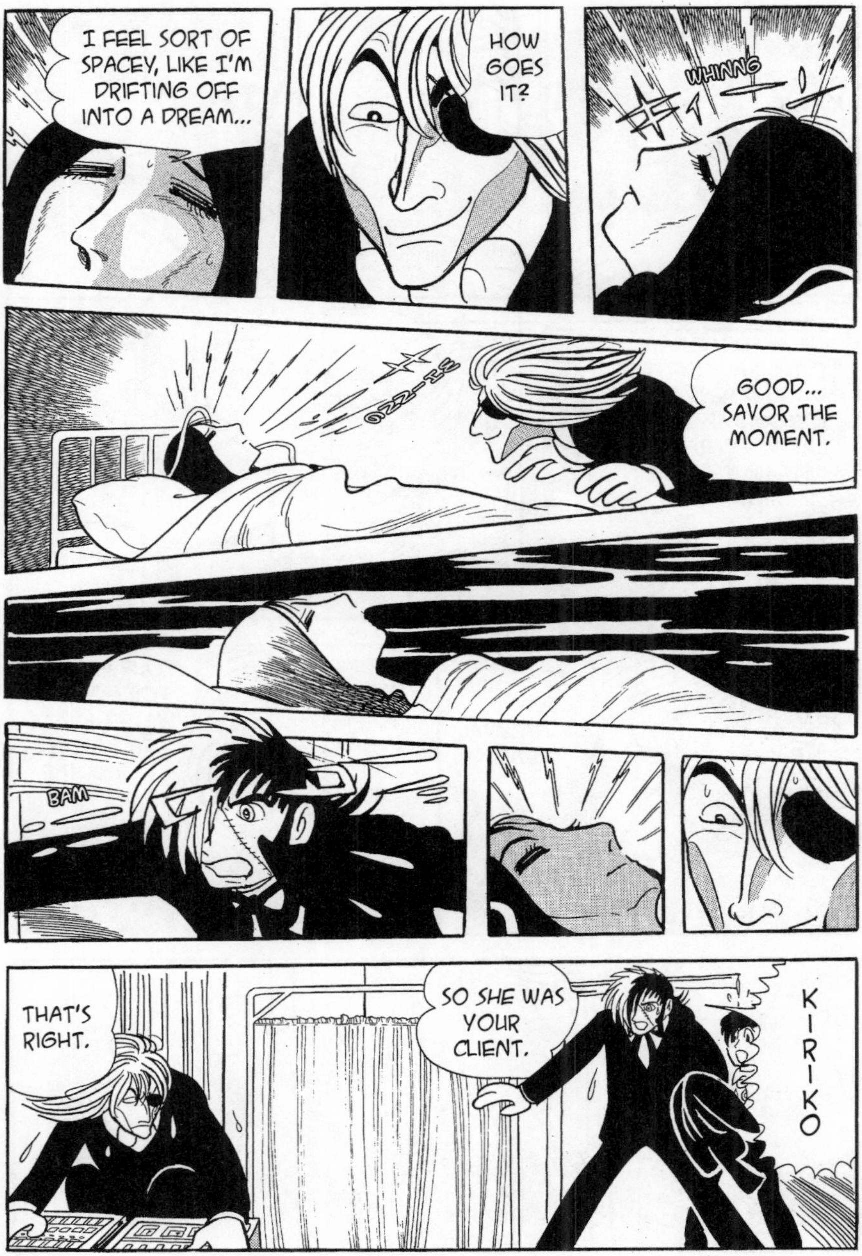
WHINNG
HOW GOES IT?
I FEEL SORT OF SPACEY, LIKE I'M DRIFTING OFF INTO A DREAM...
GOOD... SAVOR THE MOMENT.
BAM
KIRIKO
SO SHE WAS YOUR CLIENT.
THAT'S RIGHT.

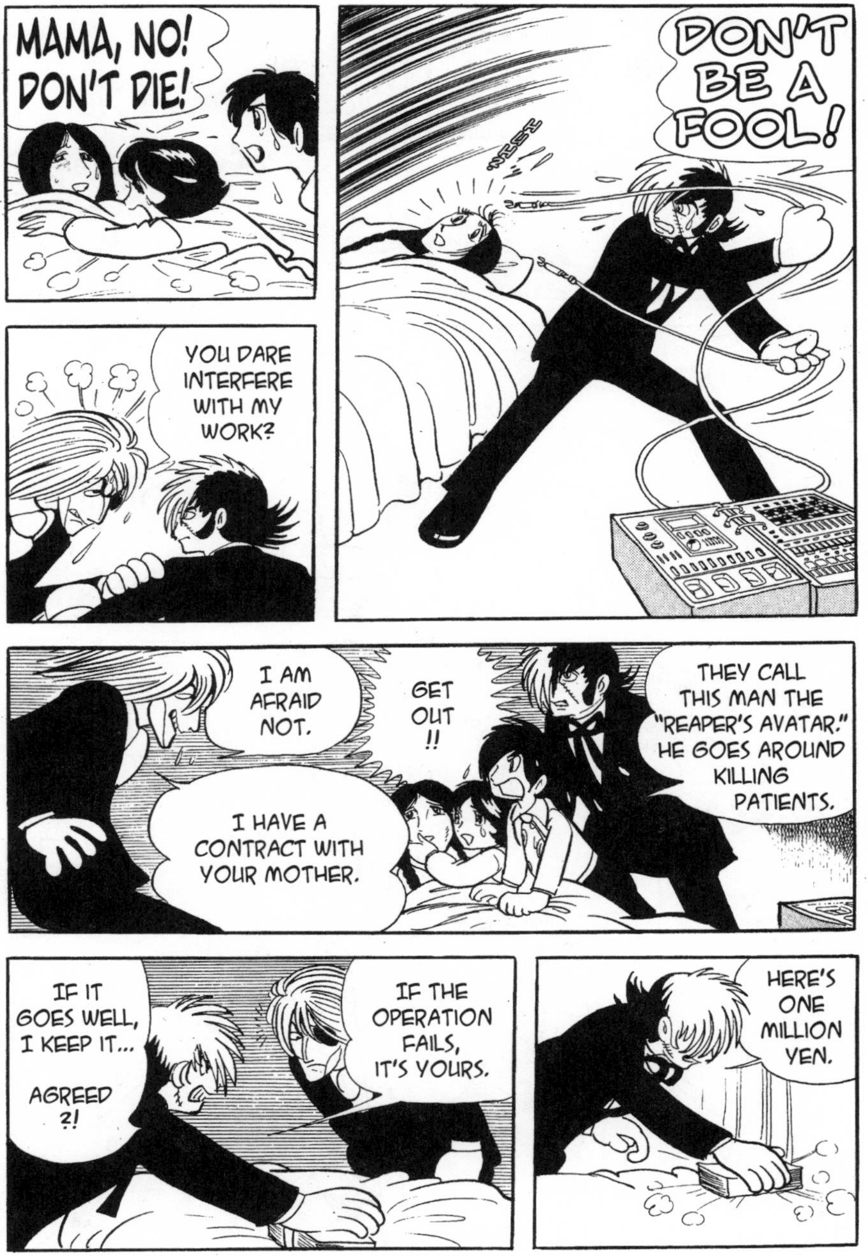
DON'T BE A FOOL!
MAMA, NO! DON'T DIE!
YOU DARE INTERFERE WITH MY WORK?
THEY CALL THIS MAN THE "REAPER'S AVATAR." HE GOES AROUND KILLING PATIENTS.
GET OUT !!
I AM AFRAID NOT.
I HAVE A CONTRACT WITH YOUR MOTHER.
HERE'S ONE MILLION YEN.
IF THE OPERATION FAILS, IT'S YOURS.
IF IT GOES WELL, I KEEP IT...
AGREED ?!

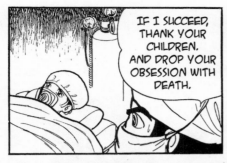

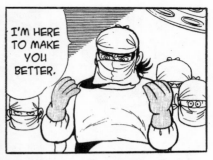

I'M HERE TO MAKE YOU BETTER.
IF I SUCCEED, THANK YOUR CHILDREN. AND DROP YOUR OBSESSION WITH DEATH.
WE'LL EXAMINE THE 3RD CERVICAL VERTEBRA, REPAIR THE SPINAL CHORD AND NERVE ROOTS
AND SEVER THE ARC OF THE 6TH CERVICAL AND 8TH DORSAL VERTEBRA.
BE CARE-FUL!
NOT TO WORRY.

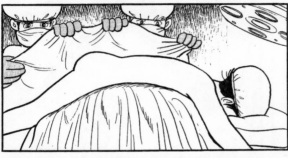

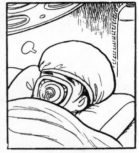

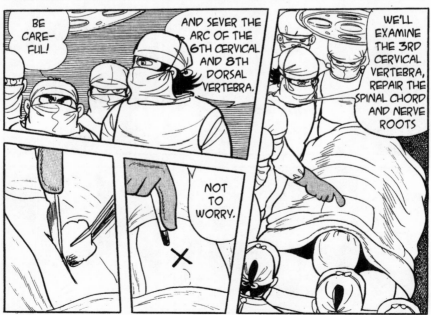

LUER FOR-CEPS!
WATCH OUT NOW...!
WILL YOU SHUT UP ?

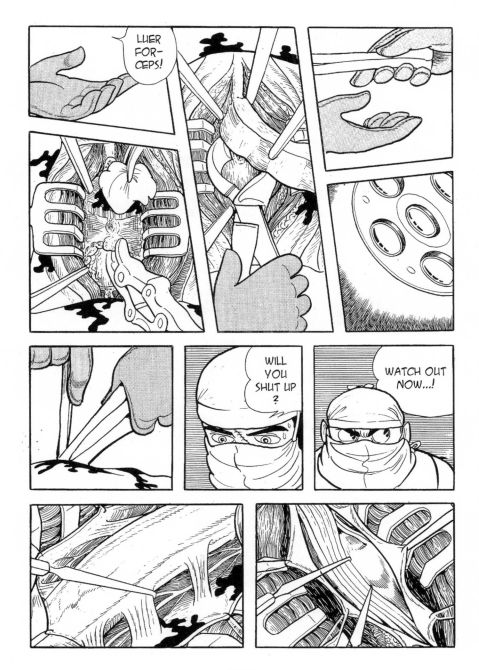

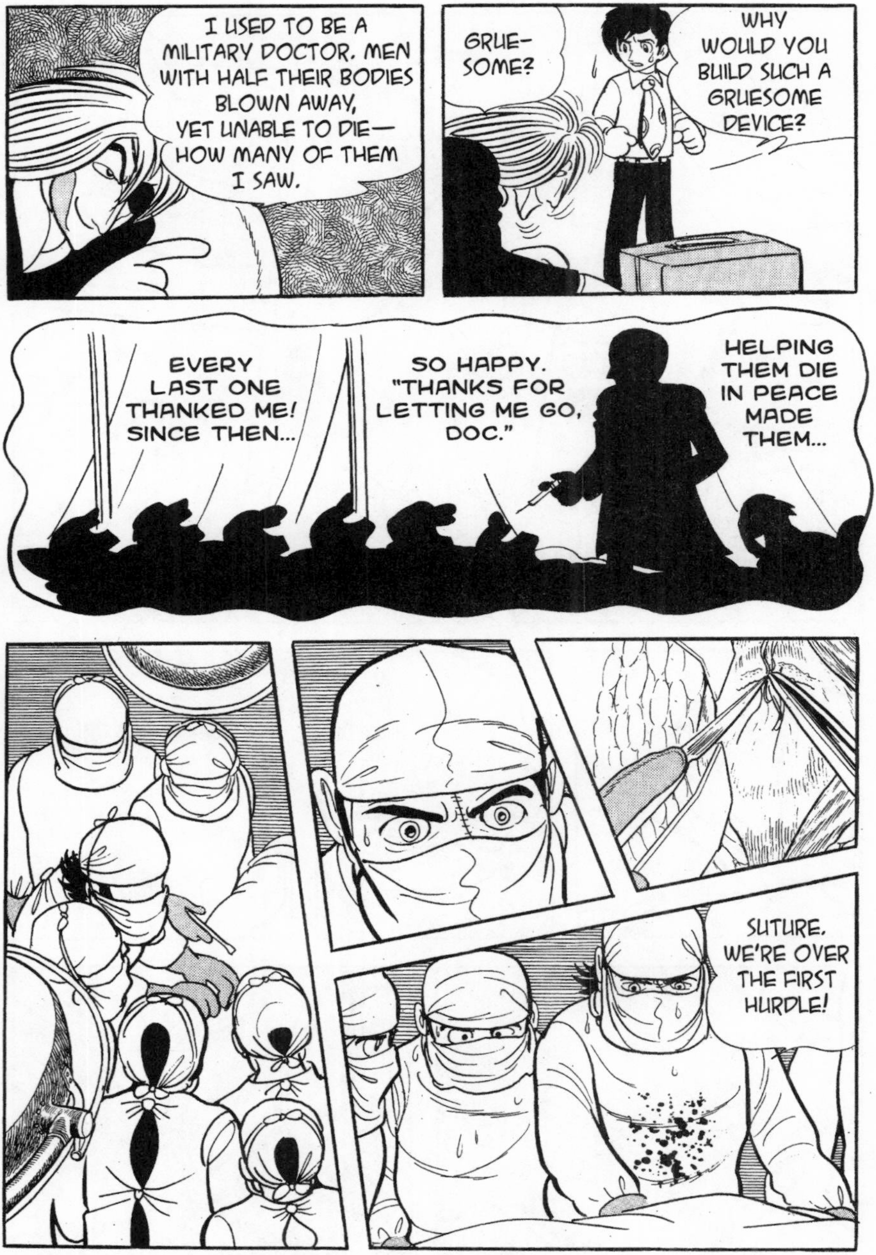
WHY WOULD YOU BUILD SUCH A GRUESOME DEVICE?
GRUE-SOME?
I USED TO BE A MILITARY DOCTOR. MEN WITH HALF THEIR BODIES BLOWN AWAY, YET UNABLE TO DIE— HOW MANY OF THEM I SAW.
HELPING THEM DIE IN PEACE MADE THEM...
SO HAPPY. "THANKS FOR LETTING ME GO, DOC."
EVERY LAST ONE THANKED ME! SINCE THEN...
SUTURE. WE'RE OVER THE FIRST HURDLE!

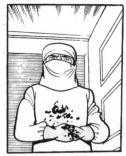

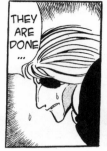

PLEASE, GOD... SAVE MY MOTHER. MAKE HER WELL.
GOD WON'T SAVE HER IF IT'S NOT MEANT TO BE.
THEY ARE DONE ...
GRIN
ニヤ
IS SHE GOING TO BE OKAY?
WHEN THE CAST COMES OFF, SHE'LL NEED TO EXERCISE.
DR. BLACK JACK !!
YOU DON'T BELONG HERE, KIRIKO. HIT THE ROAD.
I CERTAINLY DON'T ENJOY SOB-FESTS, TRUE.
BYE NOW.
BROTHER !!
IT WORKED! HE DID IT! HOORAY!

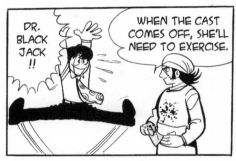

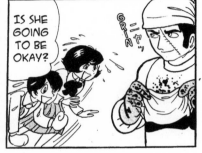

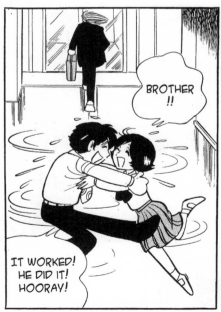

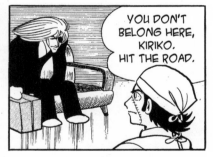

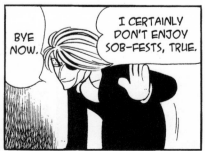

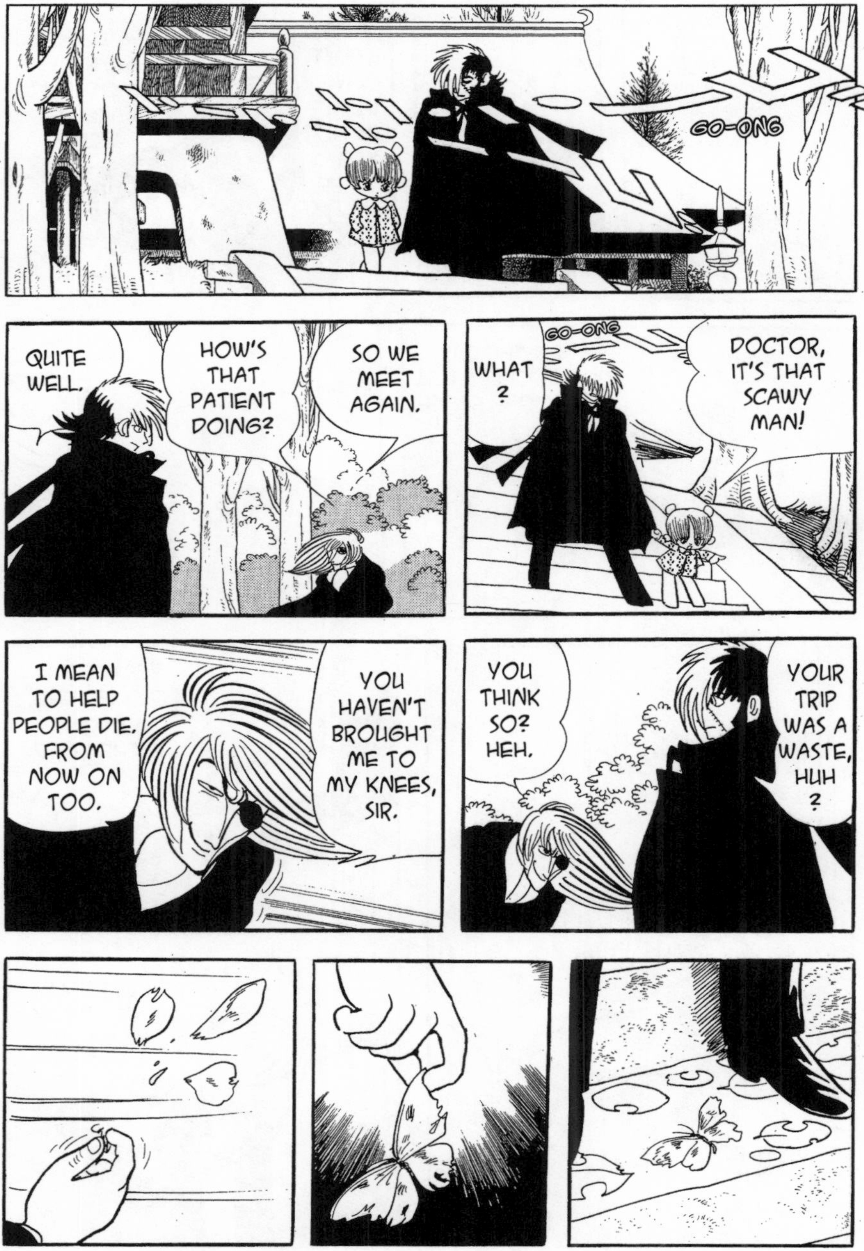
GO-ONG
GO-ONG
DOCTOR, IT'S THAT SCAWY MAN!
WHAT?
SO WE MEET AGAIN.
HOW'S THAT PATIENT DOING?
QUITE WELL.
YOUR TRIP WAS A WASTE, HUH?
YOU THINK SO? HEH.
YOU HAVEN'T BROUGHT ME TO MY KNEES, SIR.
I MEAN TO HELP PEOPLE DIE, FROM NOW ON TOO.

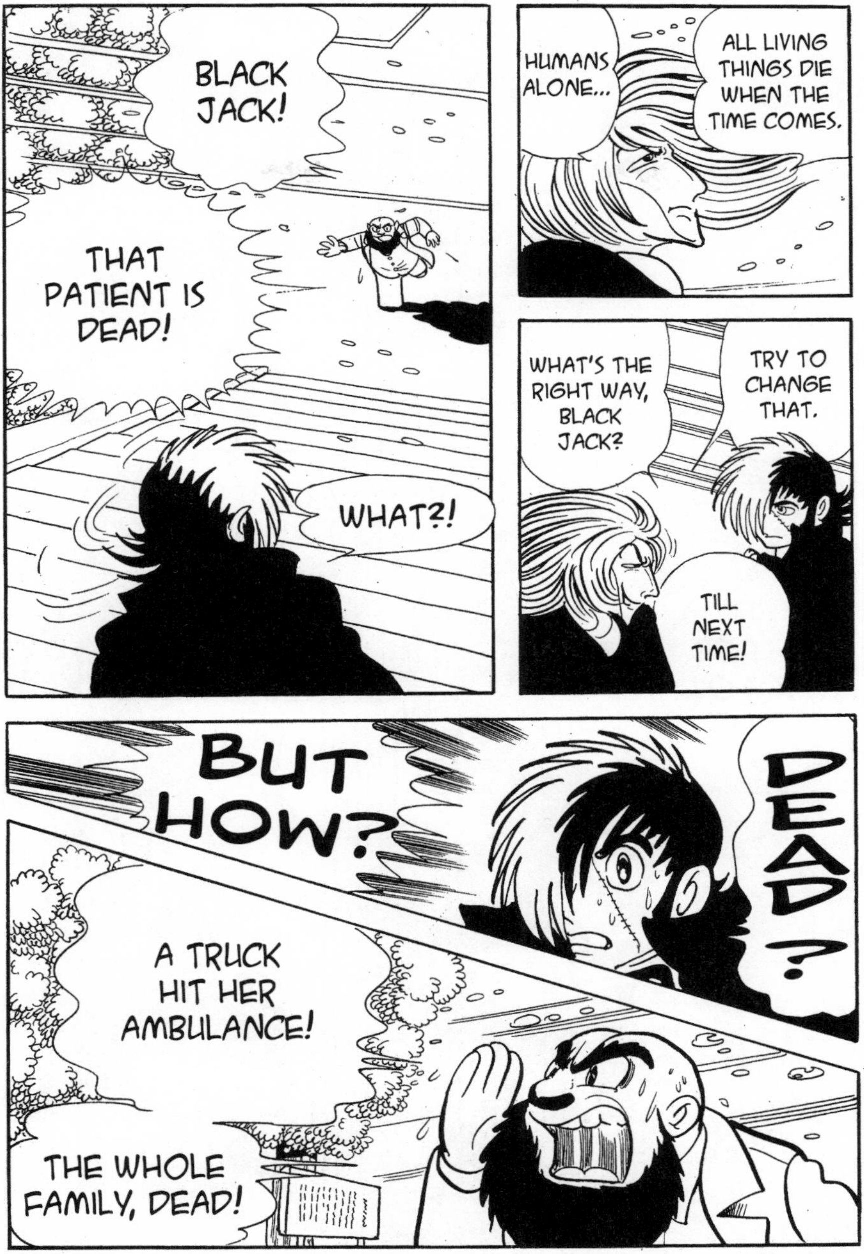
ALL LIVING THINGS DIE WHEN THE TIME COMES.
HUMANS ALONE...
TRY TO CHANGE THAT.
WHAT'S THE RIGHT WAY, BLACK JACK?
TILL NEXT TIME!
BLACK JACK!
THAT PATIENT IS DEAD!
WHAT?!
DEAD?
BUT HOW?
A TRUCK HIT HER AMBULANCE!
THE WHOLE FAMILY, DEAD!

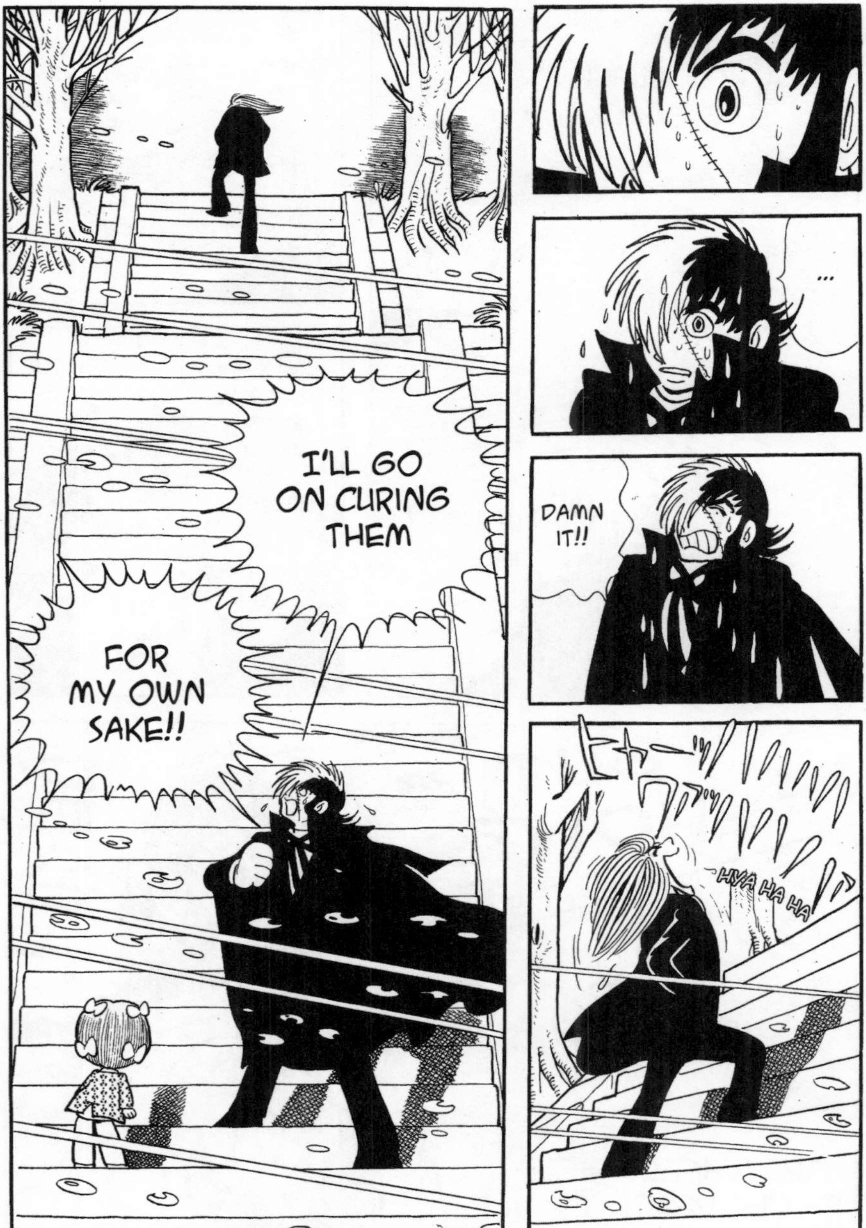
...
DAMN IT!!
ヒャーッ
HYA HA HA
I'LL GO ON CURING THEM
FOR MY OWN SAKE!!

THE RESIDENTS

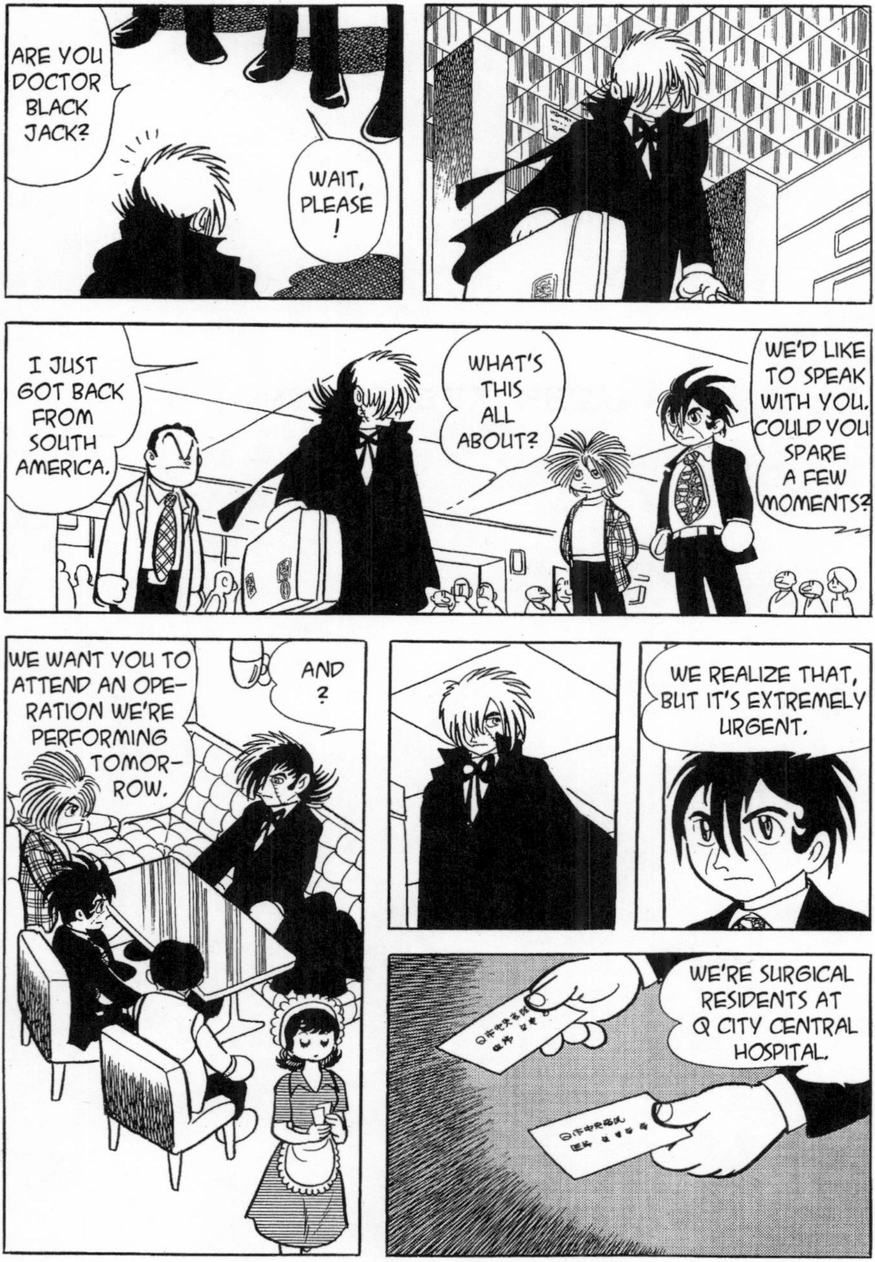
WAIT, PLEASE!
ARE YOU DOCTOR BLACK JACK?
WE'D LIKE TO SPEAK WITH YOU. COULD YOU SPARE A FEW MOMENTS?
WHAT'S THIS ALL ABOUT?
I JUST GOT BACK FROM SOUTH AMERICA.
WE REALIZE THAT, BUT IT'S EXTREMELY URGENT.
WE'RE SURGICAL RESIDENTS AT Q CITY CENTRAL HOSPITAL.
AND ?
WE WANT YOU TO ATTEND AN OPERATION WE'RE PERFORMING TOMORROW.

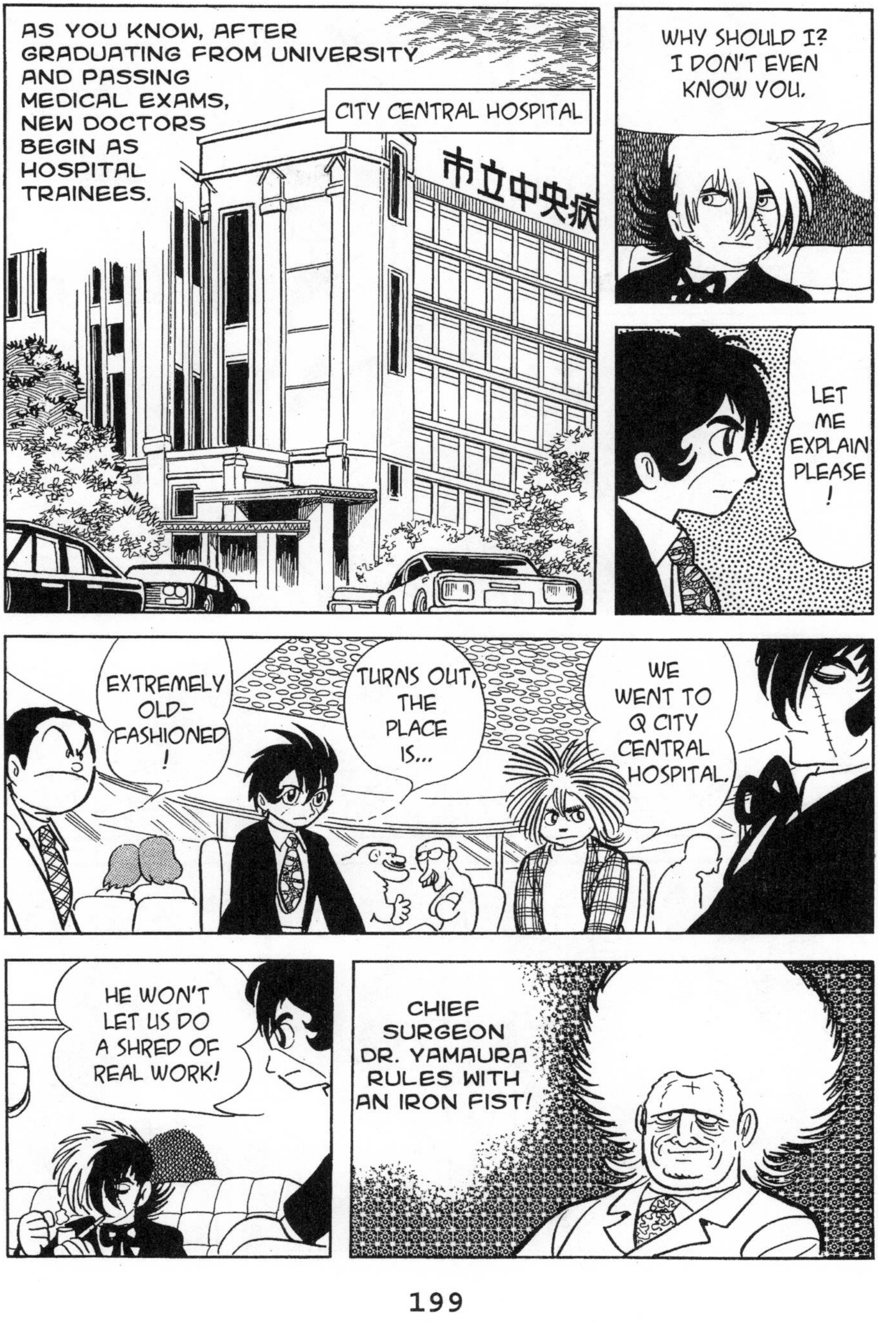
WHY SHOULD I? I DON'T EVEN KNOW YOU.
LET ME EXPLAIN PLEASE!
AS YOU KNOW, AFTER GRADUATING FROM UNIVERSITY AND PASSING MEDICAL EXAMS, NEW DOCTORS BEGIN AS HOSPITAL TRAINEES.
CITY CENTRAL HOSPITAL
WE WENT TO Q CITY CENTRAL HOSPITAL.
TURNS OUT, THE PLACE IS...
EXTREMELY OLD-FASHIONED!
CHIEF SURGEON DR. YAMAURA RULES WITH AN IRON FIST!
HE WON'T LET US DO A SHRED OF REAL WORK!

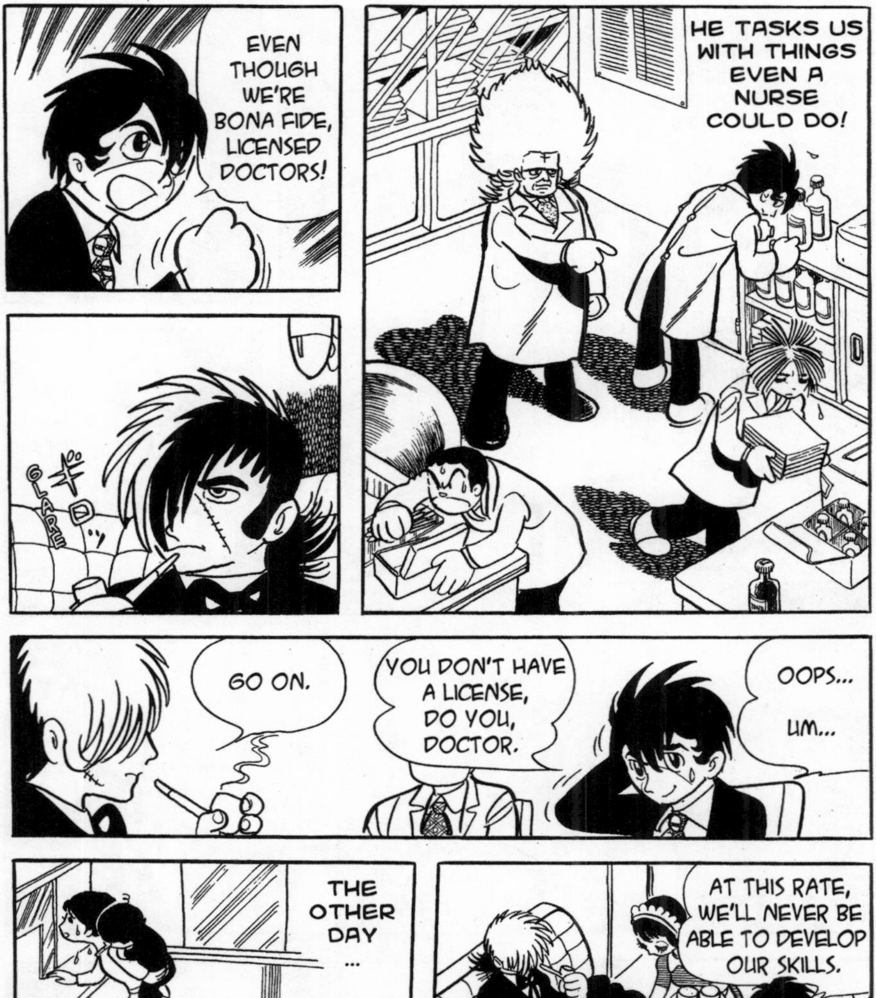
HE TASKS US WITH THINGS EVEN A NURSE COULD DO!
EVEN THOUGH WE'RE BONA FIDE, LICENSED DOCTORS!
GLARE
OOPS... UM...
YOU DON'T HAVE A LICENSE, DO YOU, DOCTOR.
GO ON.
AT THIS RATE, WE'LL NEVER BE ABLE TO DEVELOP OUR SKILLS.
CHIEF YAMAURA IS SO DENSE AND STUBBORN!
THE OTHER DAY ...

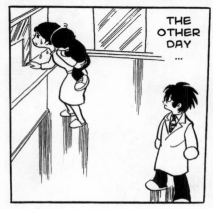

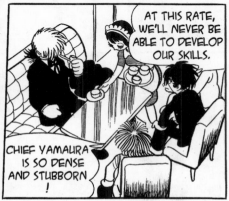

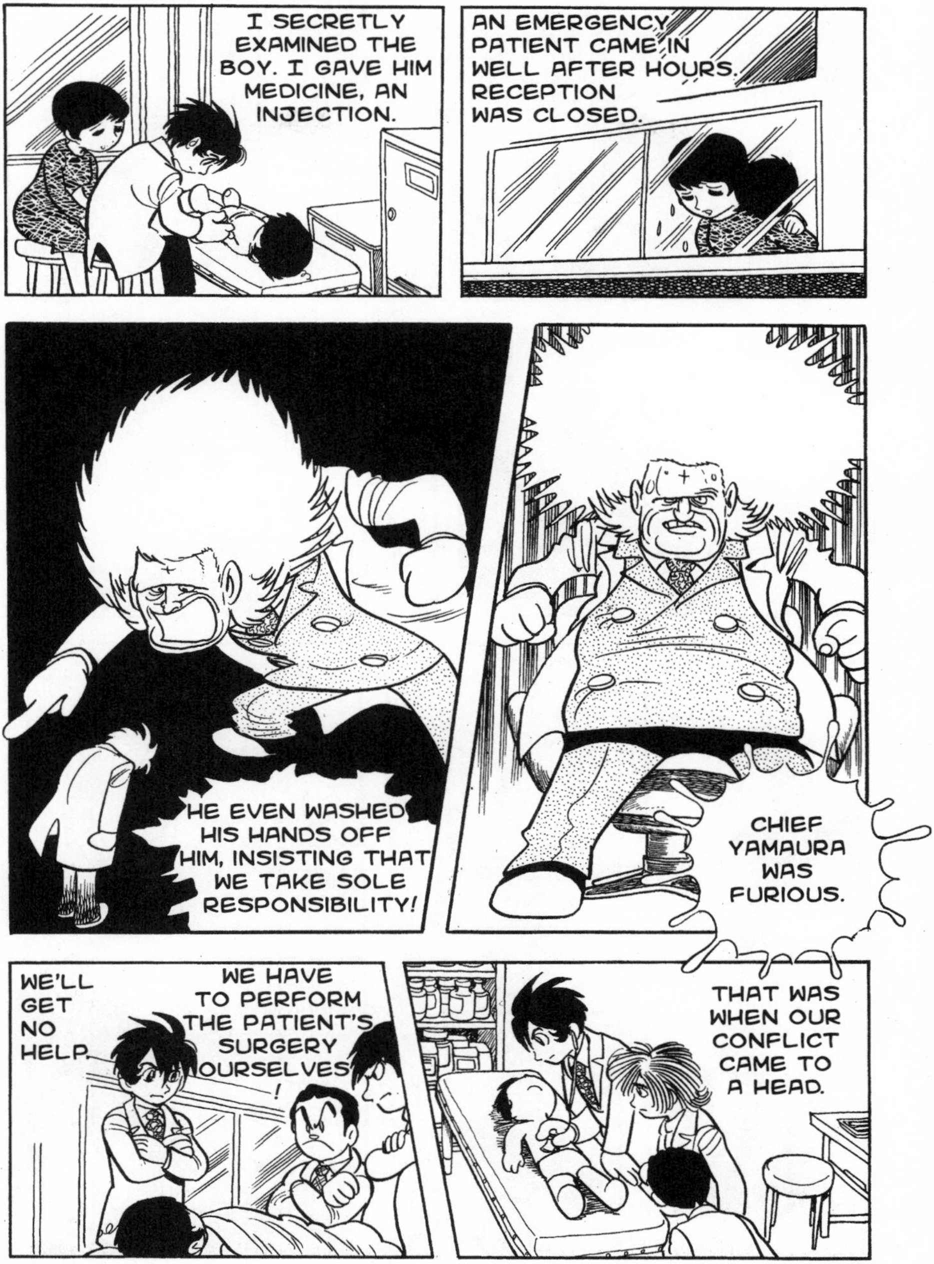
AN EMERGENCY PATIENT CAME IN WELL AFTER HOURS. RECEPTION WAS CLOSED.
I SECRETLY EXAMINED THE BOY. I GAVE HIM MEDICINE, AN INJECTION.
CHIEF YAMAURA WAS FURIOUS.
HE EVEN WASHED HIS HANDS OFF HIM, INSISTING THAT WE TAKE SOLE RESPONSIBILITY!
THAT WAS WHEN OUR CONFLICT CAME TO A HEAD.
WE HAVE TO PERFORM THE PATIENT'S SURGERY OURSELVES!
WE'LL GET NO HELP.

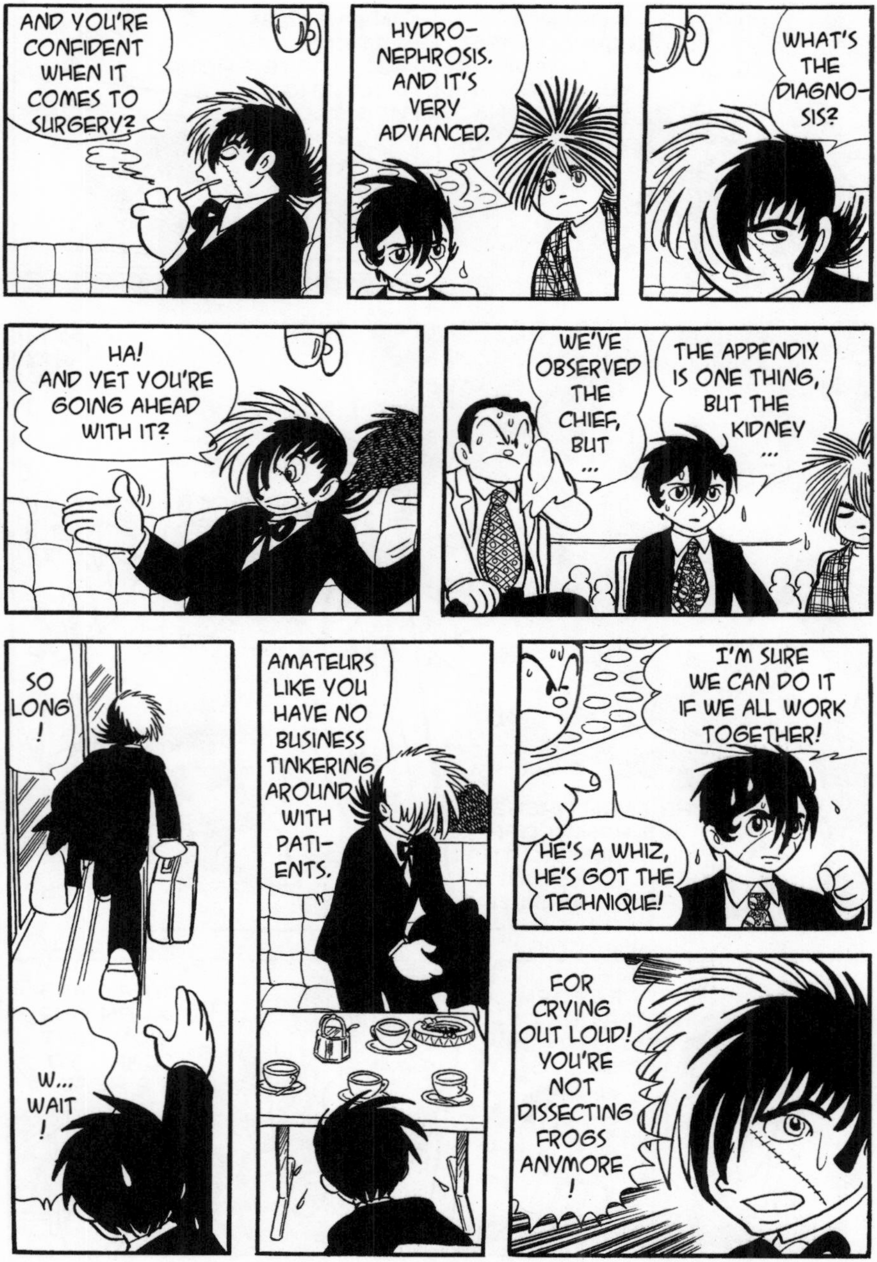
WHAT'S THE DIAGNOSIS?
HYDRONEPHROSIS. AND IT'S VERY ADVANCED.
AND YOU'RE CONFIDENT WHEN IT COMES TO SURGERY?
THE APPENDIX IS ONE THING, BUT THE KIDNEY ...
WE'VE OBSERVED THE CHIEF, BUT ...
HA! AND YET YOU'RE GOING AHEAD WITH IT?
I'M SURE WE CAN DO IT IF WE ALL WORK TOGETHER!
HE'S A WHIZ, HE'S GOT THE TECHNIQUE!
FOR CRYING OUT LOUD! YOU'RE NOT DISSECTING FROGS ANYMORE!
AMATEURS LIKE YOU HAVE NO BUSINESS TINKERING AROUND WITH PATIENTS.
SO LONG!
W... WAIT!

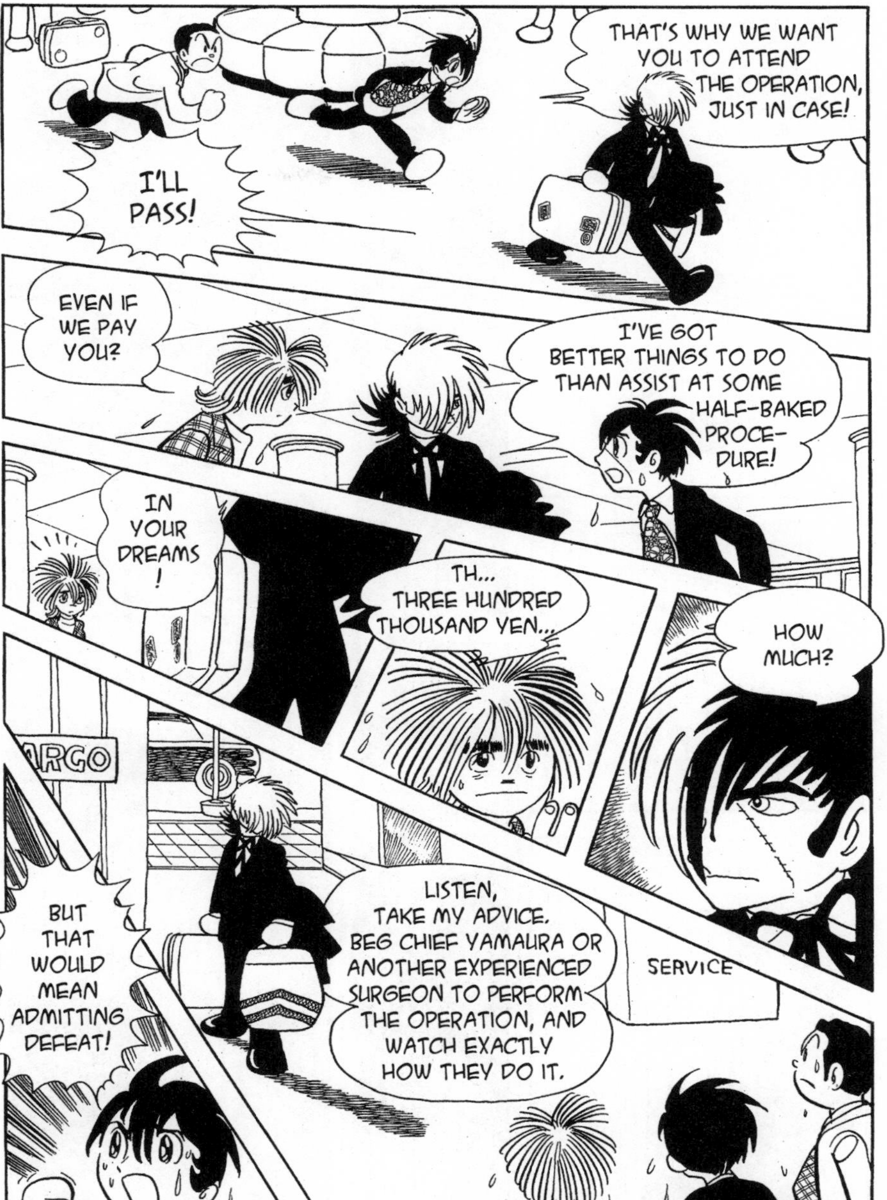
THAT'S WHY WE WANT YOU TO ATTEND THE OPERATION, JUST IN CASE!
I'LL PASS!
I'VE GOT BETTER THINGS TO DO THAN ASSIST AT SOME HALF-BAKED PROCE-DURE!
EVEN IF WE PAY YOU?
HOW MUCH?
TH... THREE HUNDRED THOUSAND YEN...
IN YOUR DREAMS!
SERVICE
ARGO
LISTEN, TAKE MY ADVICE. BEG CHIEF YAMAURA OR ANOTHER EXPERIENCED SURGEON TO PERFORM THE OPERATION, AND WATCH EXACTLY HOW THEY DO IT.
BUT THAT WOULD MEAN ADMITTING DEFEAT!

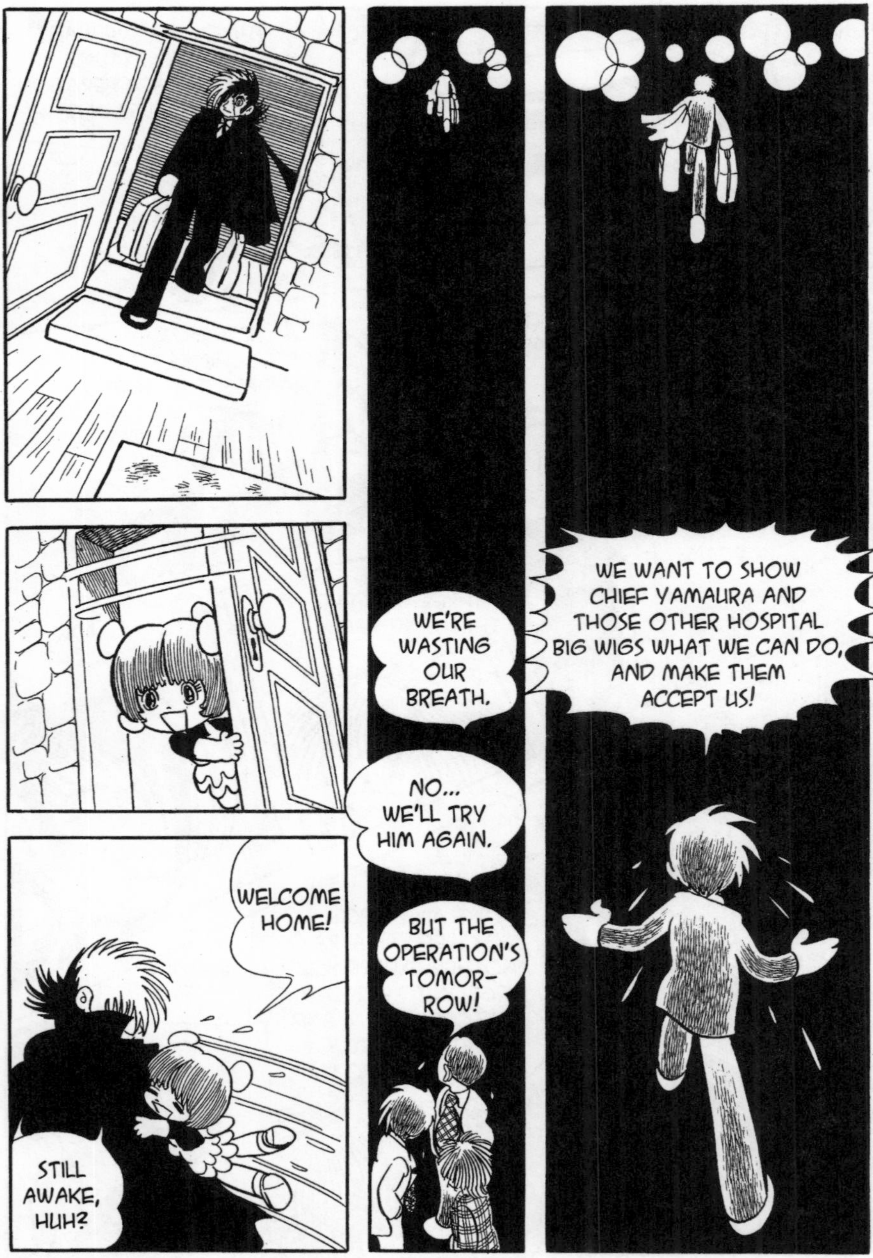
WE WANT TO SHOW CHIEF YAMAURA AND THOSE OTHER HOSPITAL BIG WIGS WHAT WE CAN DO, AND MAKE THEM ACCEPT US!
WE'RE WASTING OUR BREATH.
NO... WE'LL TRY HIM AGAIN.
BUT THE OPERATION'S TOMOR-ROW!
WELCOME HOME!
STILL AWAKE, HUH?

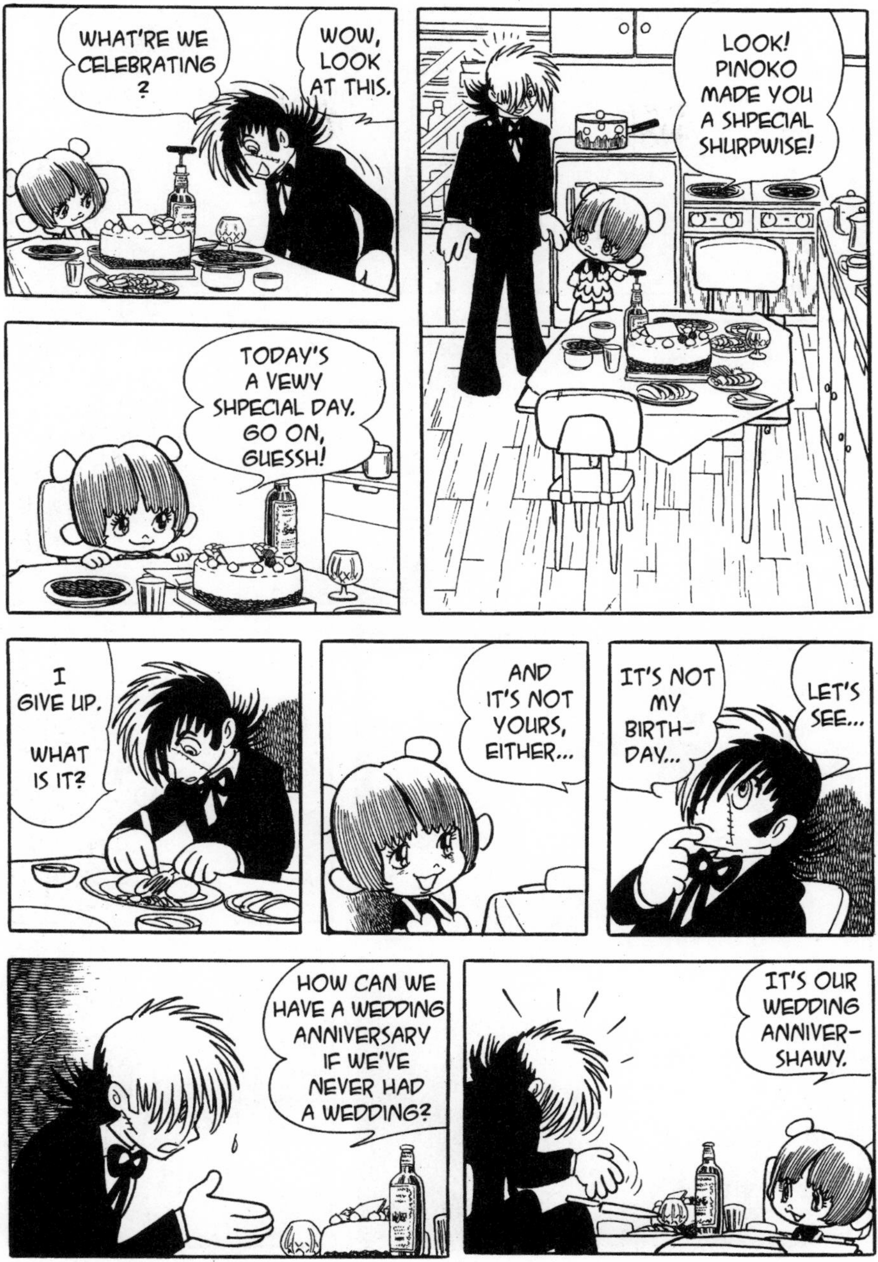
LOOK! PINOKO MADE YOU A SHPECIAL SHURPWISE!
WOW, LOOK AT THIS.
WHAT'RE WE CELEBRATING?
TODAY'S A VEWY SHPECIAL DAY. GO ON, GUESSH!
LET'S SEE...
IT'S NOT MY BIRTH-DAY...
AND IT'S NOT YOURS, EITHER...
I GIVE UP.
WHAT IS IT?
IT'S OUR WEDDING ANNIVER-SHAWY.
HOW CAN WE HAVE A WEDDING ANNIVERSARY IF WE'VE NEVER HAD A WEDDING?

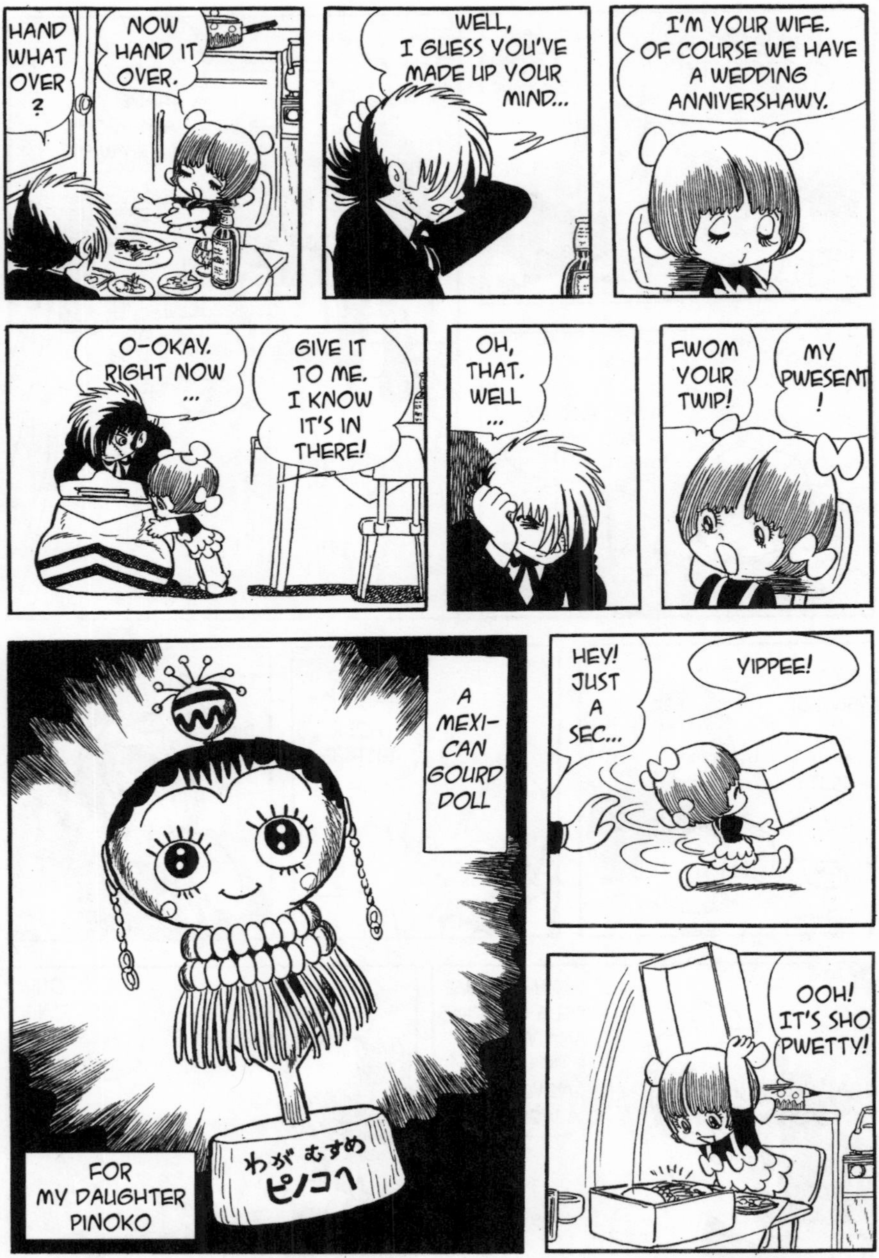
I'M YOUR WIFE. OF COURSE WE HAVE A WEDDING ANNIVERSHAWY.
WELL, I GUESS YOU'VE MADE UP YOUR MIND...
NOW HAND IT OVER.
HAND WHAT OVER ?
MY PWESENT !
FWOM YOUR TWIP!
OH, THAT. WELL ...
GIVE IT TO ME. I KNOW IT'S IN THERE!
O-OKAY. RIGHT NOW ...
YIPPEE!
HEY! JUST A SEC...
OOH! IT'S SHO PWETTY!
A MEXI-CAN GOURD DOLL
わが むすめ
ピノコへ
FOR MY DAUGHTER PINOKO

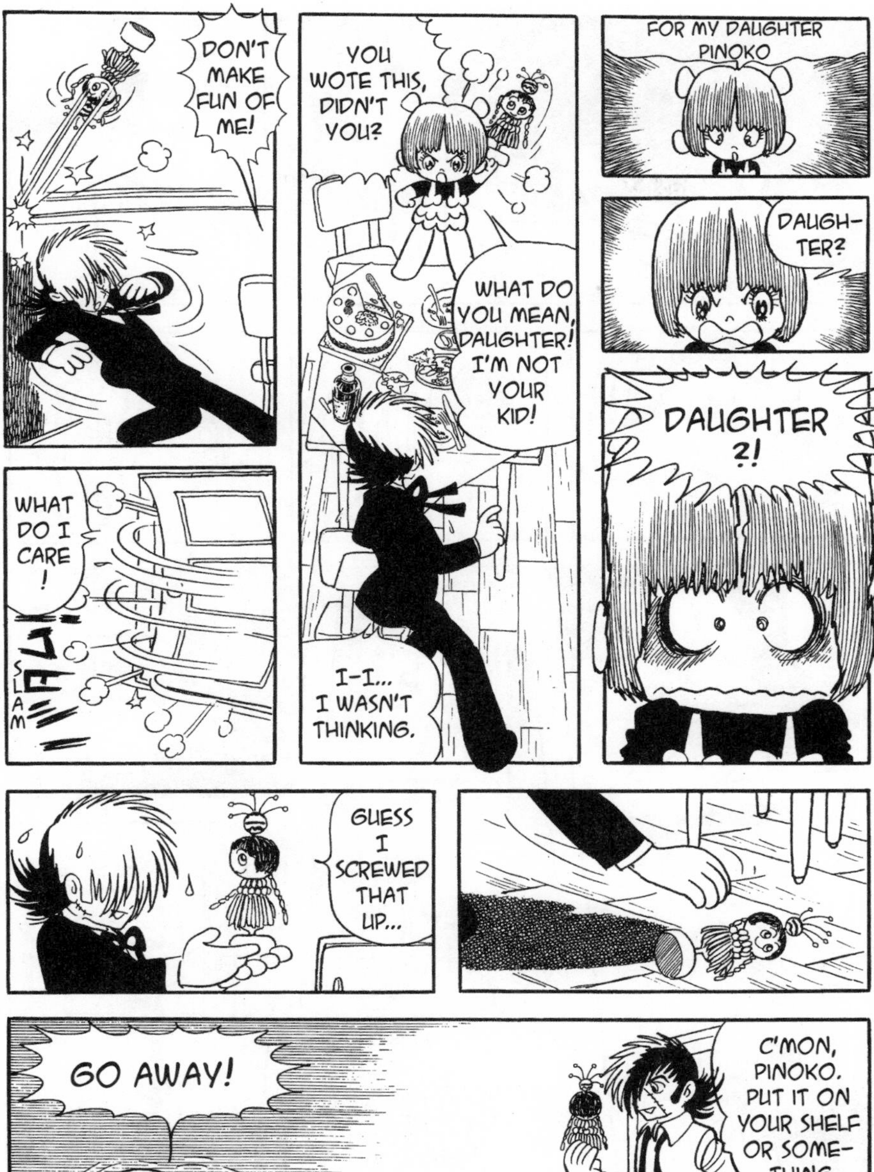
FOR MY DAUGHTER PINOKO
DAUGHTER?
DAUGHTER ?!
YOU WOTE THIS, DIDN'T YOU?
WHAT DO YOU MEAN, DAUGHTER! I'M NOT YOUR KID!
I-I... I WASN'T THINKING.
DON'T MAKE FUN OF ME!
WHAT DO I CARE!
SLAM
GUESS I SCREWED THAT UP...
C'MON, PINOKO. PUT IT ON YOUR SHELF OR SOME-THING.
GO AWAY!

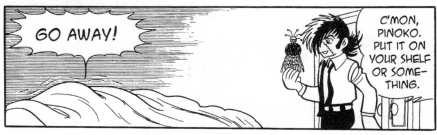

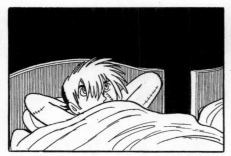

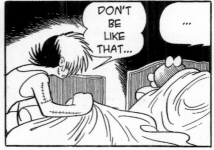

DON'T BE LIKE THAT...

...

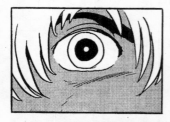

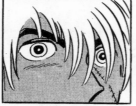

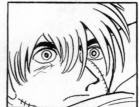

DOCTOR?

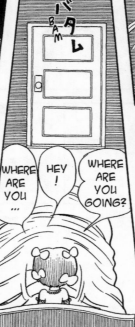

BAM

WHERE ARE YOU...

HEY!

WHERE ARE YOU GOING?

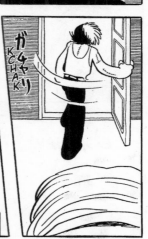

K'CHAK

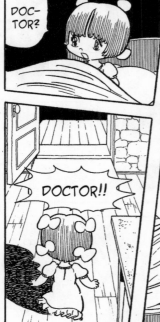

DOCTOR!!

208

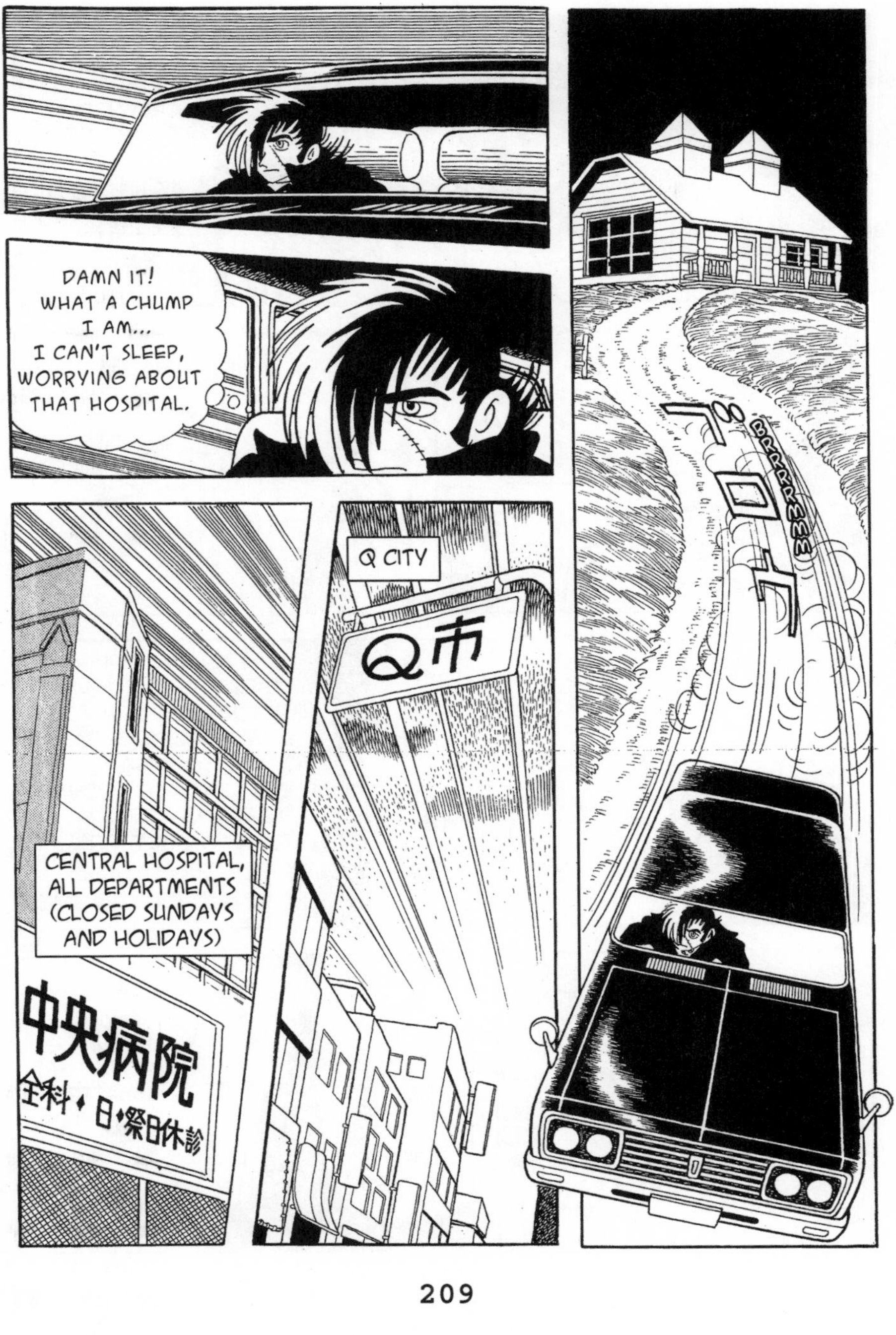

BRRRRMMM
DAMN IT! WHAT A CHUMP I AM... I CAN'T SLEEP, WORRYING ABOUT THAT HOSPITAL.
Q CITY
Q市
CENTRAL HOSPITAL, ALL DEPARTMENTS (CLOSED SUNDAYS AND HOLIDAYS)
中央病院
全科・日・祭日休診

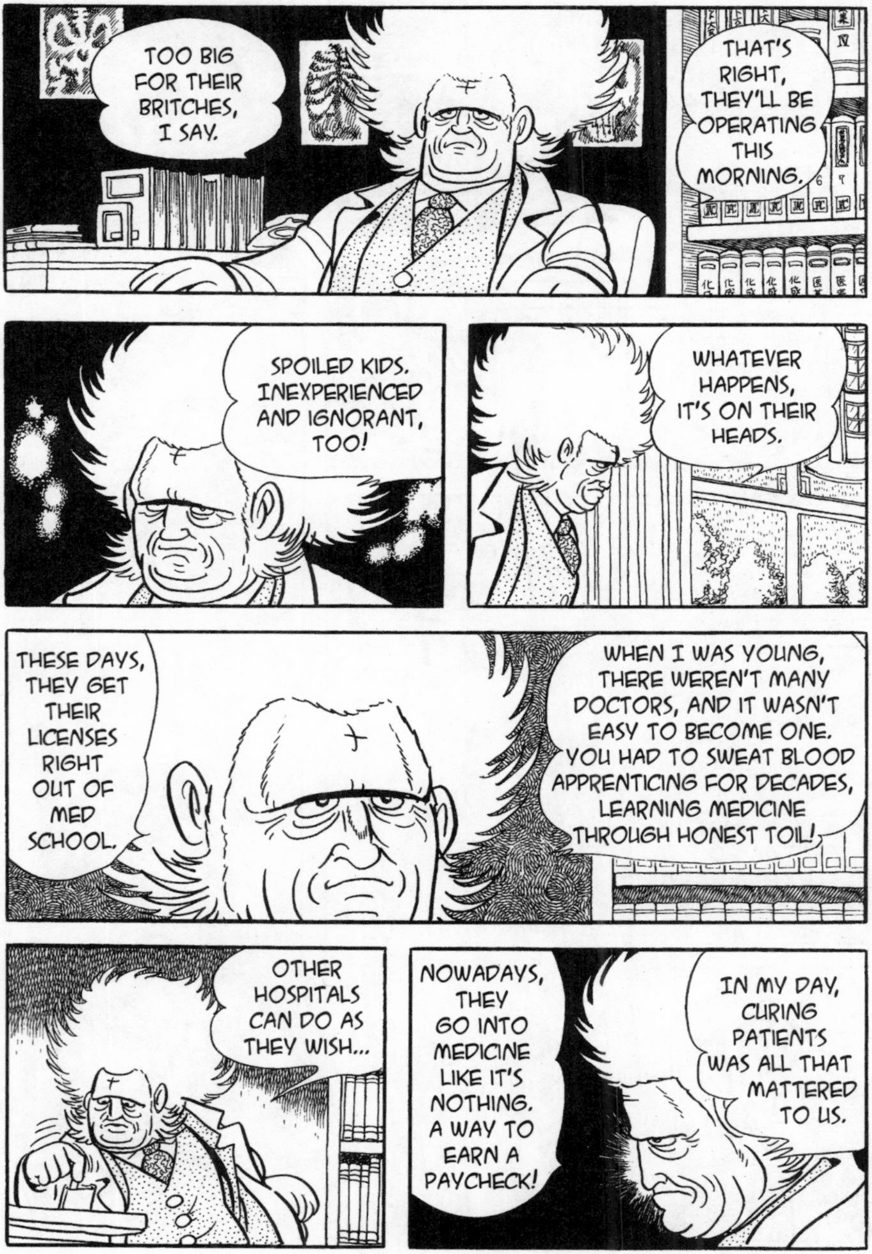
THAT'S RIGHT, THEY'LL BE OPERATING THIS MORNING.
TOO BIG FOR THEIR BRITCHES, I SAY.
WHATEVER HAPPENS, IT'S ON THEIR HEADS.
SPOILED KIDS. INEXPERIENCED AND IGNORANT, TOO!
WHEN I WAS YOUNG, THERE WEREN'T MANY DOCTORS, AND IT WASN'T EASY TO BECOME ONE. YOU HAD TO SWEAT BLOOD APPRENTICING FOR DECADES, LEARNING MEDICINE THROUGH HONEST TOIL!
THESE DAYS, THEY GET THEIR LICENSES RIGHT OUT OF MED SCHOOL.
IN MY DAY, CURING PATIENTS WAS ALL THAT MATTERED TO US.
NOWADAYS, THEY GO INTO MEDICINE LIKE IT'S NOTHING. A WAY TO EARN A PAYCHECK!
OTHER HOSPITALS CAN DO AS THEY WISH...

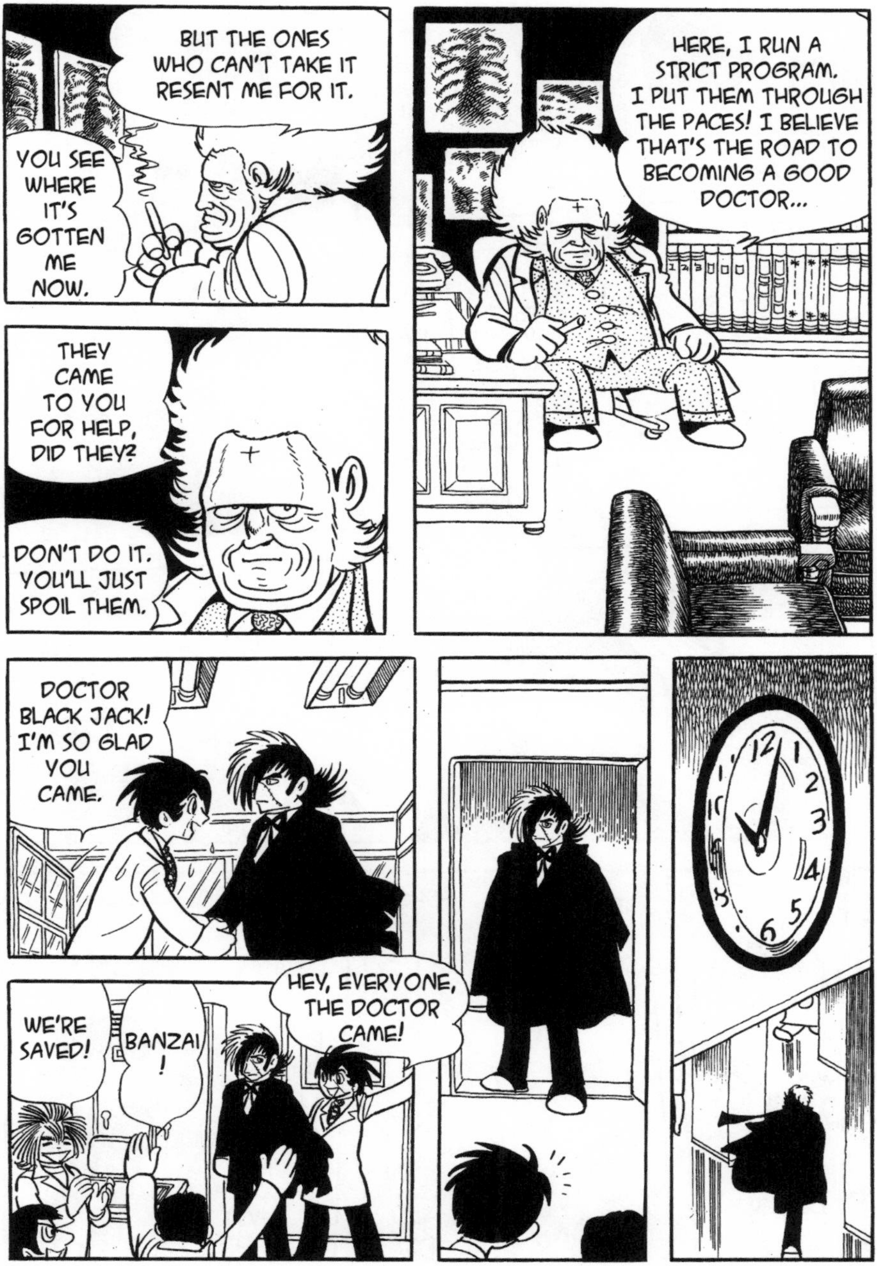
HERE, I RUN A STRICT PROGRAM. I PUT THEM THROUGH THE PACES! I BELIEVE THAT'S THE ROAD TO BECOMING A GOOD DOCTOR...
BUT THE ONES WHO CAN'T TAKE IT RESENT ME FOR IT.
YOU SEE WHERE IT'S GOTTEN ME NOW.
THEY CAME TO YOU FOR HELP, DID THEY?
DON'T DO IT. YOU'LL JUST SPOIL THEM.
DOCTOR BLACK JACK! I'M SO GLAD YOU CAME.
HEY, EVERYONE, THE DOCTOR CAME!
BANZAI!
WE'RE SAVED!

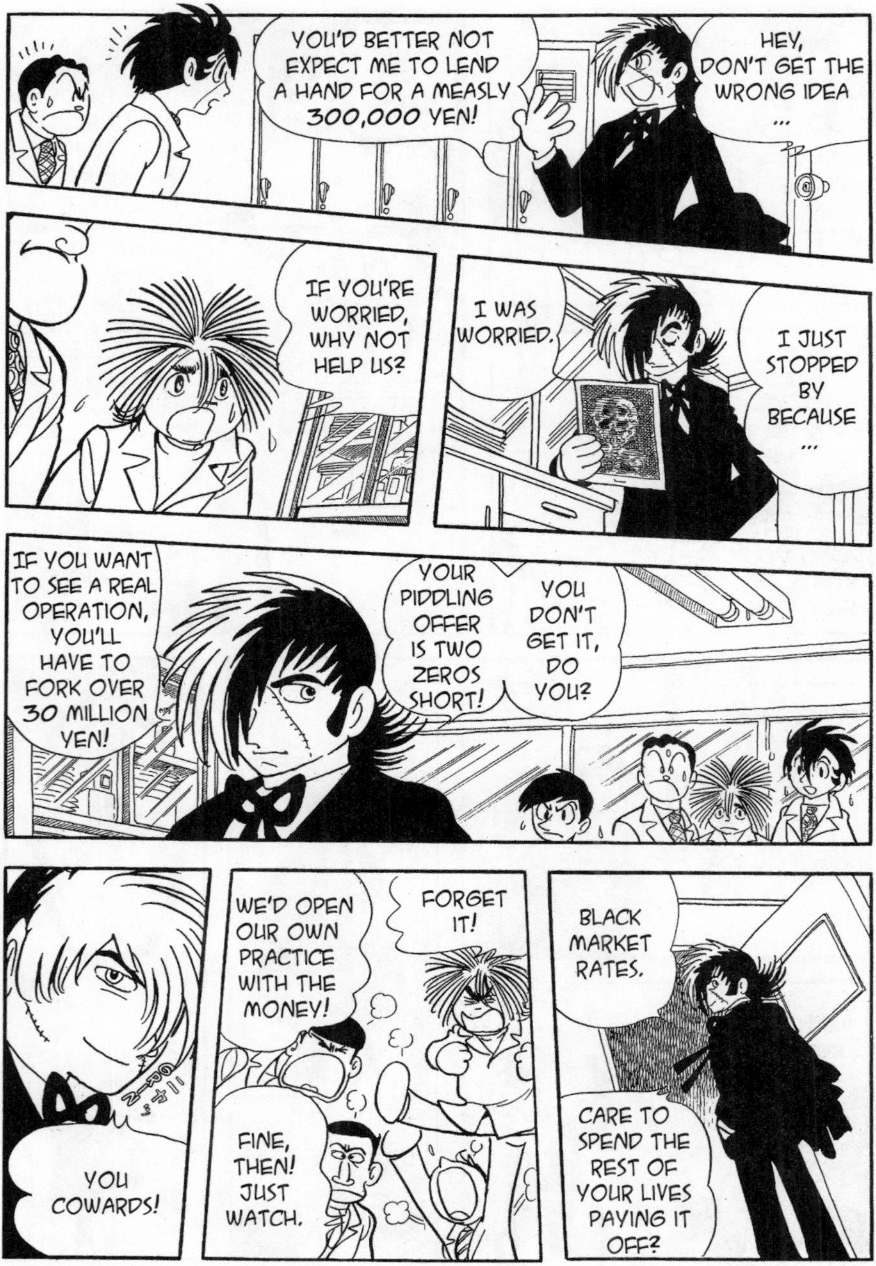
HEY, DON'T GET THE WRONG IDEA ...
YOU'D BETTER NOT EXPECT ME TO LEND A HAND FOR A MEASLY 300,000 YEN!
I JUST STOPPED BY BECAUSE ...
I WAS WORRIED.
IF YOU'RE WORRIED, WHY NOT HELP US?
YOU DON'T GET IT, DO YOU?
YOUR PIDDLING OFFER IS TWO ZEROS SHORT!
IF YOU WANT TO SEE A REAL OPERATION, YOU'LL HAVE TO FORK OVER 30 MILLION YEN!
BLACK MARKET RATES.
CARE TO SPEND THE REST OF YOUR LIVES PAYING IT OFF?
FORGET IT!
WE'D OPEN OUR OWN PRACTICE WITH THE MONEY!
FINE, THEN! JUST WATCH.
YOU COWARDS!

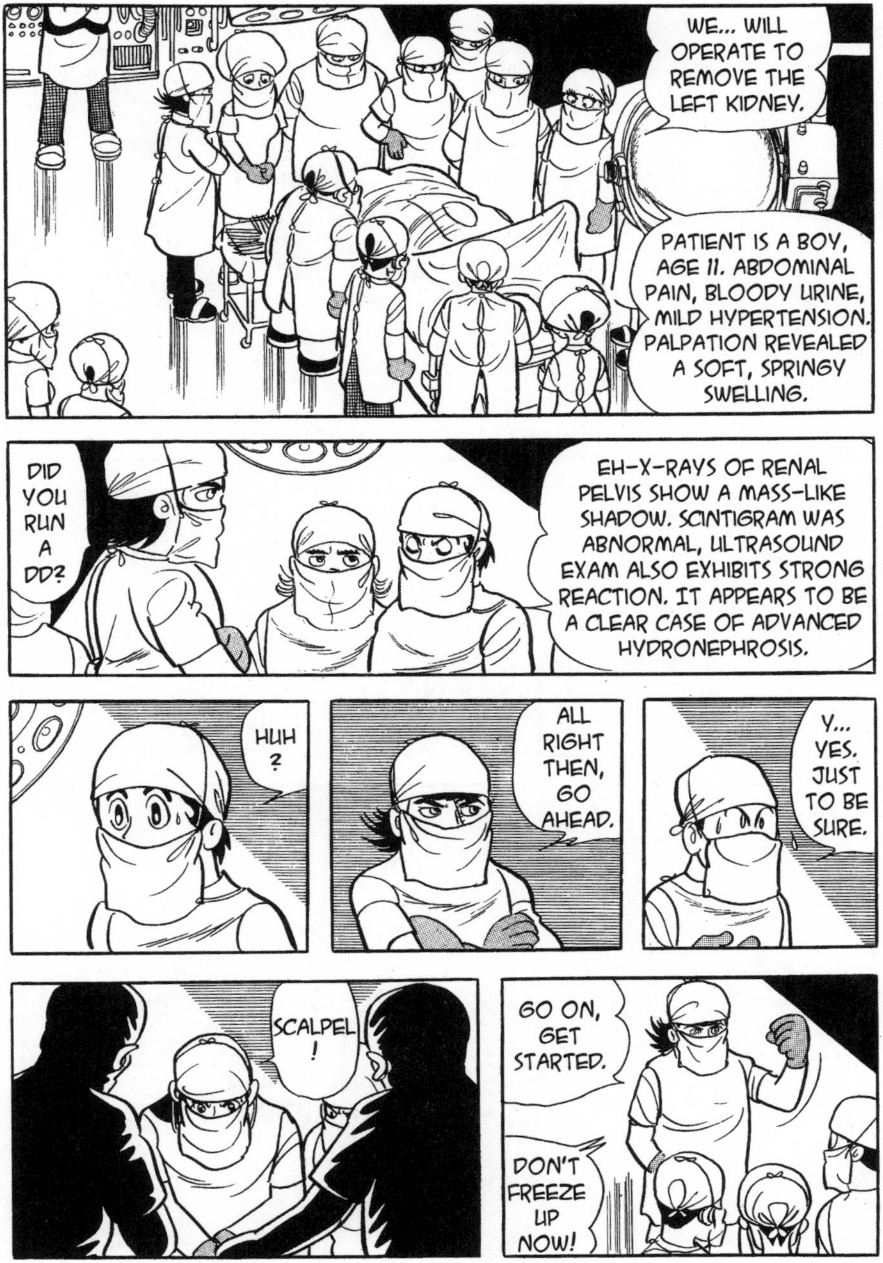
WE... WILL OPERATE TO REMOVE THE LEFT KIDNEY.
PATIENT IS A BOY, AGE 11. ABDOMINAL PAIN, BLOODY URINE, MILD HYPERTENSION. PALPATION REVEALED A SOFT, SPRINGY SWELLING.
EH–X–RAYS OF RENAL PELVIS SHOW A MASS-LIKE SHADOW. SCINTIGRAM WAS ABNORMAL, ULTRASOUND EXAM ALSO EXHIBITS STRONG REACTION. IT APPEARS TO BE A CLEAR CASE OF ADVANCED HYDRONEPHROSIS.
DID YOU RUN A DD?
Y... YES. JUST TO BE SURE.
ALL RIGHT THEN, GO AHEAD.
HUH?
GO ON, GET STARTED.
DON'T FREEZE UP NOW!
SCALPEL!

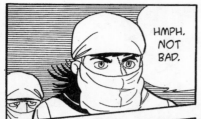

HMPH. NOT BAD.
THE KIDNEY ...
LIGA-TURE!
WAIT ...
THIS ISN'T HYDRO-NEPHROSIS!
IS IT A TUMOR?
WHAT IS THIS THING?
IT'S A WILMS' TUMOR.
A W-WILMS' TUMOR...?
THAT'S RIGHT! A FULL-BLOWN TUMOR!
LOOKS LIKE YOUR DIAGNOSIS WAS OFF THE MARK.

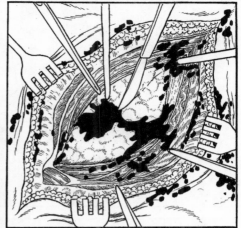

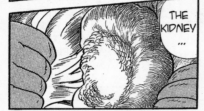

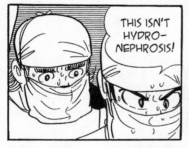

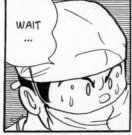

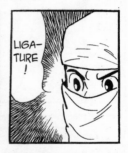

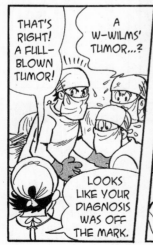

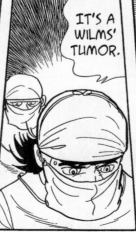

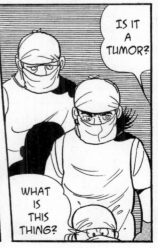

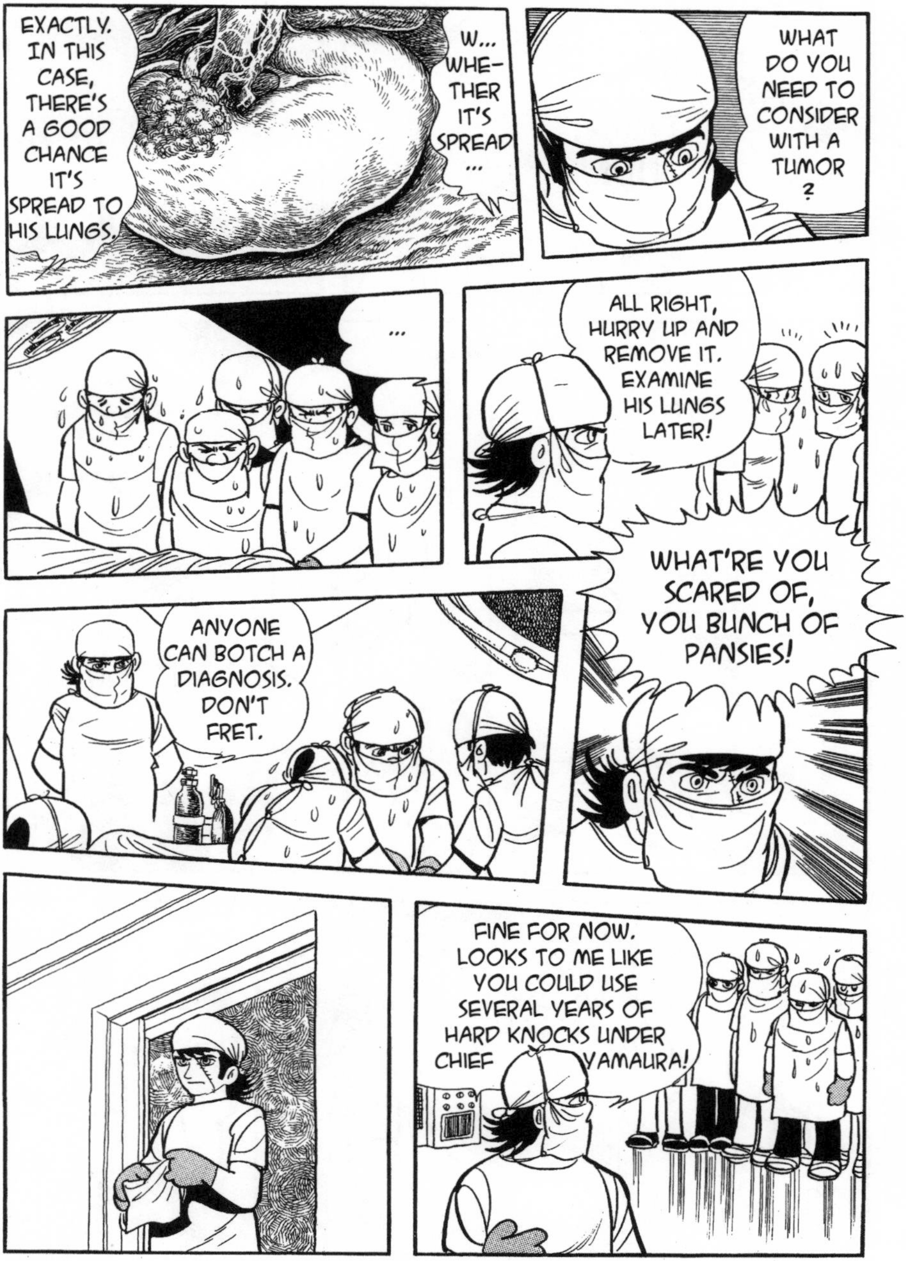
WHAT DO YOU NEED TO CONSIDER WITH A TUMOR?
W... WHE-THER IT'S SPREAD...
EXACTLY. IN THIS CASE, THERE'S A GOOD CHANCE IT'S SPREAD TO HIS LUNGS.
ALL RIGHT, HURRY UP AND REMOVE IT. EXAMINE HIS LUNGS LATER!
...
WHAT'RE YOU SCARED OF, YOU BUNCH OF PANSIES!
ANYONE CAN BOTCH A DIAGNOSIS. DON'T FRET.
FINE FOR NOW. LOOKS TO ME LIKE YOU COULD USE SEVERAL YEARS OF HARD KNOCKS UNDER CHIEF YAMAURA!

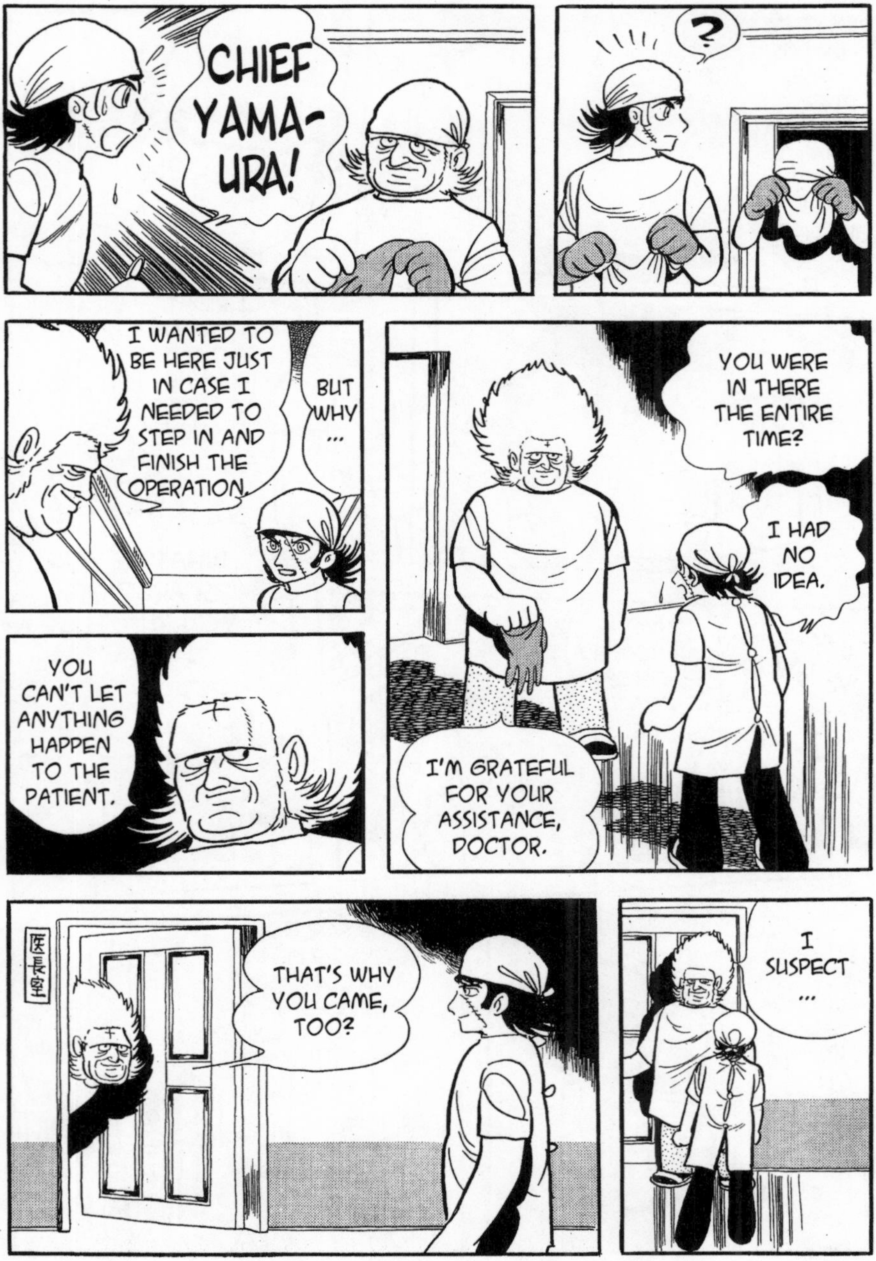
?
CHIEF YAMA-URA!
YOU WERE IN THERE THE ENTIRE TIME?
I HAD NO IDEA.
I'M GRATEFUL FOR YOUR ASSISTANCE, DOCTOR.
BUT WHY ...
I WANTED TO BE HERE JUST IN CASE I NEEDED TO STEP IN AND FINISH THE OPERATION.
YOU CAN'T LET ANYTHING HAPPEN TO THE PATIENT.
I SUSPECT ...
THAT'S WHY YOU CAME, TOO?
医長室

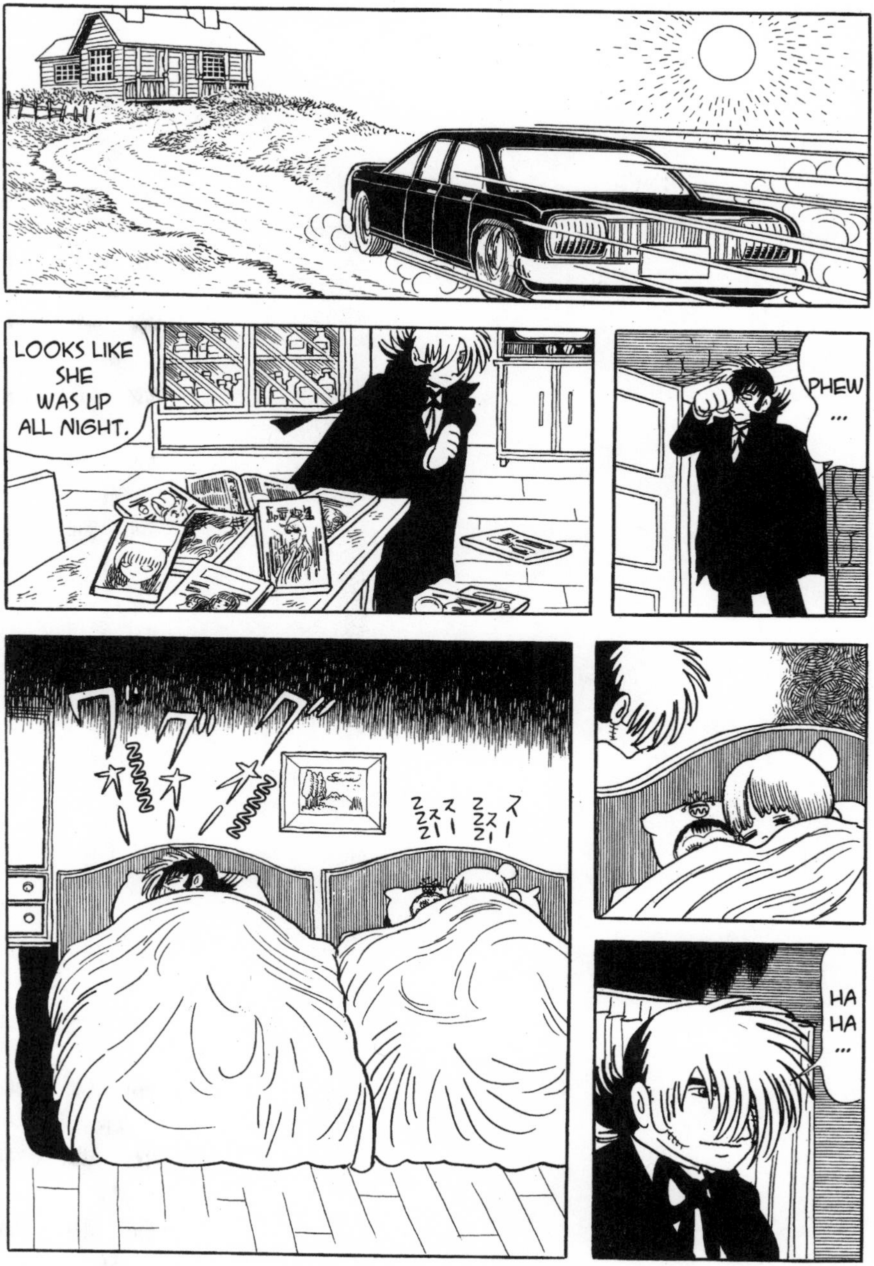
PHEW ...
LOOKS LIKE SHE WAS UP ALL NIGHT.
HA HA ...

RECOLLECTIONS OF A SPINSTER

SOMEONE ONCE SAID THAT A HUMAN IS LIKE A SPECK OF DUST IN THE VAST UNIVERSE...
AND YET, WE ARE BORN INTO HISTORY, FATED EVENTUALLY TO DIE...
IF YOU CAN SAVE A PERSON'S LIFE, PERHAPS YOU CAN CHANGE HISTORY. THAT IS THE ROLE OF DOCTORS AND NURSES.
IT'S BEEN FIFTY YEARS SINCE THAT DAY...
BACK WHEN I WAS A NURSE AT A CERTAIN HOSPITAL.
PÉAN FORCEPS!

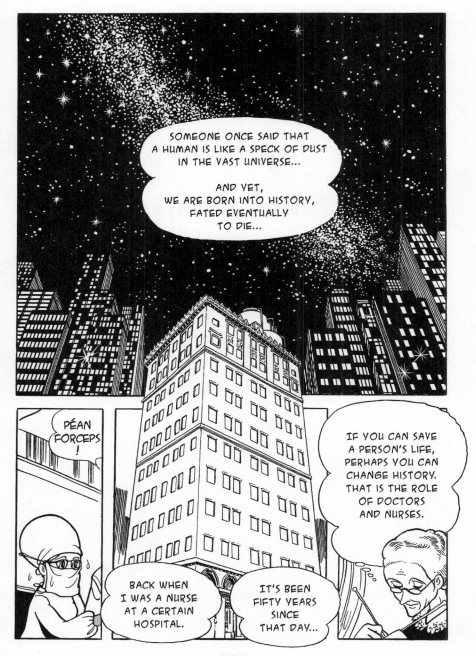

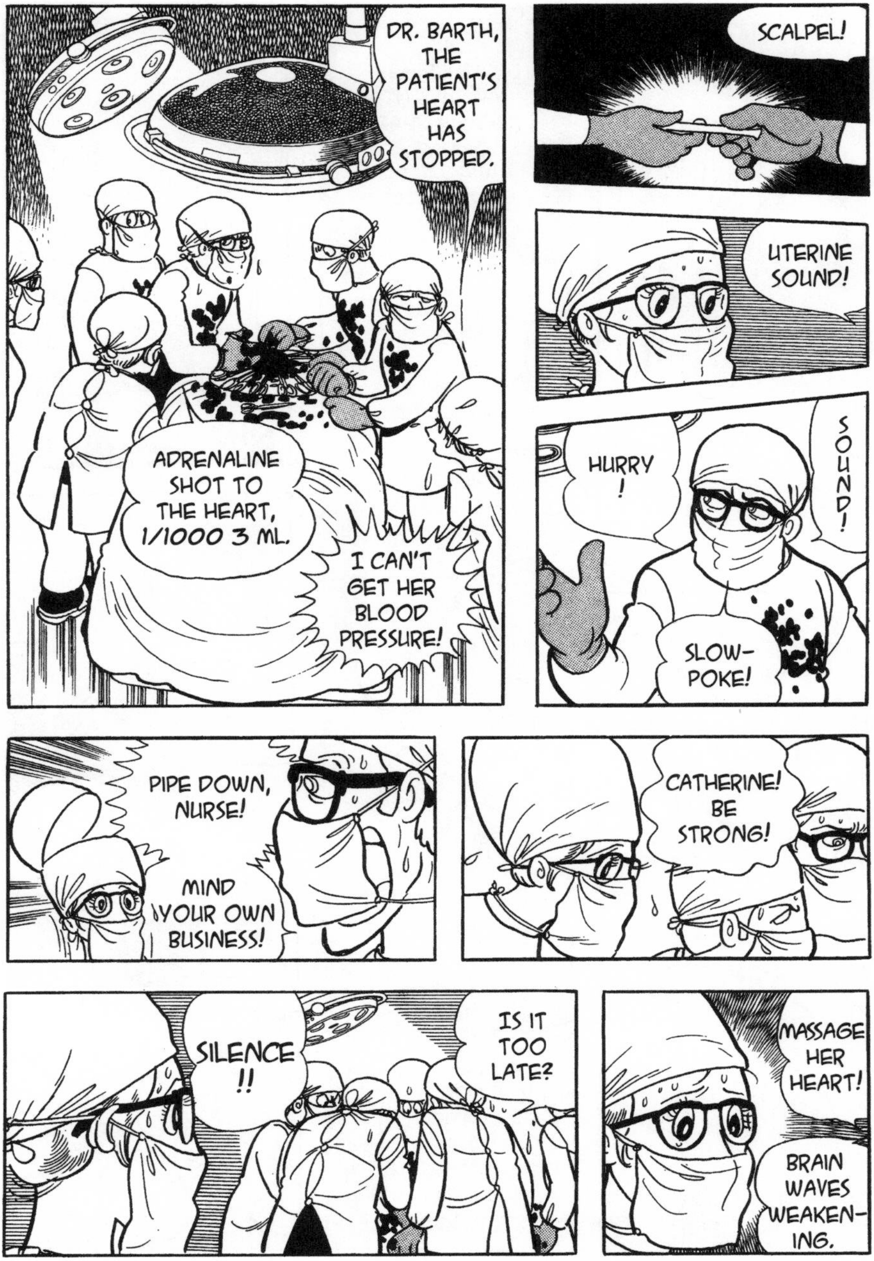
SCALPEL!
UTERINE SOUND!
SOUND!
HURRY!
SLOW-POKE!
DR. BARTH, THE PATIENT'S HEART HAS STOPPED.
ADRENALINE SHOT TO THE HEART, 1/1000 3 ML.
I CAN'T GET HER BLOOD PRESSURE!
CATHERINE! BE STRONG!
PIPE DOWN, NURSE!
MIND YOUR OWN BUSINESS!
MASSAGE HER HEART!
BRAIN WAVES WEAKENING.
IS IT TOO LATE?
SILENCE !!

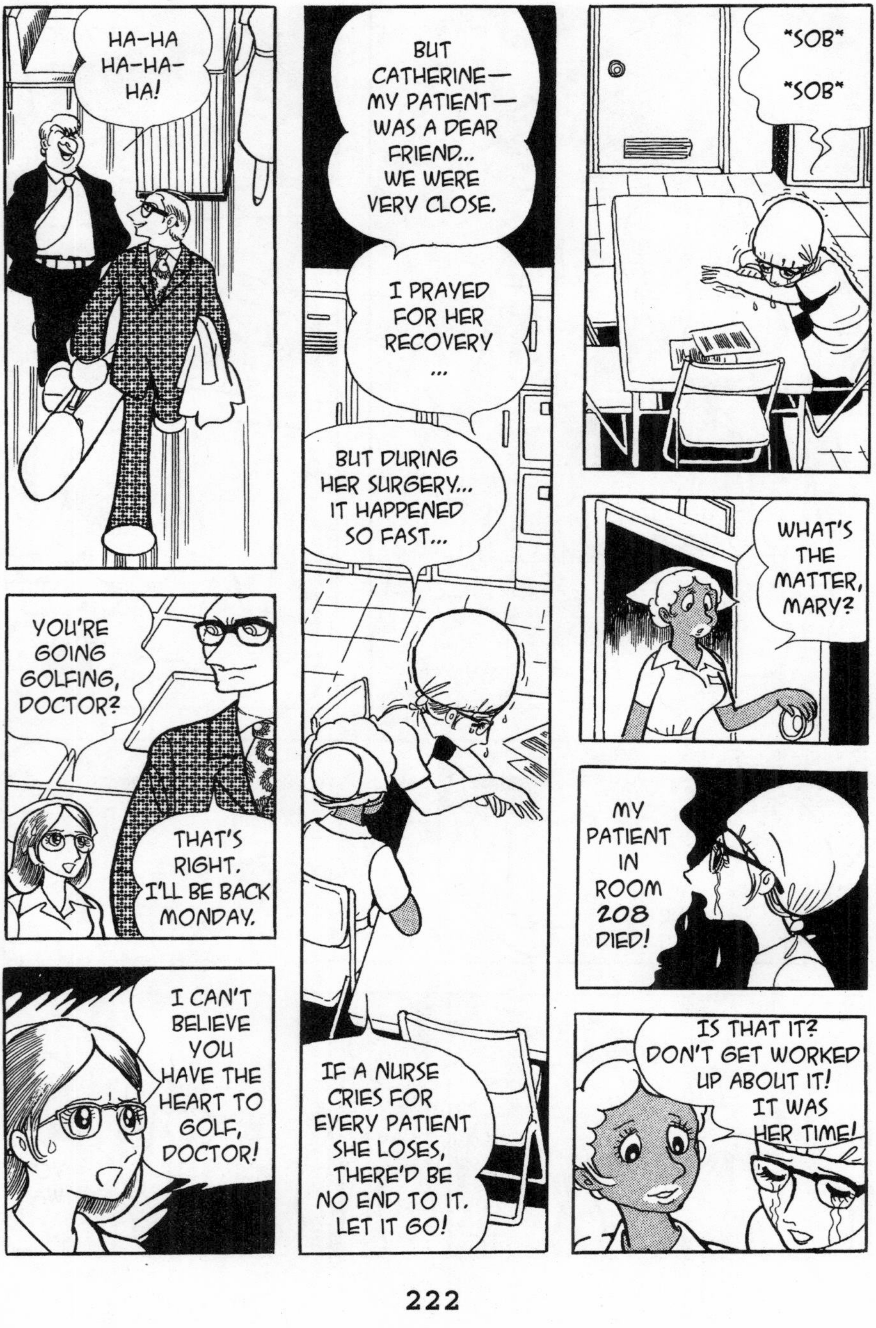
SOB
SOB
WHAT'S THE MATTER, MARY?
MY PATIENT IN ROOM 208 DIED!
IS THAT IT? DON'T GET WORKED UP ABOUT IT!
IT WAS HER TIME!
BUT CATHERINE— MY PATIENT— WAS A DEAR FRIEND... WE WERE VERY CLOSE.
I PRAYED FOR HER RECOVERY ...
BUT DURING HER SURGERY... IT HAPPENED SO FAST...
IF A NURSE CRIES FOR EVERY PATIENT SHE LOSES, THERE'D BE NO END TO IT. LET IT GO!
HA-HA HA-HA-HA!
YOU'RE GOING GOLFING, DOCTOR?
THAT'S RIGHT. I'LL BE BACK MONDAY.
I CAN'T BELIEVE YOU HAVE THE HEART TO GOLF, DOCTOR!

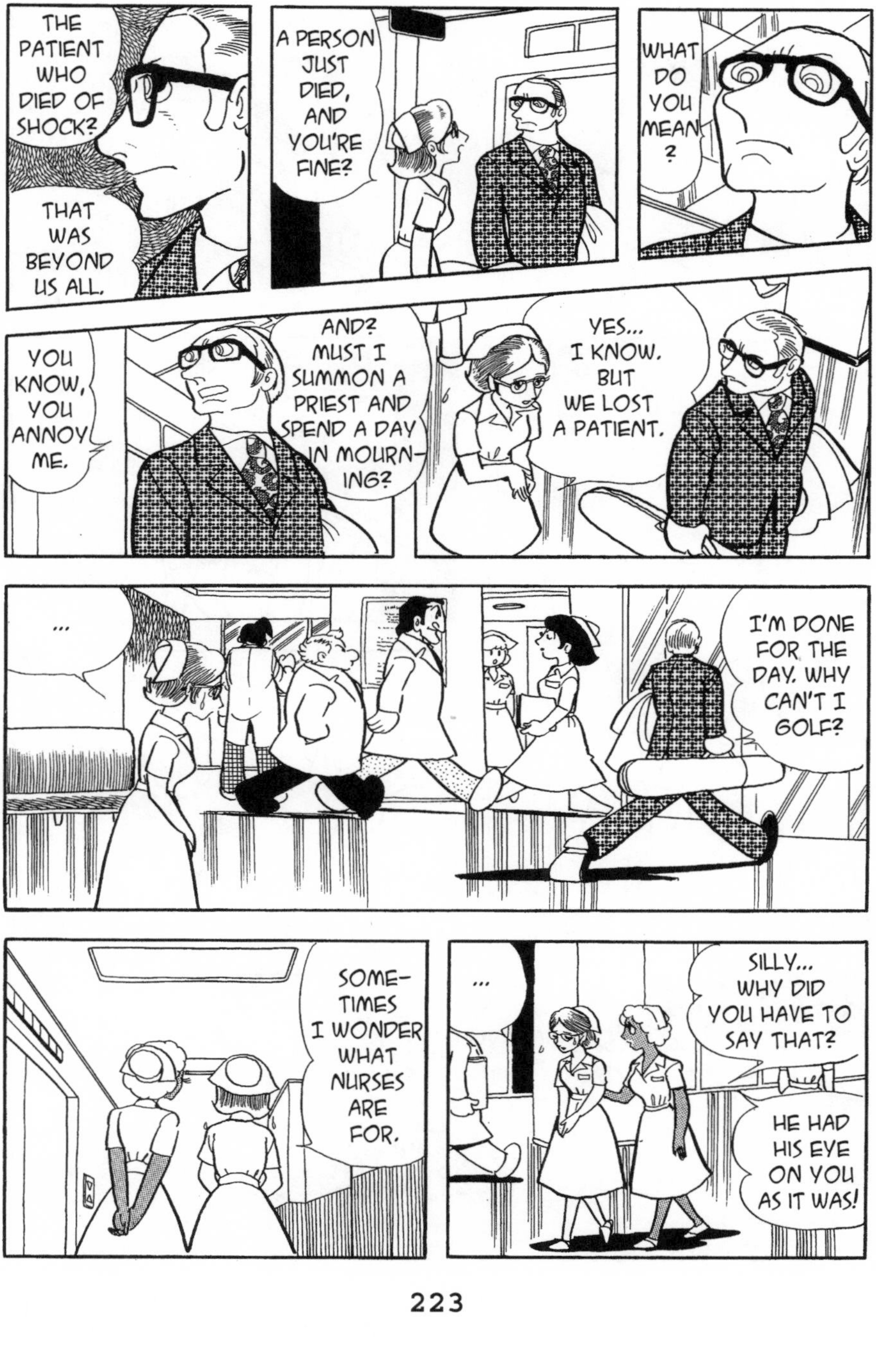
WHAT DO YOU MEAN?
A PERSON JUST DIED, AND YOU'RE FINE?
THE PATIENT WHO DIED OF SHOCK?
THAT WAS BEYOND US ALL.
YES... I KNOW. BUT WE LOST A PATIENT.
AND? MUST I SUMMON A PRIEST AND SPEND A DAY IN MOURNING?
YOU KNOW, YOU ANNOY ME.
I'M DONE FOR THE DAY. WHY CAN'T I GOLF?
...
SILLY... WHY DID YOU HAVE TO SAY THAT?
HE HAD HIS EYE ON YOU AS IT WAS!
...
SOMETIMES I WONDER WHAT NURSES ARE FOR.

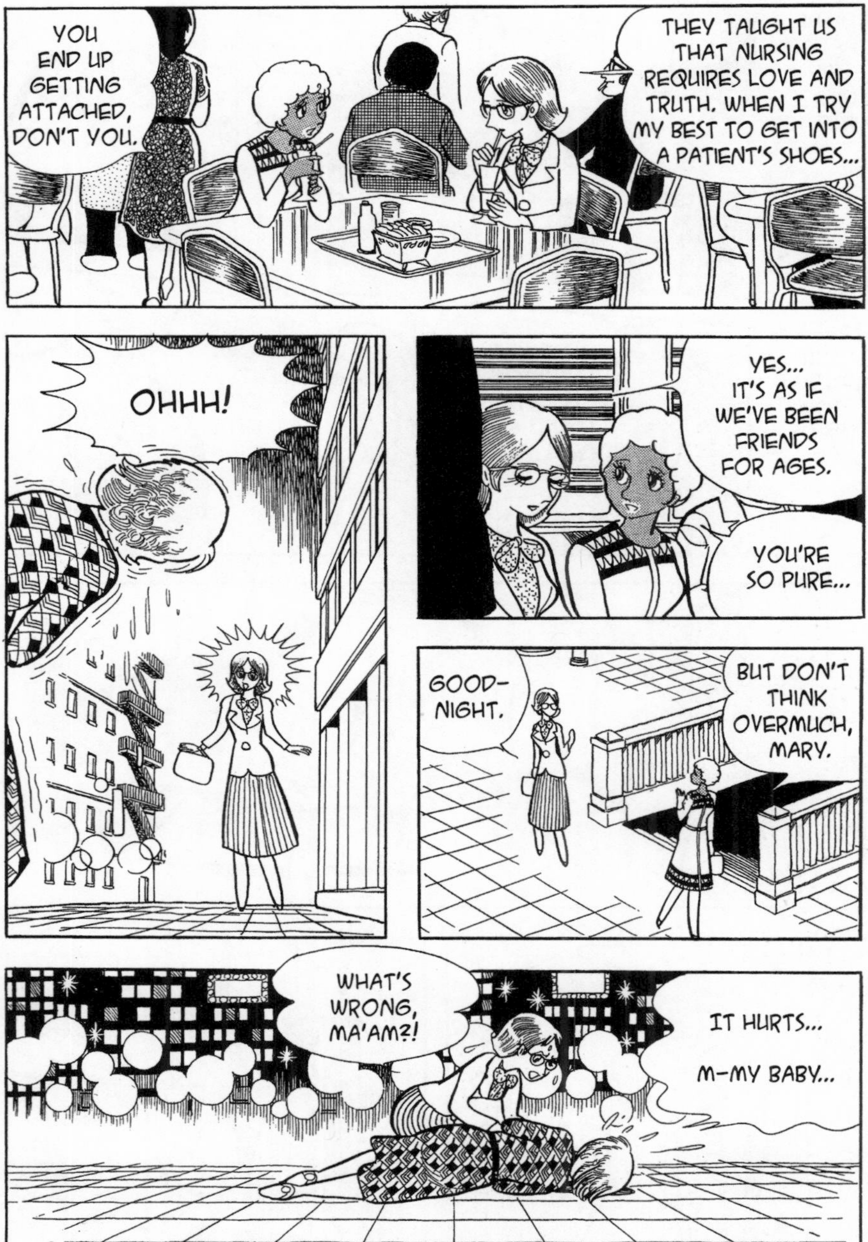
THEY TAUGHT US THAT NURSING REQUIRES LOVE AND TRUTH. WHEN I TRY MY BEST TO GET INTO A PATIENT'S SHOES...
YOU END UP GETTING ATTACHED, DON'T YOU.
YES... IT'S AS IF WE'VE BEEN FRIENDS FOR AGES.
YOU'RE SO PURE...
BUT DON'T THINK OVERMUCH, MARY.
GOOD-NIGHT.
OHHH!
IT HURTS...
M-MY BABY...
WHAT'S WRONG, MA'AM?!

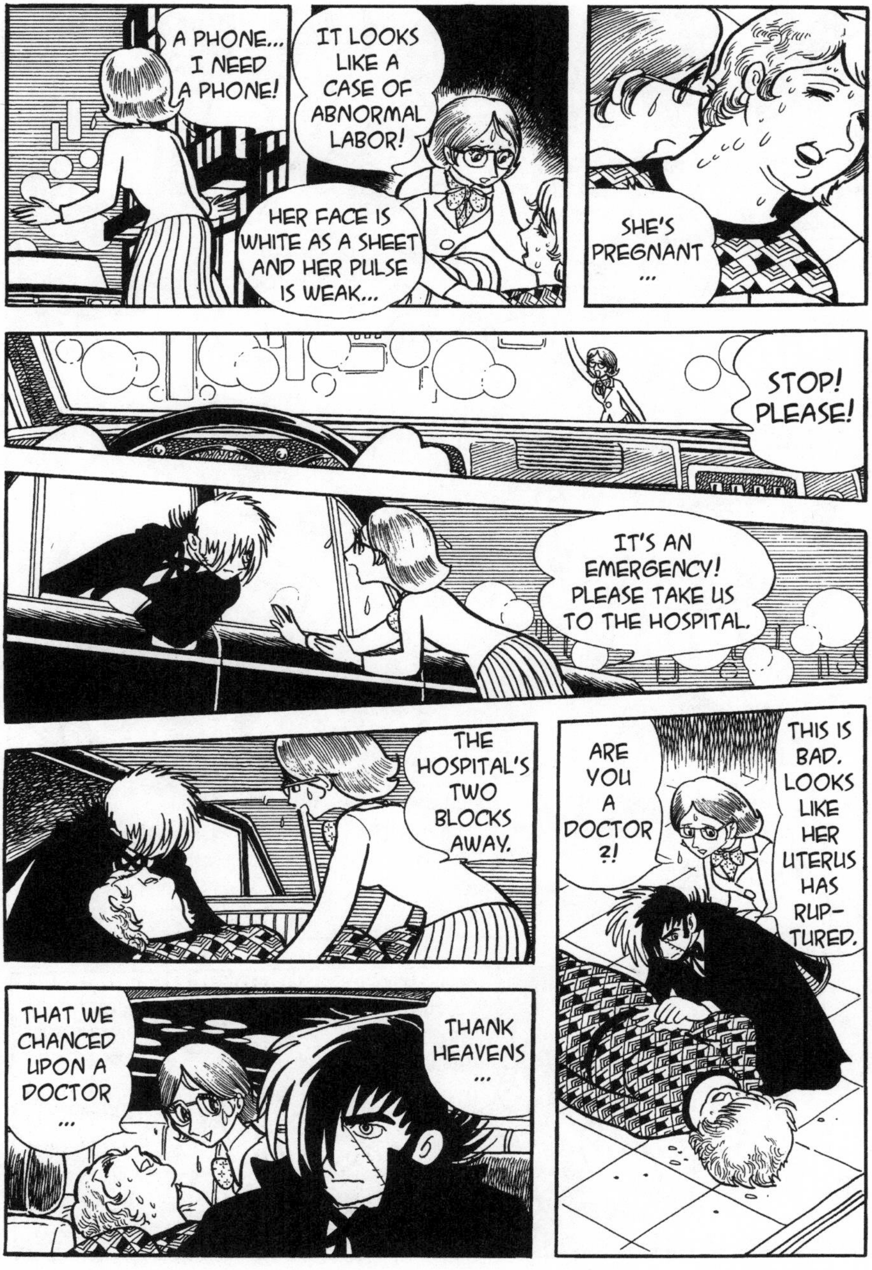
SHE'S PREGNANT ...
IT LOOKS LIKE A CASE OF ABNORMAL LABOR!
HER FACE IS WHITE AS A SHEET AND HER PULSE IS WEAK...
A PHONE... I NEED A PHONE!
STOP! PLEASE!
IT'S AN EMERGENCY! PLEASE TAKE US TO THE HOSPITAL.
THIS IS BAD. LOOKS LIKE HER UTERUS HAS RUP-TURED.
ARE YOU A DOCTOR?!
THE HOSPITAL'S TWO BLOCKS AWAY.
THANK HEAVENS ...
THAT WE CHANCED UPON A DOCTOR ...

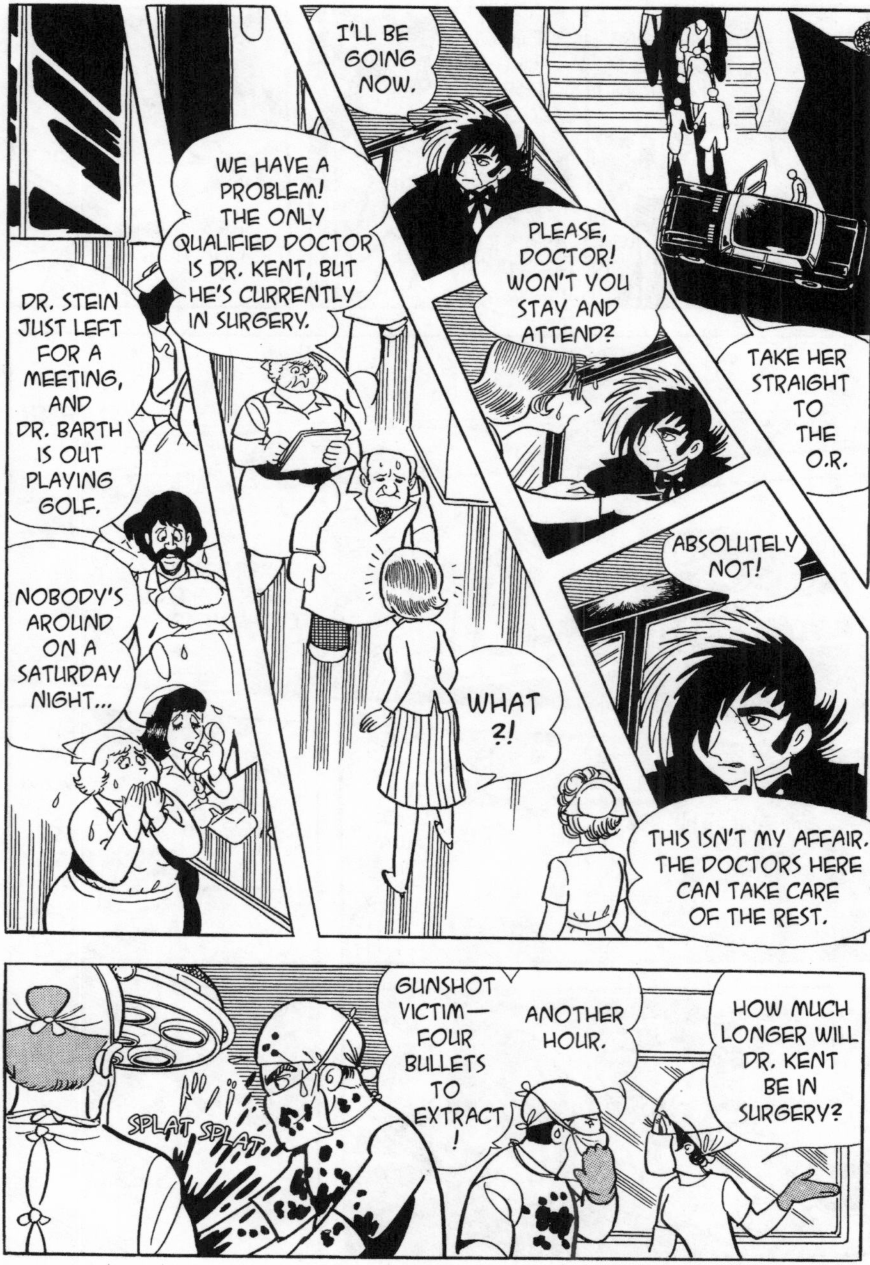

I'LL BE GOING NOW.
PLEASE, DOCTOR! WON'T YOU STAY AND ATTEND?
TAKE HER STRAIGHT TO THE O.R.
ABSOLUTELY NOT!
THIS ISN'T MY AFFAIR. THE DOCTORS HERE CAN TAKE CARE OF THE REST.
WHAT ?!
WE HAVE A PROBLEM! THE ONLY QUALIFIED DOCTOR IS DR. KENT, BUT HE'S CURRENTLY IN SURGERY.
DR. STEIN JUST LEFT FOR A MEETING, AND DR. BARTH IS OUT PLAYING GOLF.
NOBODY'S AROUND ON A SATURDAY NIGHT...
HOW MUCH LONGER WILL DR. KENT BE IN SURGERY?
ANOTHER HOUR.
GUNSHOT VICTIM— FOUR BULLETS TO EXTRACT !
SPLAT SPLAT

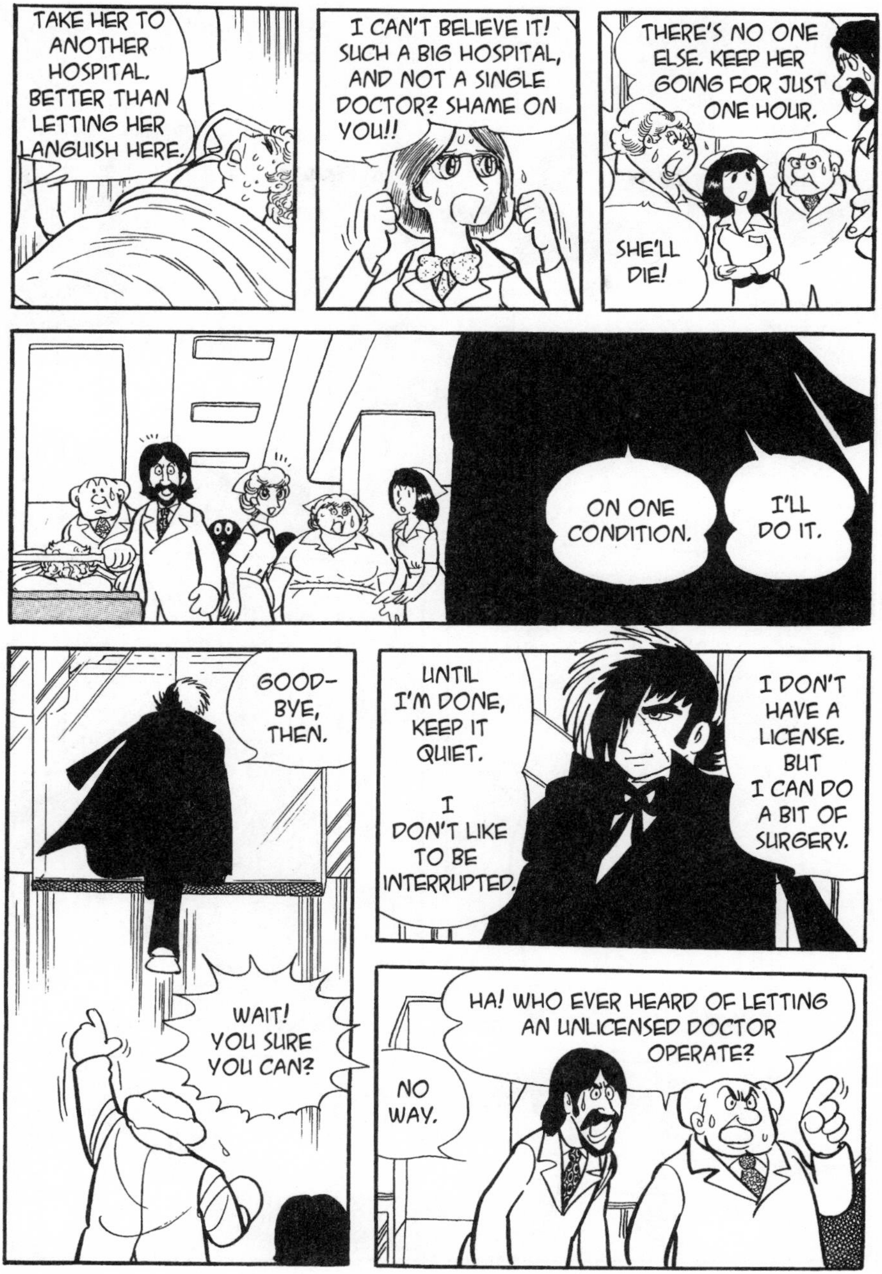
THERE'S NO ONE ELSE. KEEP HER GOING FOR JUST ONE HOUR.
SHE'LL DIE!
I CAN'T BELIEVE IT! SUCH A BIG HOSPITAL, AND NOT A SINGLE DOCTOR? SHAME ON YOU!!
TAKE HER TO ANOTHER HOSPITAL. BETTER THAN LETTING HER LANGUISH HERE.
I'LL DO IT.
ON ONE CONDITION.
I DON'T HAVE A LICENSE. BUT I CAN DO A BIT OF SURGERY.
UNTIL I'M DONE, KEEP IT QUIET.
I DON'T LIKE TO BE INTERRUPTED.
HA! WHO EVER HEARD OF LETTING AN UNLICENSED DOCTOR OPERATE?
NO WAY.
GOOD-BYE, THEN.
WAIT! YOU SURE YOU CAN?

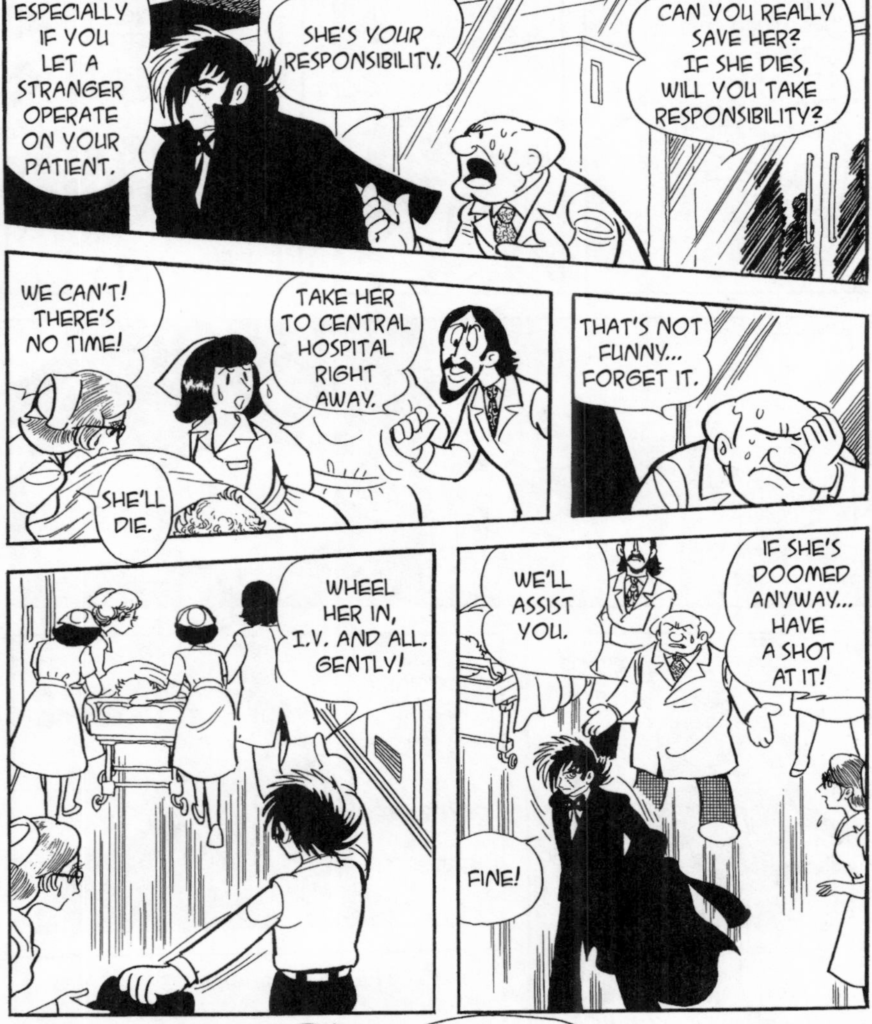
CAN YOU REALLY SAVE HER? IF SHE DIES, WILL YOU TAKE RESPONSIBILITY?
SHE'S YOUR RESPONSIBILITY.
ESPECIALLY IF YOU LET A STRANGER OPERATE ON YOUR PATIENT.
THAT'S NOT FUNNY... FORGET IT.
TAKE HER TO CENTRAL HOSPITAL RIGHT AWAY.
WE CAN'T! THERE'S NO TIME!
SHE'LL DIE.
IF SHE'S DOOMED ANYWAY... HAVE A SHOT AT IT!
WE'LL ASSIST YOU.
FINE!
WHEEL HER IN, I.V. AND ALL. GENTLY!
WILL SHE BE ALL RIGHT, DOCTOR?
GET AN INCUBATOR READY!

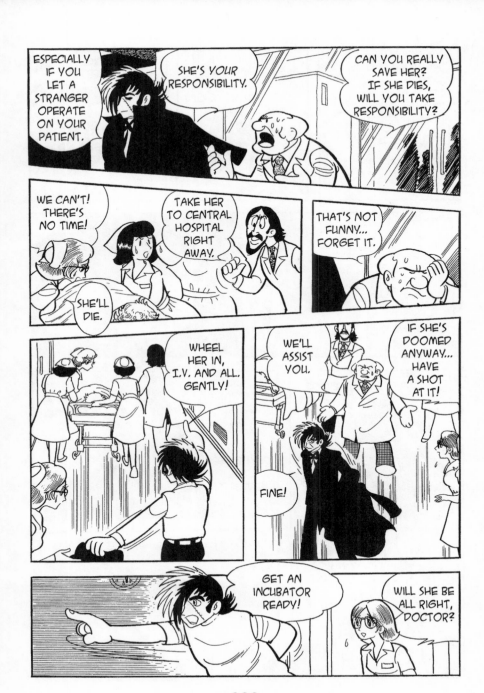

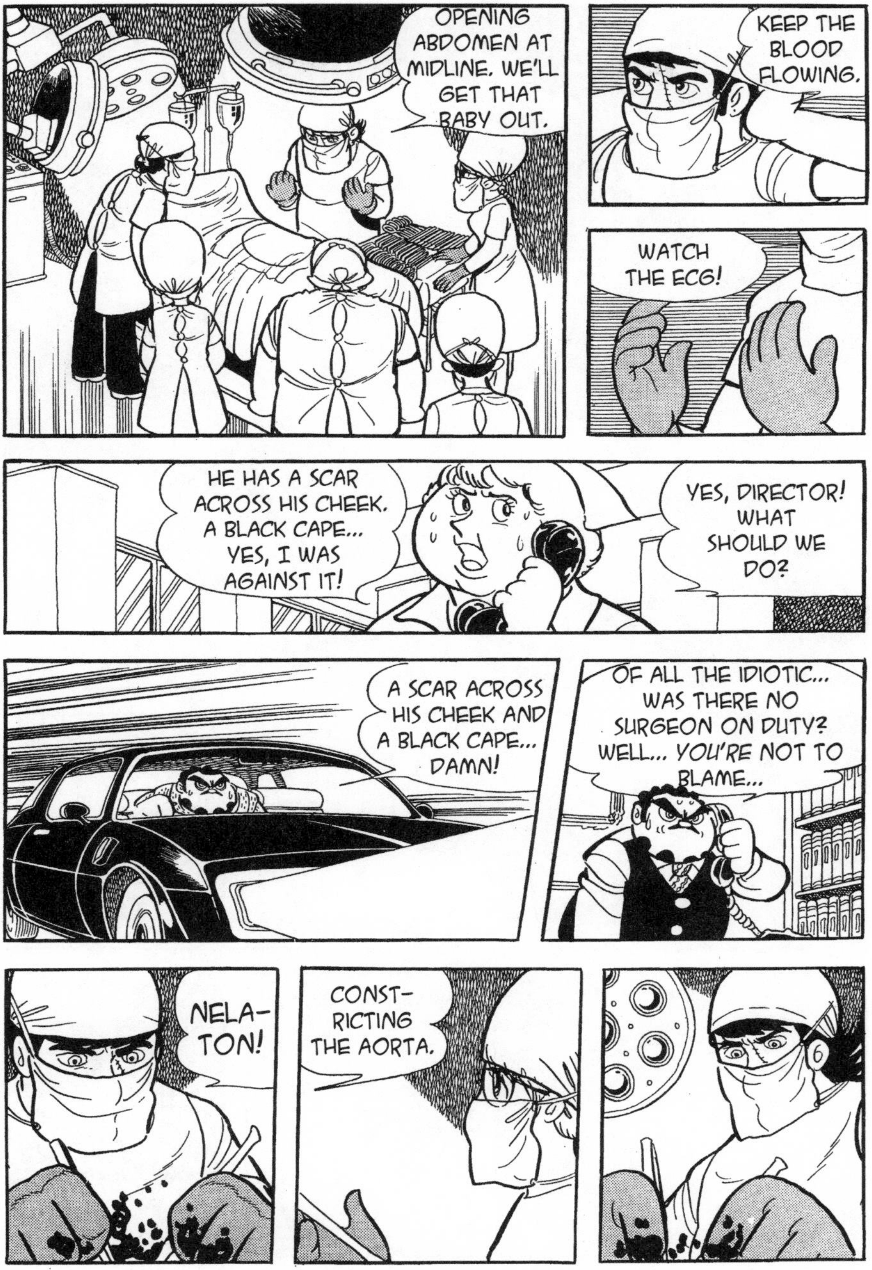
KEEP THE BLOOD FLOWING.
WATCH THE ECG!
OPENING ABDOMEN AT MIDLINE. WE'LL GET THAT BABY OUT.
YES, DIRECTOR! WHAT SHOULD WE DO?
HE HAS A SCAR ACROSS HIS CHEEK. A BLACK CAPE... YES, I WAS AGAINST IT!
OF ALL THE IDIOTIC... WAS THERE NO SURGEON ON DUTY? WELL... *YOU'RE* NOT TO BLAME...
A SCAR ACROSS HIS CHEEK AND A BLACK CAPE... DAMN!
CONST-RICTING THE AORTA.
NELA-TON!

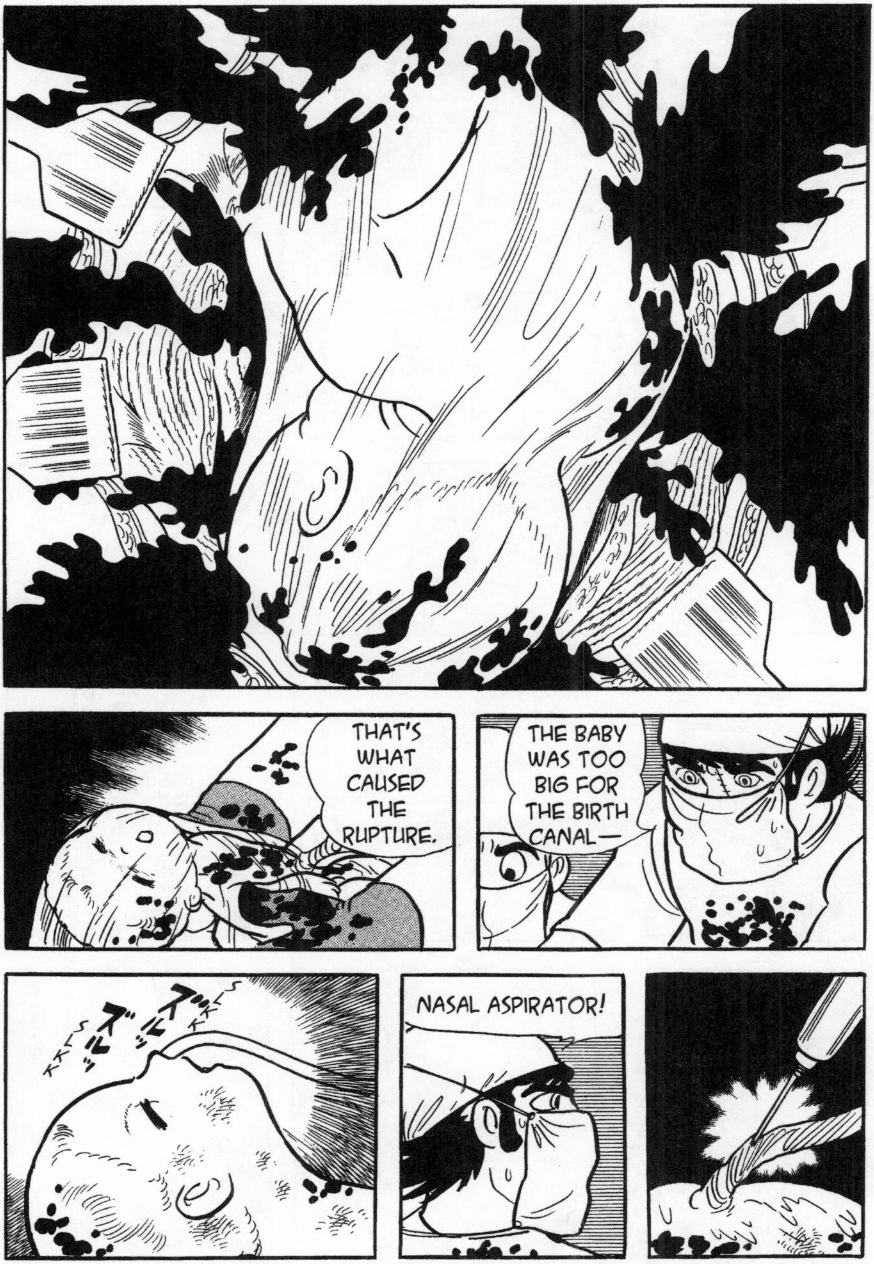
THE BABY WAS TOO BIG FOR THE BIRTH CANAL—
THAT'S WHAT CAUSED THE RUPTURE.
NASAL ASPIRATOR!
ズルッ
SLKK
ズルッ
SLKK

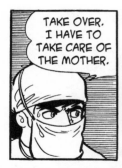

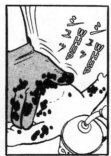

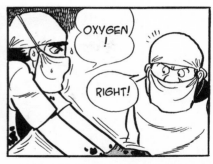

OXYGEN!
RIGHT!
WHUP WHUP
WHUP WHUP
TAKE OVER. I HAVE TO TAKE CARE OF THE MOTHER.
HER BLOOD PRESSURE'S PLUMMETING! SHE'S IN DANGER!
KEEP UP TRANSFUSION. VASOPRESSOR NOT NEEDED.
THAT'S ENOUGH, BLACK JACK!
GET OUT!! I'M PERFORMING SURGERY HERE!
I'M THE DIRECTOR OF THIS HOSPITAL.
I DON'T CARE IF YOU'RE THE KING! JUST DON'T INTERFERE.
SOMEONE GET HIM OUT OF HERE.
WHO GAVE THIS MAN PERMISSION TO OPE-RATE?
YOU'RE THE ONE WHO'S GETTING THE BOOT, BLACK JACK!

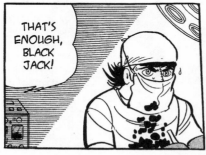

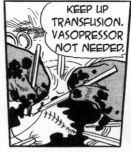

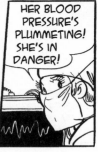

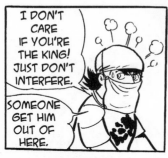

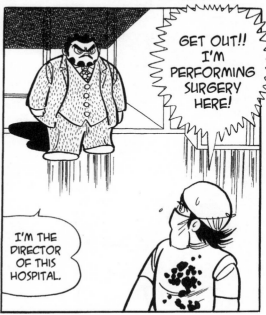

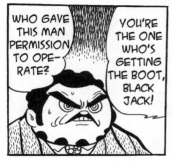

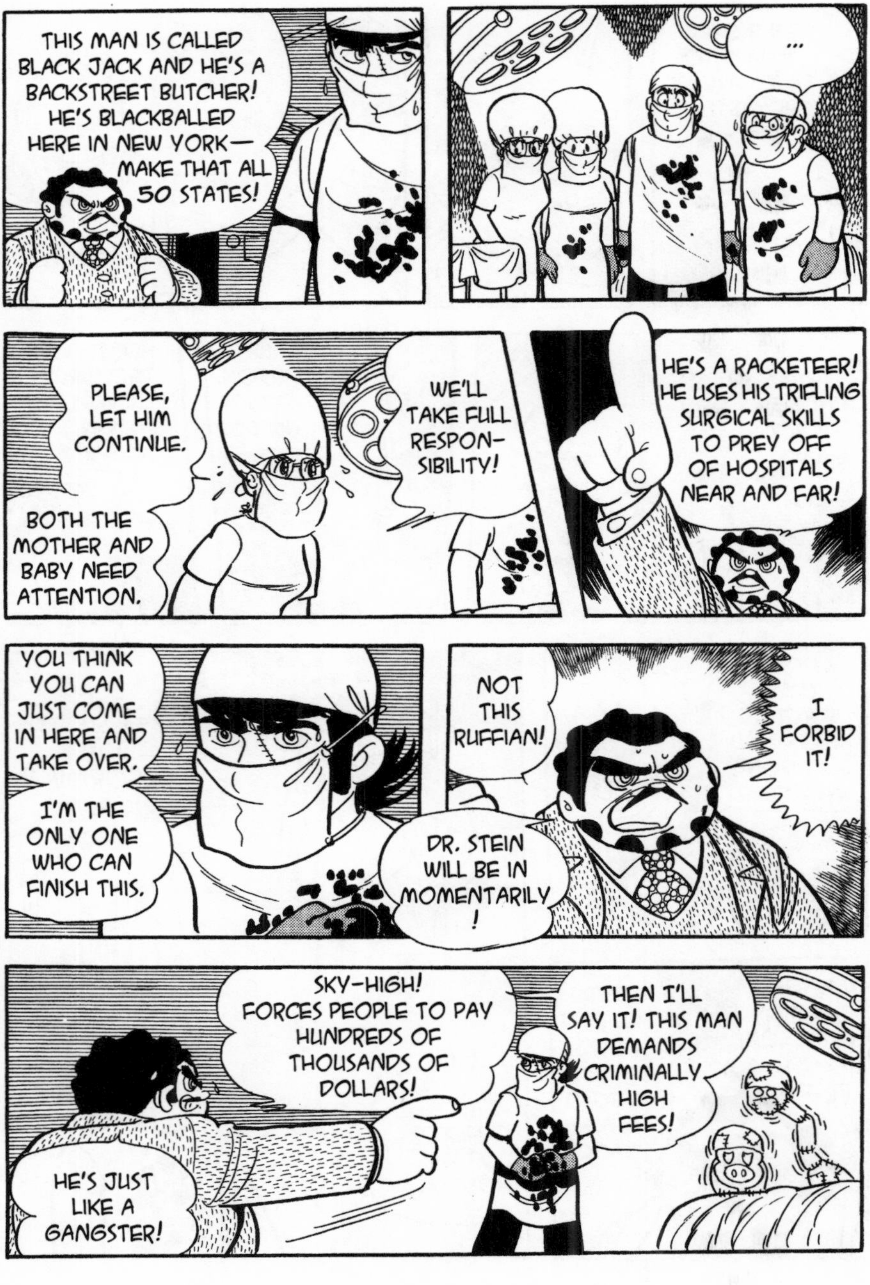
...
THIS MAN IS CALLED BLACK JACK AND HE'S A BACKSTREET BUTCHER! HE'S BLACKBALLED HERE IN NEW YORK—MAKE THAT ALL 50 STATES!
HE'S A RACKETEER! HE USES HIS TRIFLING SURGICAL SKILLS TO PREY OFF OF HOSPITALS NEAR AND FAR!
WE'LL TAKE FULL RESPON-SIBILITY!
PLEASE, LET HIM CONTINUE.
BOTH THE MOTHER AND BABY NEED ATTENTION.
I FORBID IT!
NOT THIS RUFFIAN!
DR. STEIN WILL BE IN MOMENTARILY!
YOU THINK YOU CAN JUST COME IN HERE AND TAKE OVER.
I'M THE ONLY ONE WHO CAN FINISH THIS.
THEN I'LL SAY IT! THIS MAN DEMANDS CRIMINALLY HIGH FEES!
SKY-HIGH! FORCES PEOPLE TO PAY HUNDREDS OF THOUSANDS OF DOLLARS!
HE'S JUST LIKE A GANGSTER!

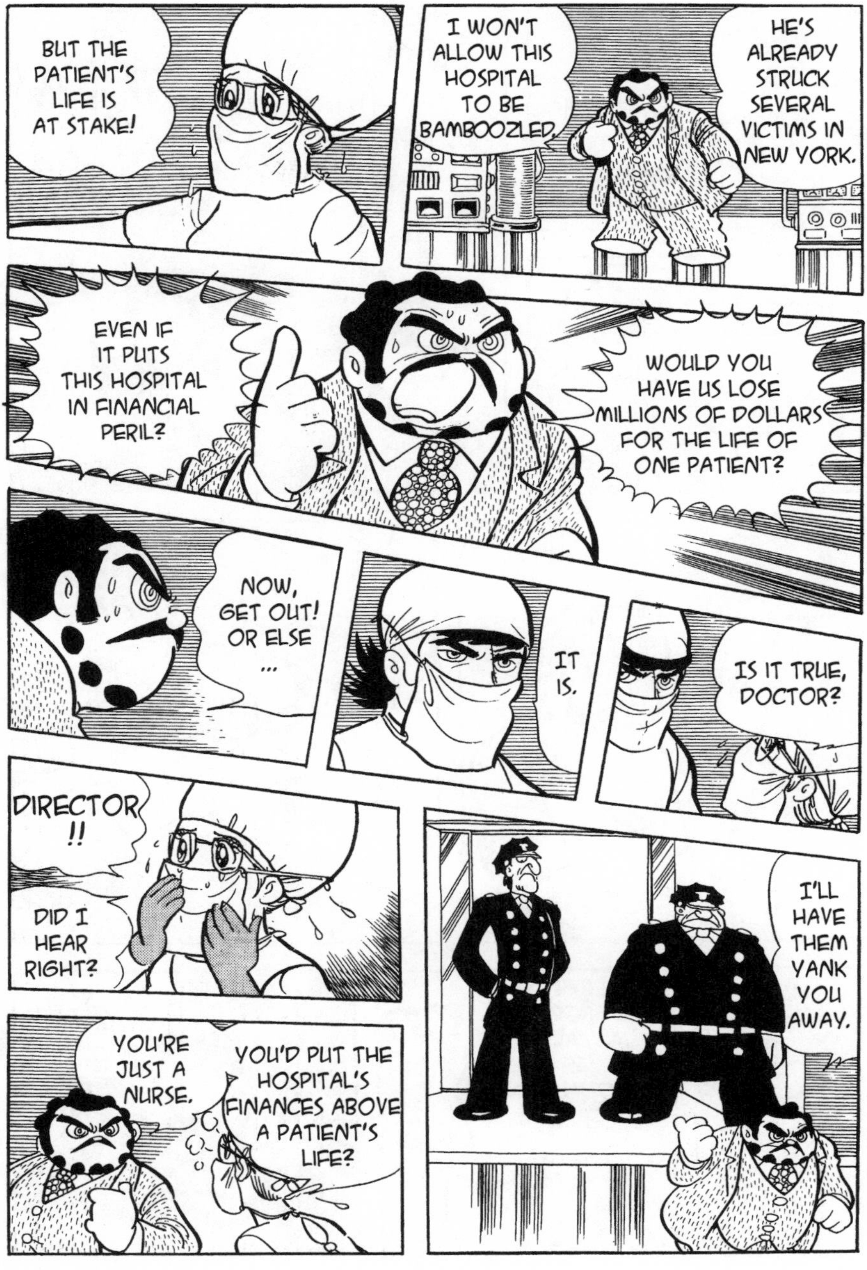
HE'S ALREADY STRUCK SEVERAL VICTIMS IN NEW YORK.
I WON'T ALLOW THIS HOSPITAL TO BE BAMBOOZLED.
BUT THE PATIENT'S LIFE IS AT STAKE!
WOULD YOU HAVE US LOSE MILLIONS OF DOLLARS FOR THE LIFE OF ONE PATIENT?
EVEN IF IT PUTS THIS HOSPITAL IN FINANCIAL PERIL?
IS IT TRUE, DOCTOR?
IT IS.
NOW, GET OUT! OR ELSE ...
I'LL HAVE THEM YANK YOU AWAY.
DIRECTOR !!
DID I HEAR RIGHT?
YOU'D PUT THE HOSPITAL'S FINANCES ABOVE A PATIENT'S LIFE?
YOU'RE JUST A NURSE.

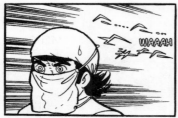

WAAAH
WAAAAH
WAAAH
WAAAH
THE BABY'S BREATHING, DOCTOR.
WAAAAH
WAAAAH
AH, NOW... THAT'S A GOOD BOY.
YOUR BABY'S BEEN BORN, MA'AM. YOU'LL SEE HIM SOON.
URR...

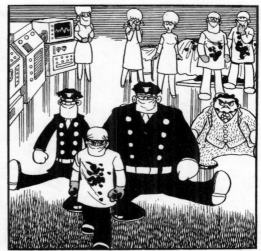

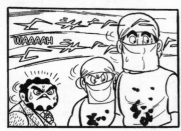

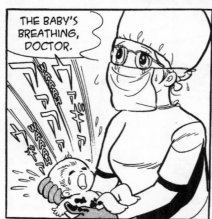

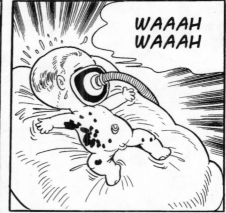

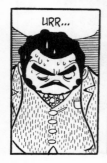

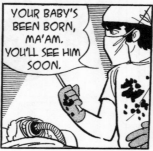

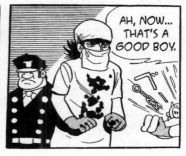

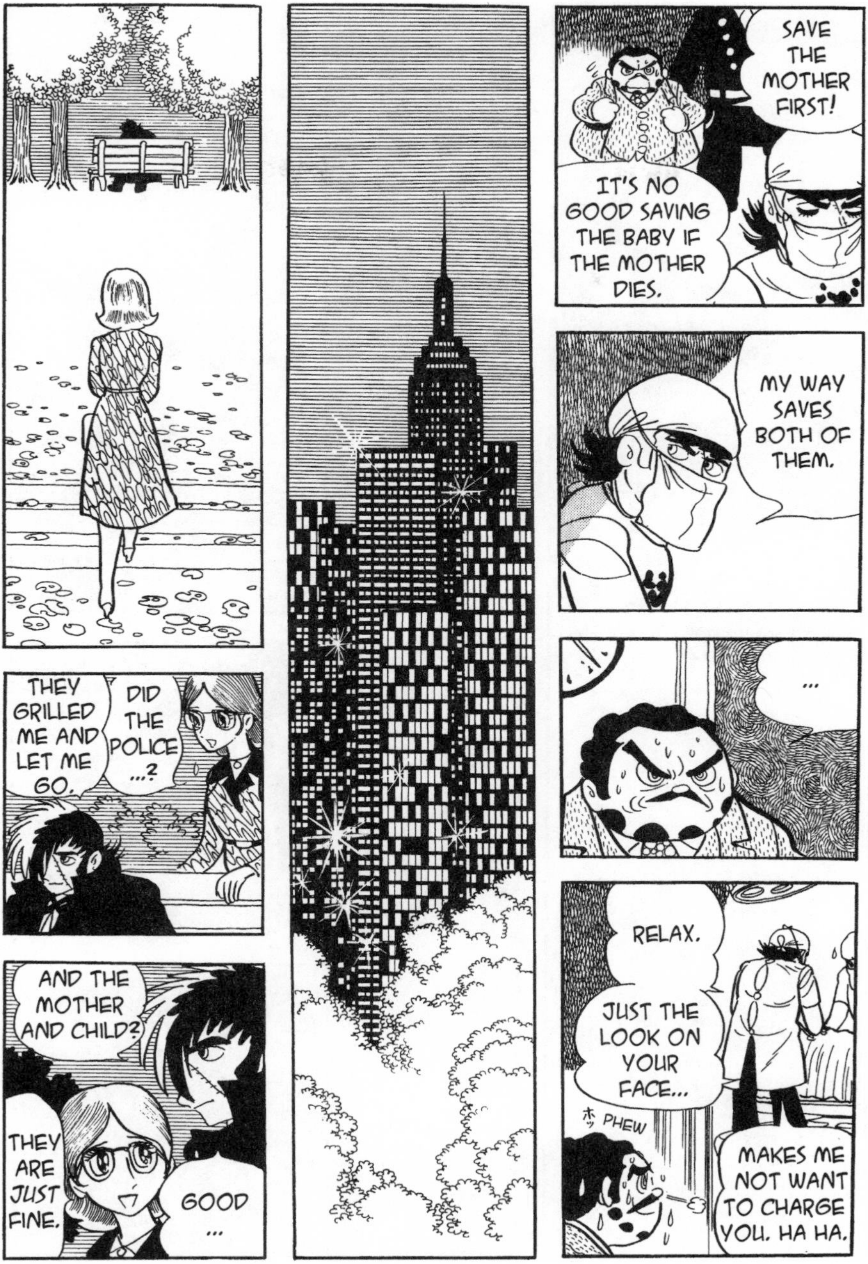
SAVE THE MOTHER FIRST!
IT'S NO GOOD SAVING THE BABY IF THE MOTHER DIES.
MY WAY SAVES BOTH OF THEM.
...
RELAX.
JUST THE LOOK ON YOUR FACE...
ホッ PHEW
MAKES ME NOT WANT TO CHARGE YOU. HA HA.
DID THE POLICE ...?
THEY GRILLED ME AND LET ME GO.
AND THE MOTHER AND CHILD?
THEY ARE JUST FINE.
GOOD ...

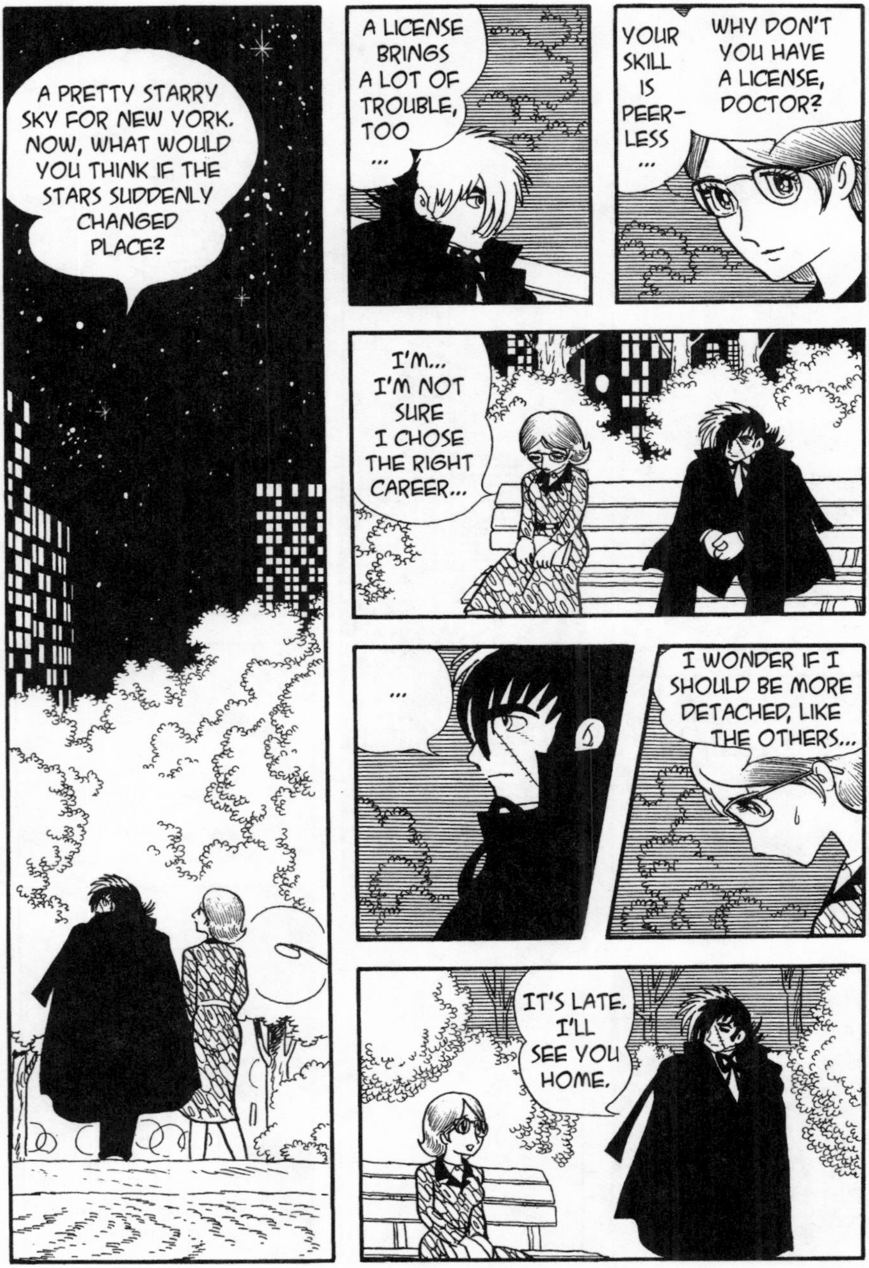
WHY DON'T YOU HAVE A LICENSE, DOCTOR?
YOUR SKILL IS PEER-LESS ...
A LICENSE BRINGS A LOT OF TROUBLE, TOO ...
I'M... I'M NOT SURE I CHOSE THE RIGHT CAREER...
I WONDER IF I SHOULD BE MORE DETACHED, LIKE THE OTHERS...
...
IT'S LATE. I'LL SEE YOU HOME.
A PRETTY STARRY SKY FOR NEW YORK. NOW, WHAT WOULD YOU THINK IF THE STARS SUDDENLY CHANGED PLACE?

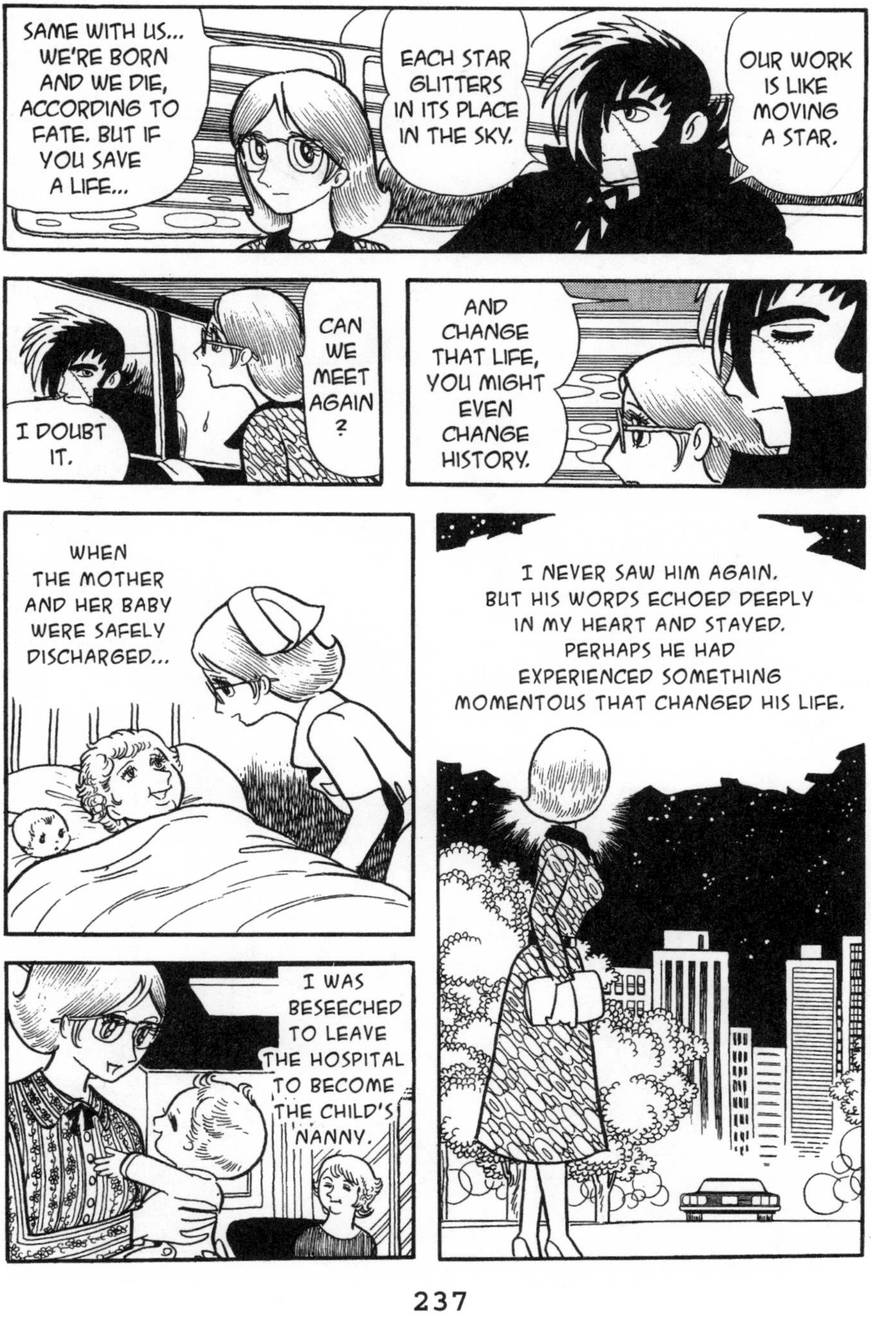
OUR WORK IS LIKE MOVING A STAR.
EACH STAR GLITTERS IN ITS PLACE IN THE SKY.
SAME WITH US... WE'RE BORN AND WE DIE, ACCORDING TO FATE. BUT IF YOU SAVE A LIFE...
AND CHANGE THAT LIFE, YOU MIGHT EVEN CHANGE HISTORY.
CAN WE MEET AGAIN?
I DOUBT IT.
I NEVER SAW HIM AGAIN. BUT HIS WORDS ECHOED DEEPLY IN MY HEART AND STAYED. PERHAPS HE HAD EXPERIENCED SOMETHING MOMENTOUS THAT CHANGED HIS LIFE.
WHEN THE MOTHER AND HER BABY WERE SAFELY DISCHARGED...
I WAS BESEECHED TO LEAVE THE HOSPITAL TO BECOME THE CHILD'S NANNY.

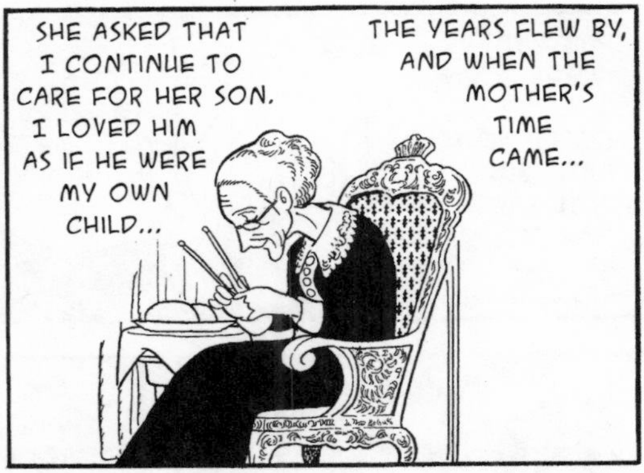
THE YEARS FLEW BY, AND WHEN THE MOTHER'S TIME CAME...
SHE ASKED THAT I CONTINUE TO CARE FOR HER SON. I LOVED HIM AS IF HE WERE MY OWN CHILD...
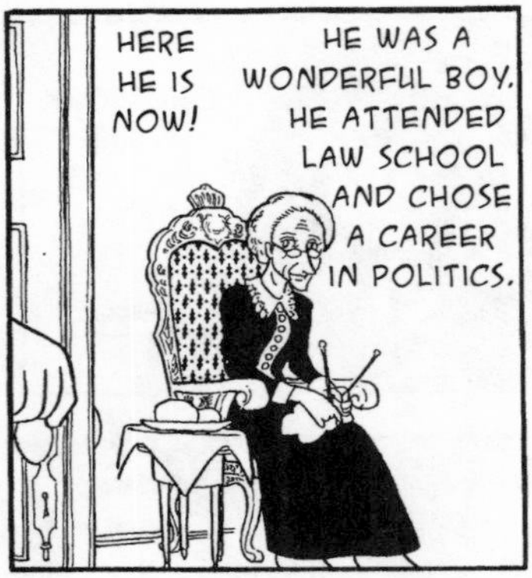
HE WAS A WONDERFUL BOY. HE ATTENDED LAW SCHOOL AND CHOSE A CAREER IN POLITICS.
HERE HE IS NOW!
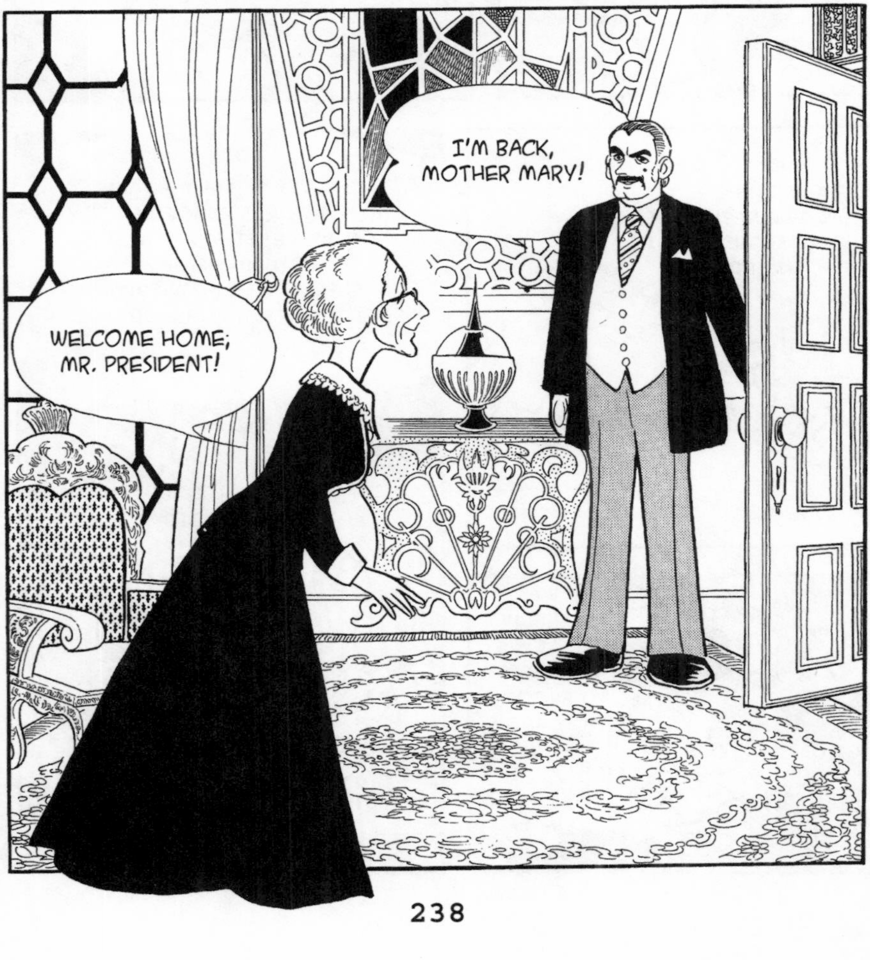
I'M BACK, MOTHER MARY!
WELCOME HOME; MR. PRESIDENT!

PINOKO LOVES YOU

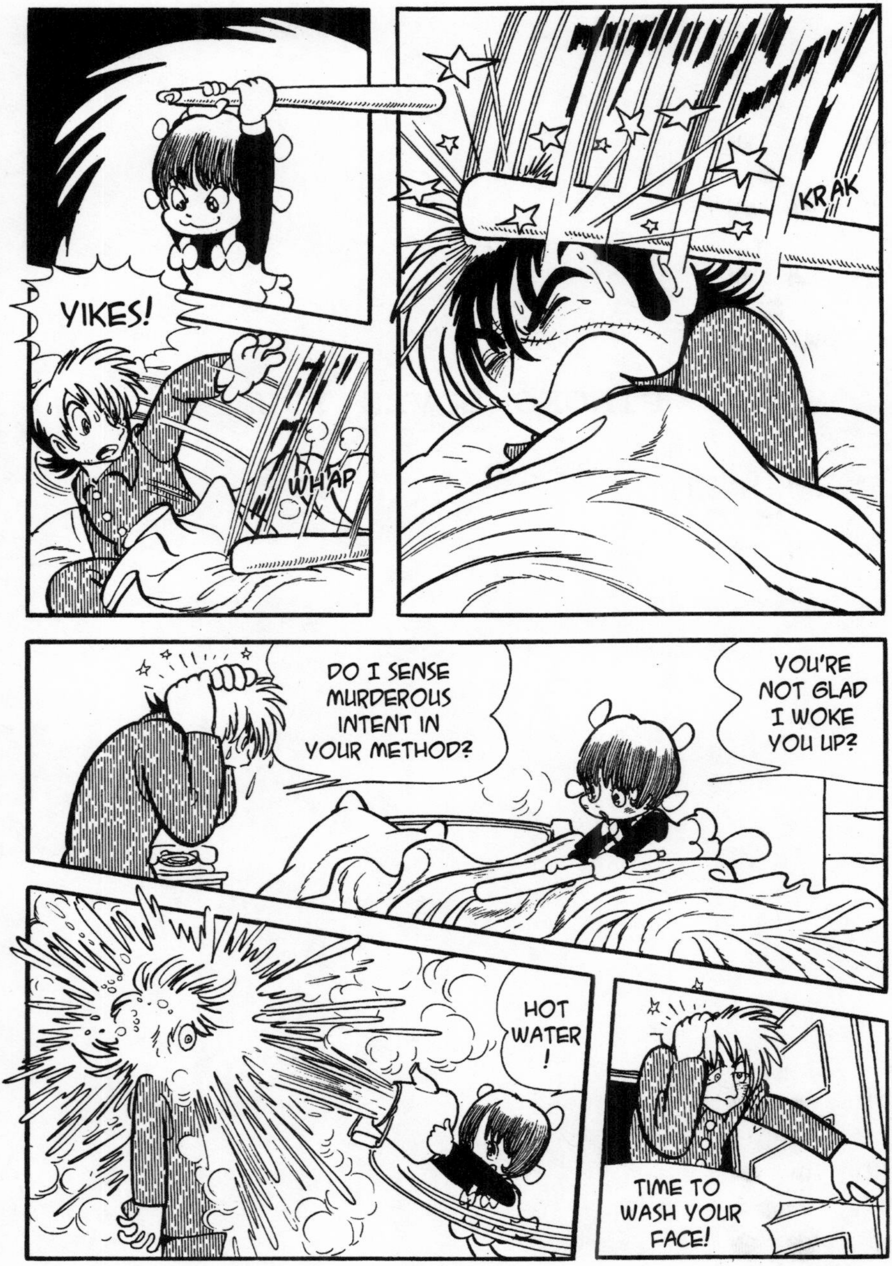
KRAK
YIKES!
WH'AP
YOU'RE NOT GLAD I WOKE YOU UP?
DO I SENSE MURDEROUS INTENT IN YOUR METHOD?
TIME TO WASH YOUR FACE!
HOT WATER!

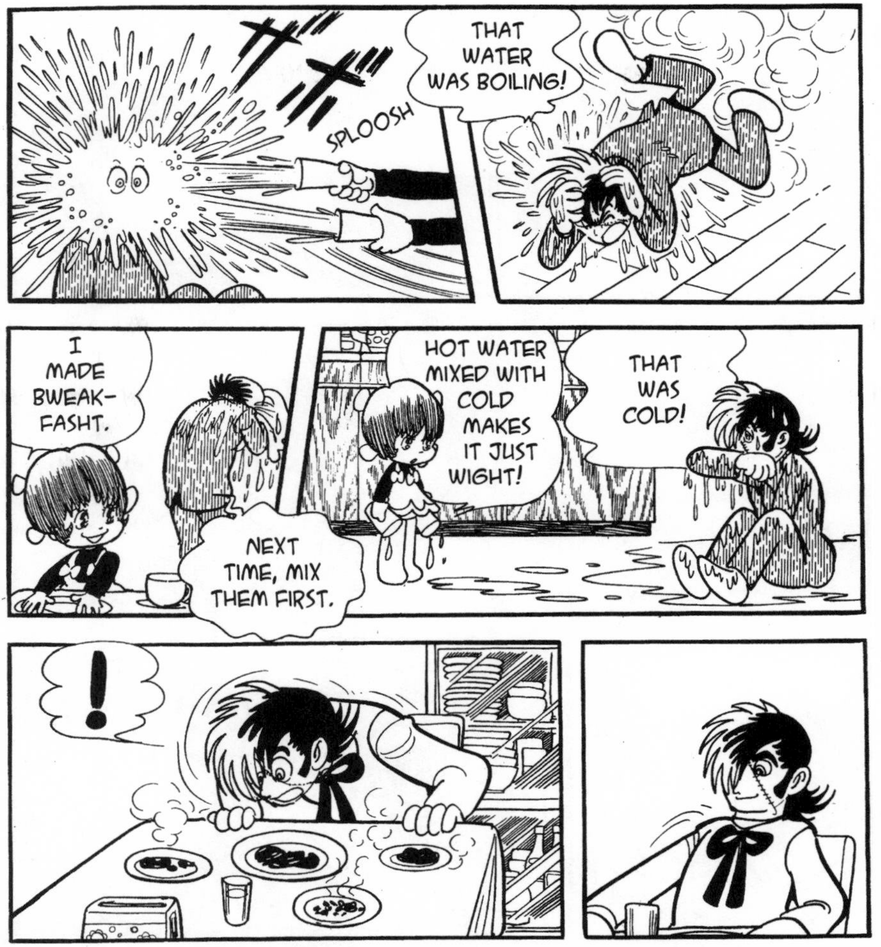
THAT WATER WAS BOILING!
SPLOOSH
THAT WAS COLD!
HOT WATER MIXED WITH COLD MAKES IT JUST WIGHT!
NEXT TIME, MIX THEM FIRST.
I MADE BWEAK-FASHT.
!
TH-THIS IS CHARCOAL!
YOU EXPECT ME TO EAT THAT?
IT'S BWEAD!
I BAKED IT FOR SHIX HOURS!

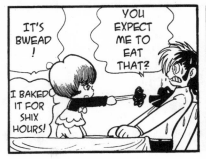

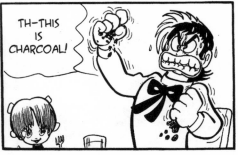

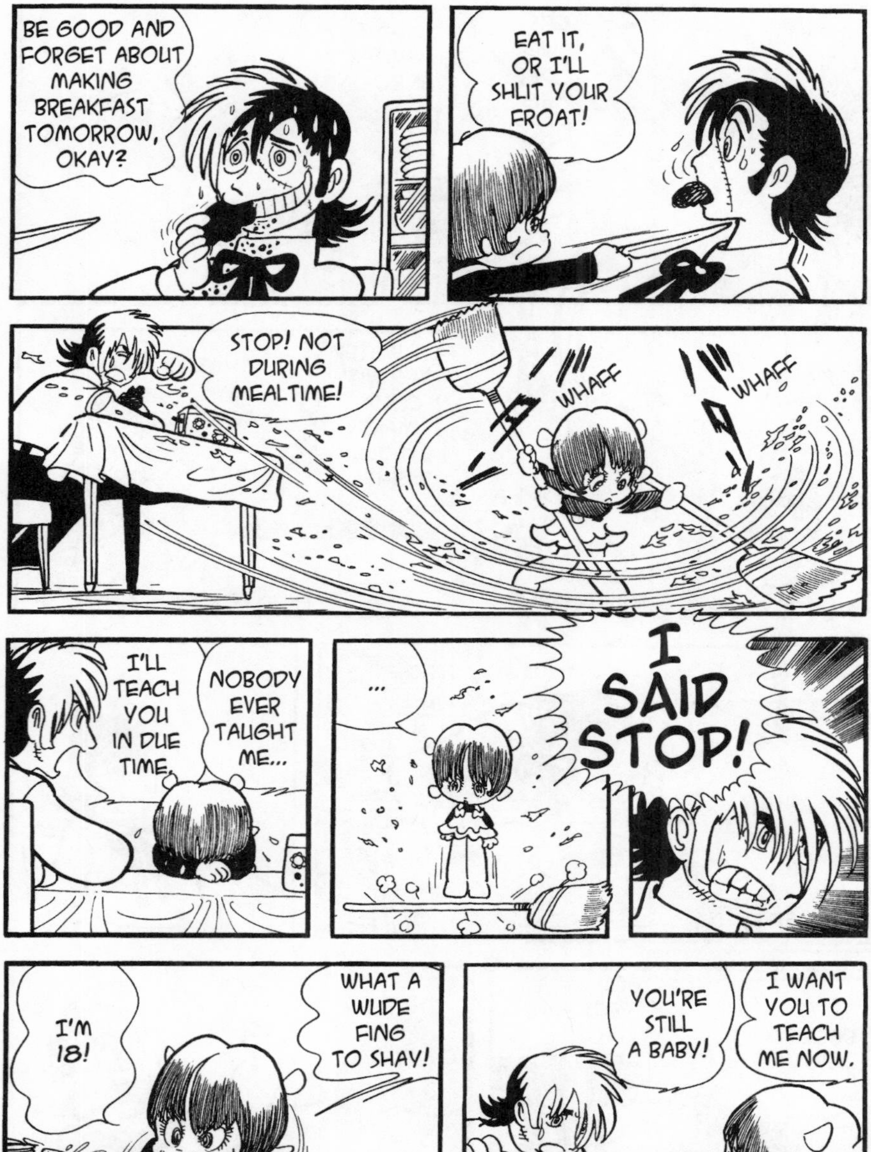
EAT IT, OR I'LL SHLIT YOUR FROAT!
BE GOOD AND FORGET ABOUT MAKING BREAKFAST TOMORROW, OKAY?
WHAFF
WHAFF
STOP! NOT DURING MEALTIME!
I SAID STOP!
...
NOBODY EVER TAUGHT ME...
I'LL TEACH YOU IN DUE TIME.
I WANT YOU TO TEACH ME NOW.
YOU'RE STILL A BABY!
WHAT A WUDE FING TO SHAY!
I'M 18!

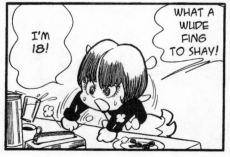

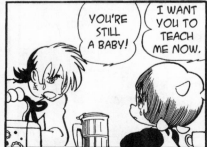

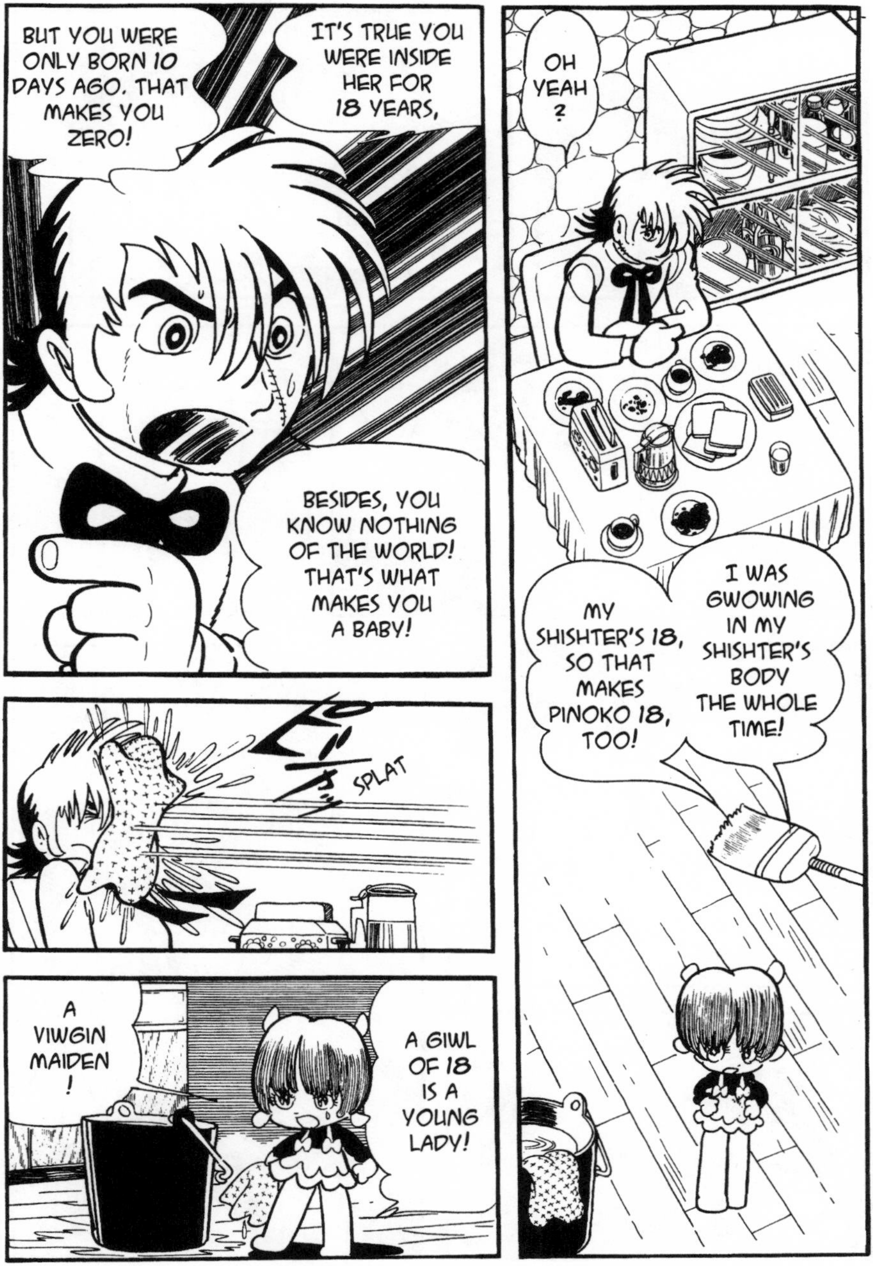
OH YEAH?
I WAS GWOWING IN MY SHISHTER'S BODY THE WHOLE TIME!
MY SHISHTER'S 18, SO THAT MAKES PINOKO 18, TOO!
IT'S TRUE YOU WERE INSIDE HER FOR 18 YEARS,
BUT YOU WERE ONLY BORN 10 DAYS AGO. THAT MAKES YOU ZERO!
BESIDES, YOU KNOW NOTHING OF THE WORLD! THAT'S WHAT MAKES YOU A BABY!
SPLAT
A GIWL OF 18 IS A YOUNG LADY!
A VIWGIN MAIDEN!

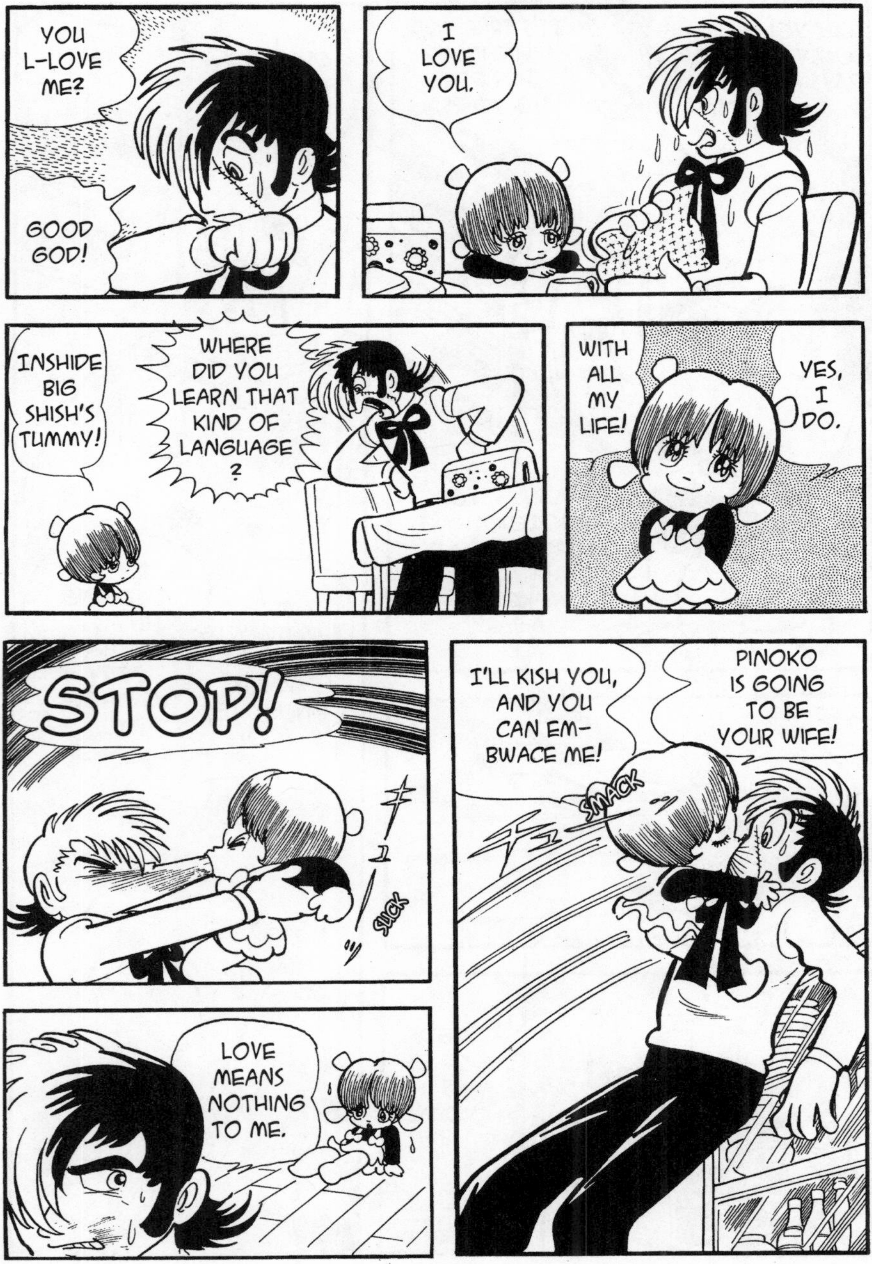

I LOVE YOU.
YOU L-LOVE ME?
GOOD GOD!
YES, I DO.
WITH ALL MY LIFE!
WHERE DID YOU LEARN THAT KIND OF LANGUAGE ?
INSHIDE BIG SHISH'S TUMMY!
PINOKO IS GOING TO BE YOUR WIFE!
I'LL KISH YOU, AND YOU CAN EM-BWACE ME!
SMACK
チュ
STOP!
SLICK
LOVE MEANS NOTHING TO ME.

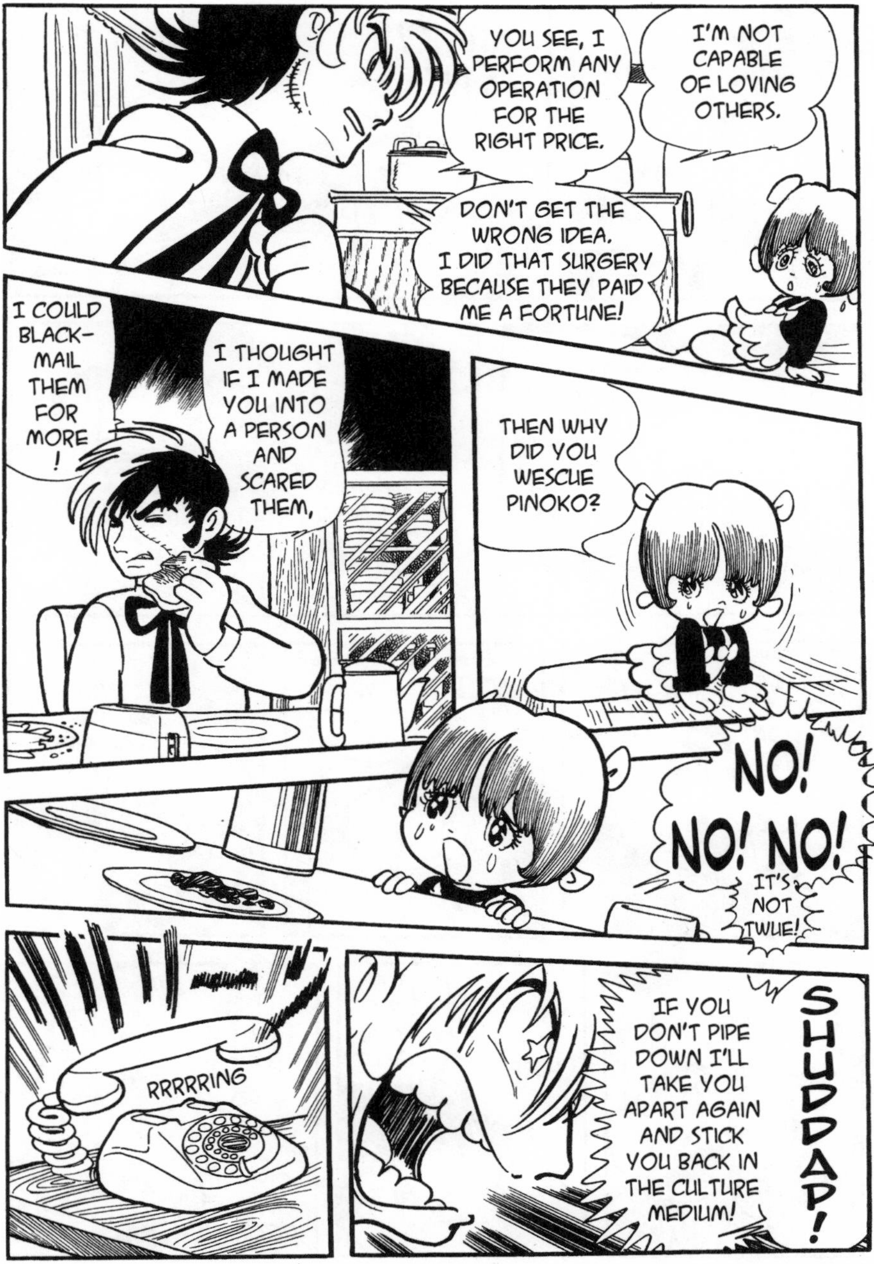
I'M NOT CAPABLE OF LOVING OTHERS.
YOU SEE, I PERFORM ANY OPERATION FOR THE RIGHT PRICE.
DON'T GET THE WRONG IDEA. I DID THAT SURGERY BECAUSE THEY PAID ME A FORTUNE!
THEN WHY DID YOU WESCUE PINOKO?
I THOUGHT IF I MADE YOU INTO A PERSON AND SCARED THEM,
I COULD BLACK-MAIL THEM FOR MORE!
NO! NO! NO!
IT'S NOT TWUE!
SHUDDAP!
IF YOU DON'T PIPE DOWN I'LL TAKE YOU APART AGAIN AND STICK YOU BACK IN THE CULTURE MEDIUM!
RRRRRING

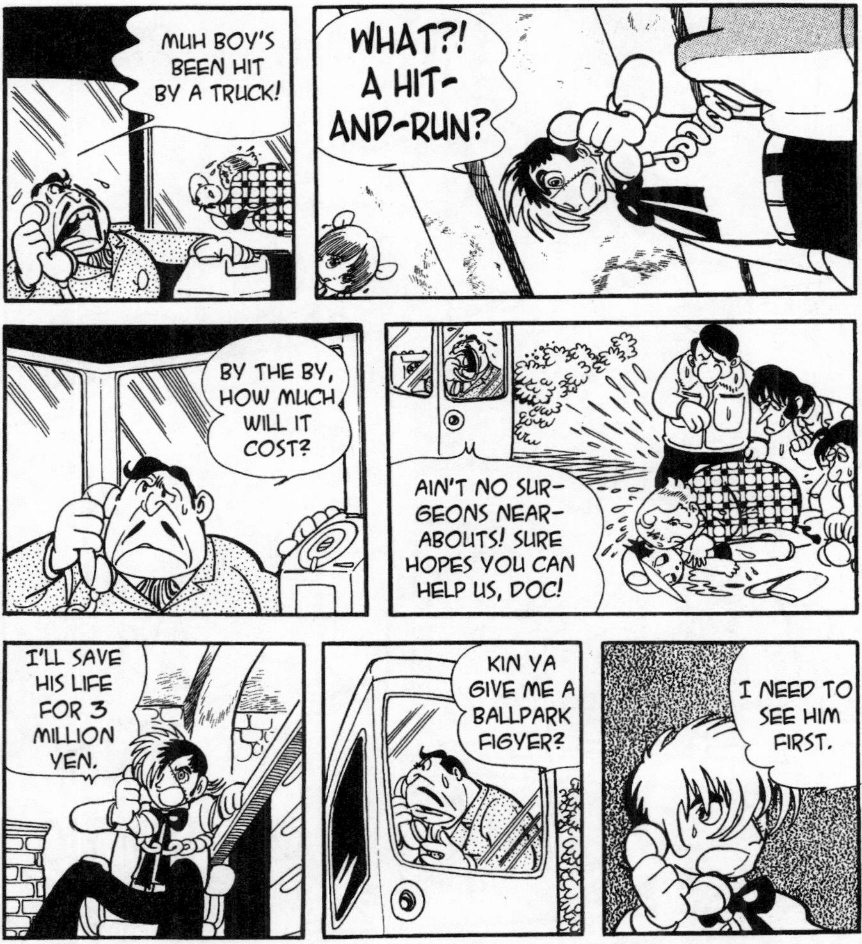

WHAT?! A HIT-AND-RUN?
MUH BOY'S BEEN HIT BY A TRUCK!
AIN'T NO SURGEONS NEARABOUTS! SURE HOPES YOU CAN HELP US, DOC!
BY THE BY, HOW MUCH WILL IT COST?
I NEED TO SEE HIM FIRST.
KIN YA GIVE ME A BALLPARK FIGYER?
I'LL SAVE HIS LIFE FOR 3 MILLION YEN.
THREE MILLYUN
HOW 'BOUT A DISCOUNT, DOC?
THE LIFE OF YOUR CHILD
IS AT STAKE HERE!
BUT THREE MILLYUN!!
JUS' A LIL DISCOUNT?

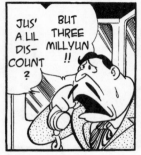

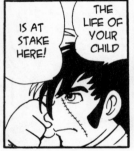

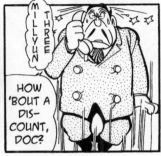

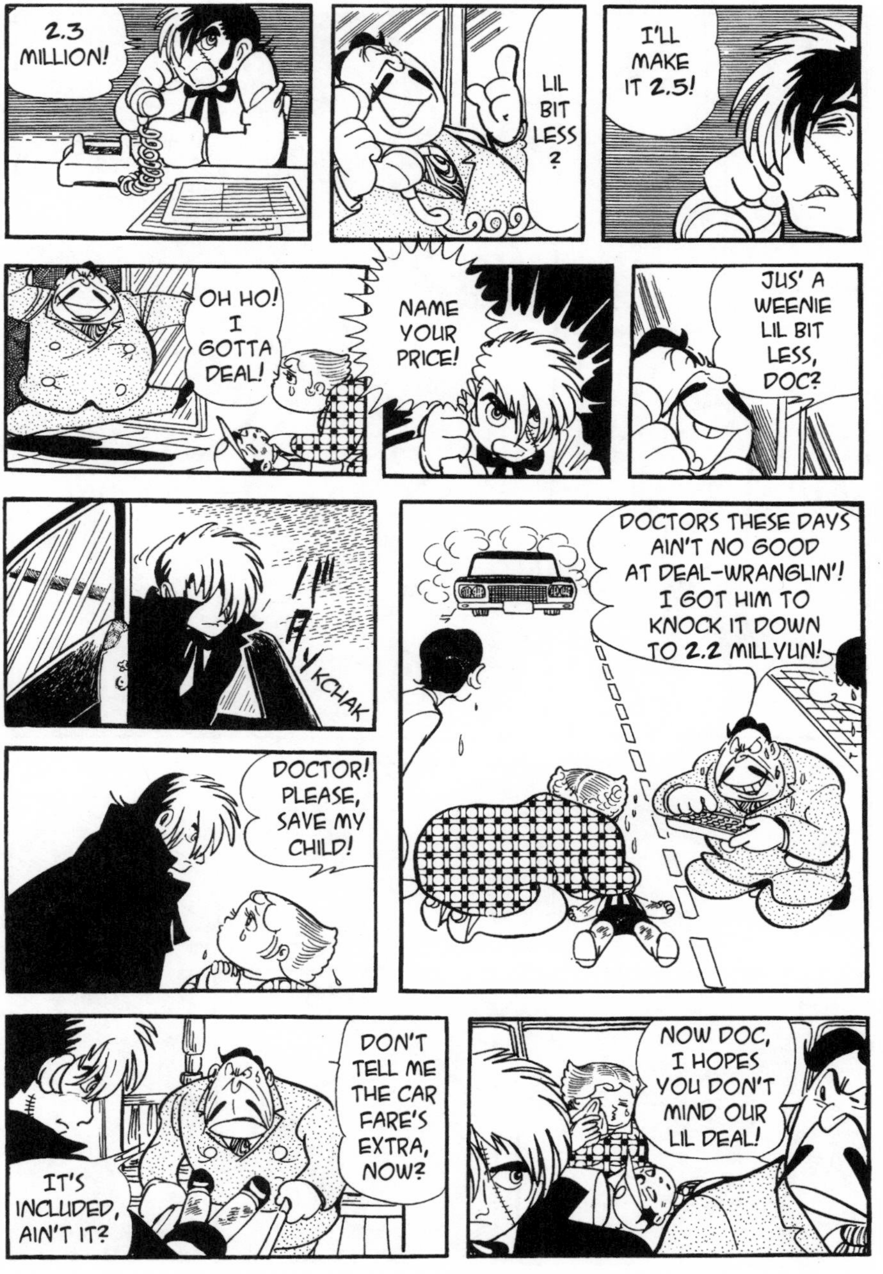
I'LL MAKE IT 2.5!
LIL BIT LESS?
2.3 MILLION!
JUS' A WEENIE LIL BIT LESS, DOC?
NAME YOUR PRICE!
OH HO! I GOTTA DEAL!
DOCTORS THESE DAYS AIN'T NO GOOD AT DEAL-WRANGLIN'! I GOT HIM TO KNOCK IT DOWN TO 2.2 MILLYUN!
KCHAK
DOCTOR! PLEASE, SAVE MY CHILD!
NOW DOC, I HOPES YOU DON'T MIND OUR LIL DEAL!
DON'T TELL ME THE CAR FARE'S EXTRA, NOW?
IT'S INCLUDED, AIN'T IT?

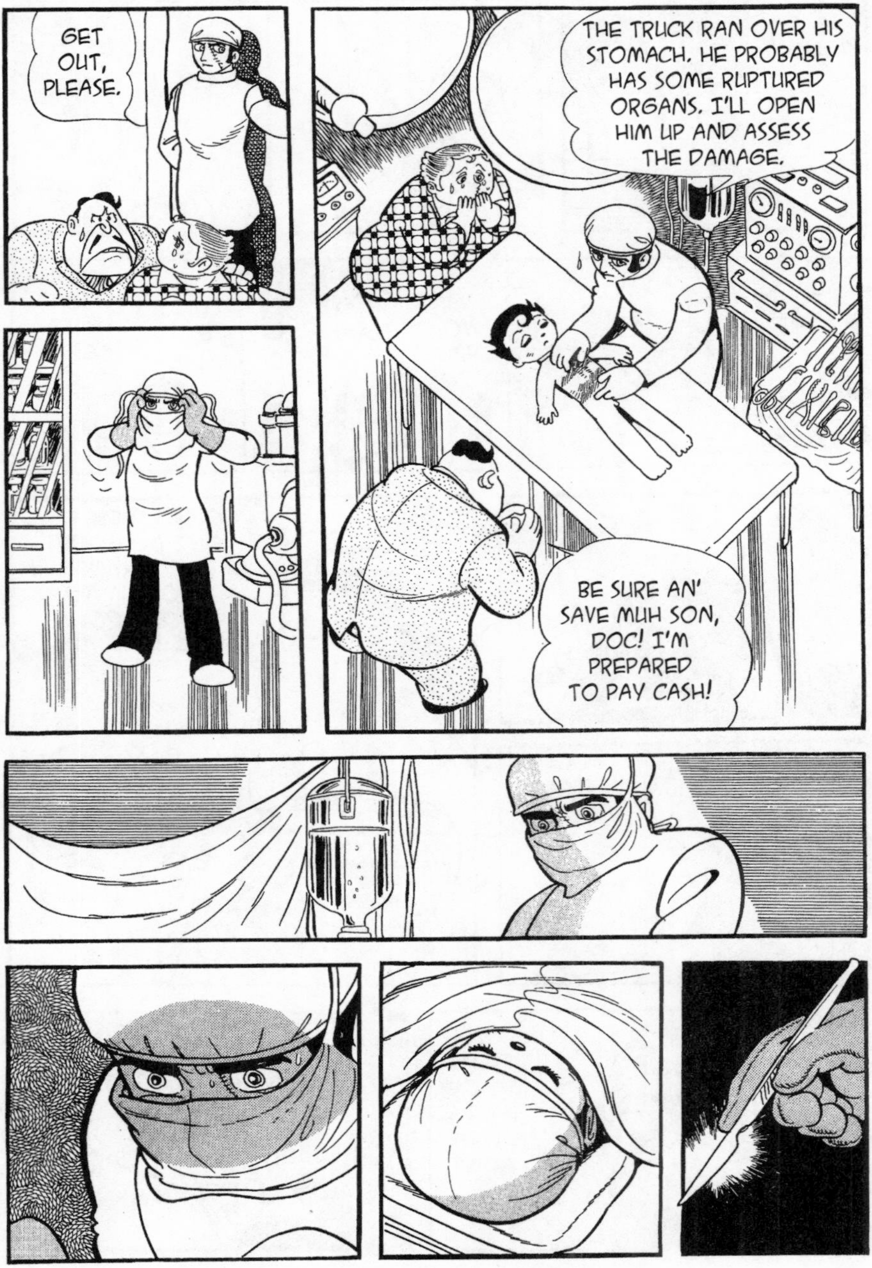
THE TRUCK RAN OVER HIS STOMACH. HE PROBABLY HAS SOME RUPTURED ORGANS. I'LL OPEN HIM UP AND ASSESS THE DAMAGE.
BE SURE AN' SAVE MUH SON, DOC! I'M PREPARED TO PAY CASH!
GET OUT, PLEASE.

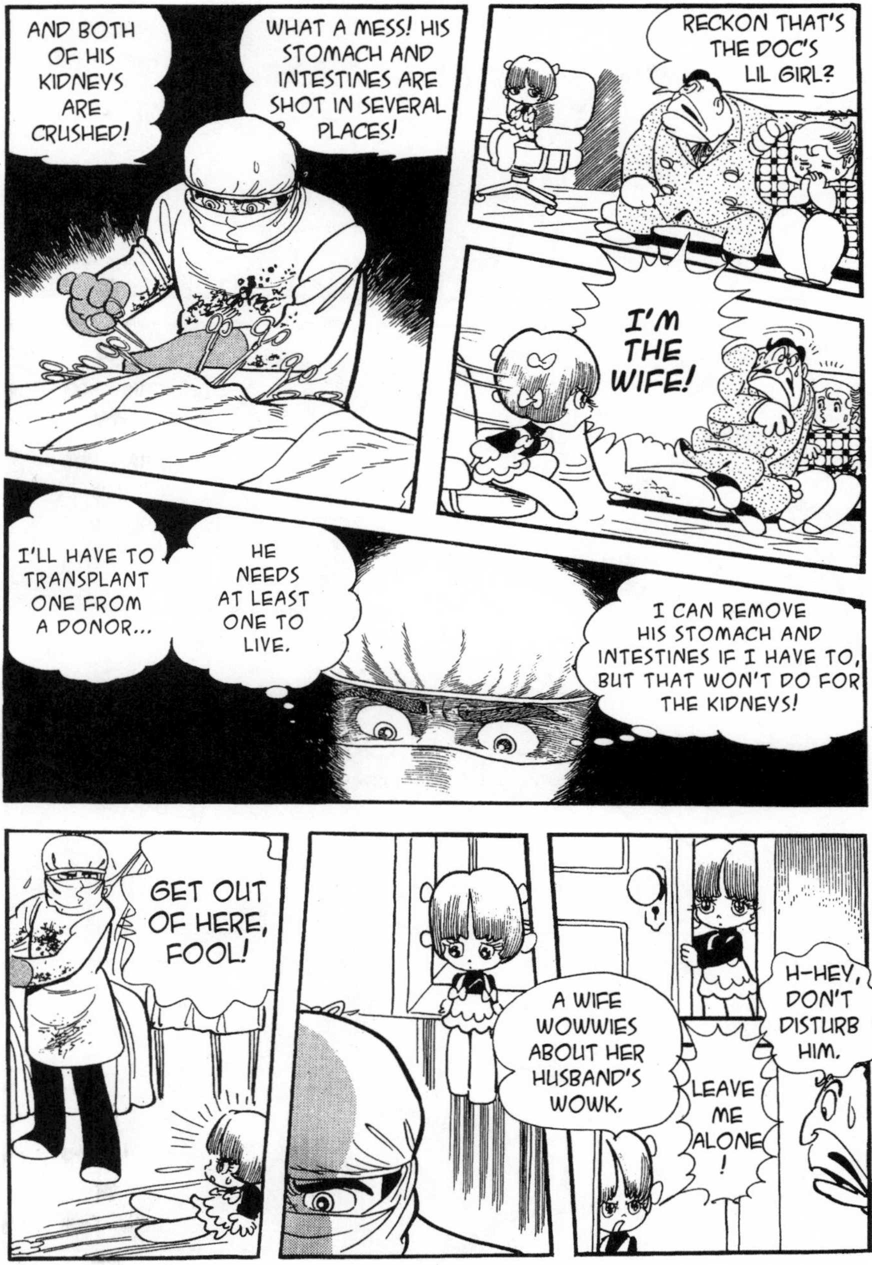
RECKON THAT'S THE DOC'S LIL GIRL?
I'M THE WIFE!
WHAT A MESS! HIS STOMACH AND INTESTINES ARE SHOT IN SEVERAL PLACES!
AND BOTH OF HIS KIDNEYS ARE CRUSHED!
I CAN REMOVE HIS STOMACH AND INTESTINES IF I HAVE TO, BUT THAT WON'T DO FOR THE KIDNEYS!
HE NEEDS AT LEAST ONE TO LIVE.
I'LL HAVE TO TRANSPLANT ONE FROM A DONOR...
H-HEY, DON'T DISTURB HIM.
LEAVE ME ALONE!
A WIFE WOWWIES ABOUT HER HUSBAND'S WOWK.
GET OUT OF HERE, FOOL!

HE NEEDS ANOTHER BODY, WIGHT, DOCTOR?
YES.
YOU CAN USE PINOKO'S BODY.
WHAT?
YOU SHAID YOU'LL TAKE ME APART AND PUT ME BACK IN THAT FING.
I DON'T MIND. GO AHEAD, PLEASE.
IT'S TRUE, THAT WOULD SOLVE EVERY-THING!
A KIDNEY!
YES !!
I NEED YOUR KIDNEY!
OKAY, GO WIGHT AHEAD.

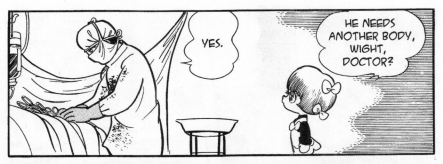

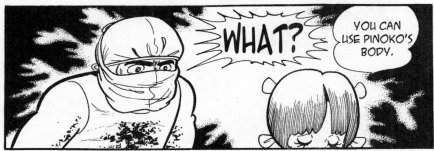

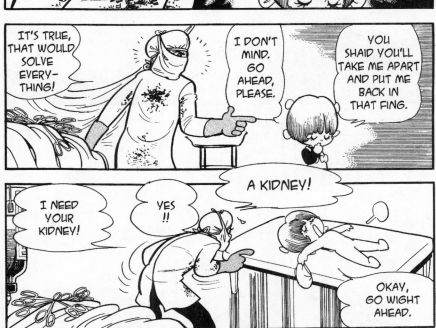

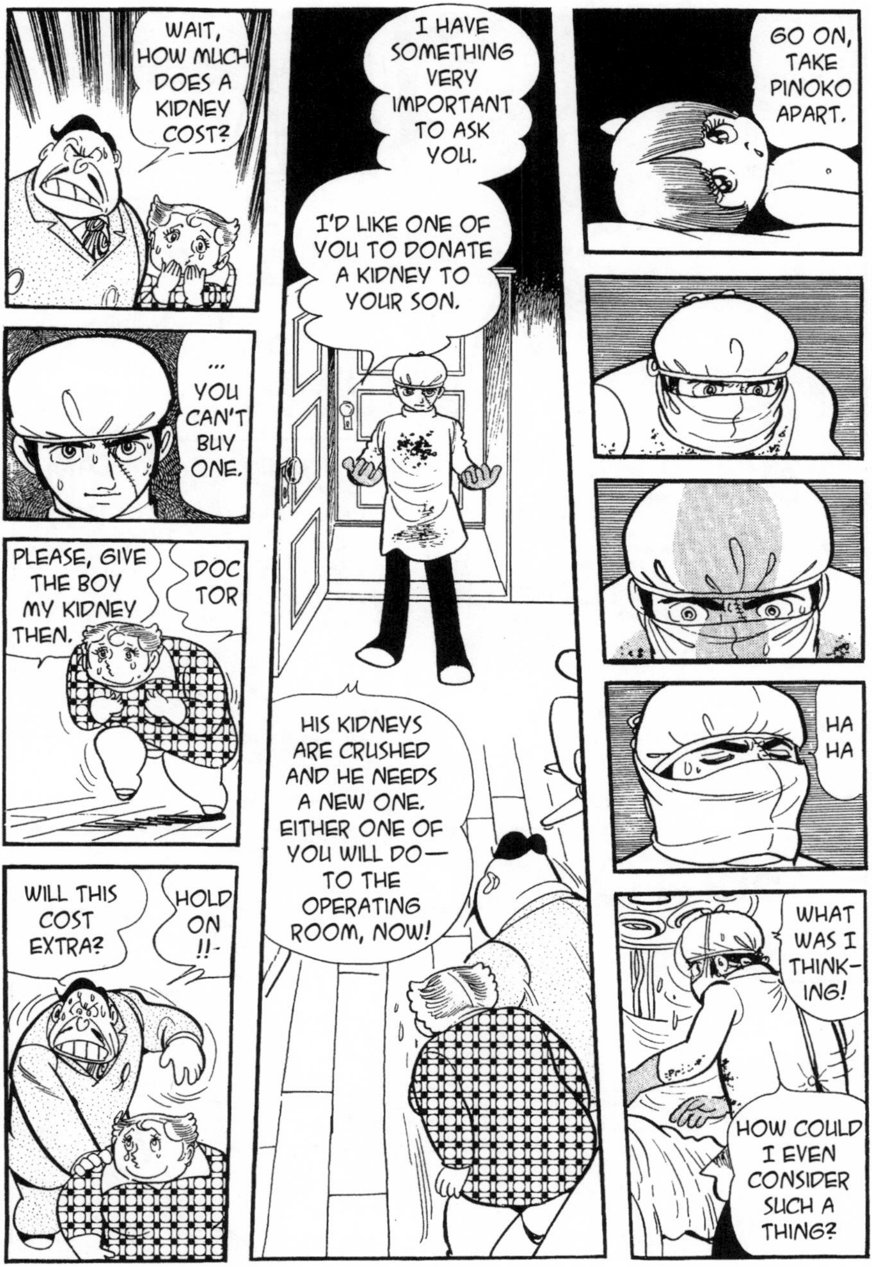
GO ON, TAKE PINOKO APART.
HA HA
WHAT WAS I THINK-ING!
HOW COULD I EVEN CONSIDER SUCH A THING?
I HAVE SOMETHING VERY IMPORTANT TO ASK YOU.
I'D LIKE ONE OF YOU TO DONATE A KIDNEY TO YOUR SON.
HIS KIDNEYS ARE CRUSHED AND HE NEEDS A NEW ONE. EITHER ONE OF YOU WILL DO— TO THE OPERATING ROOM, NOW!
WAIT, HOW MUCH DOES A KIDNEY COST?
... YOU CAN'T BUY ONE.
DOC TOR
PLEASE, GIVE THE BOY MY KIDNEY THEN.
HOLD ON !!-
WILL THIS COST EXTRA?

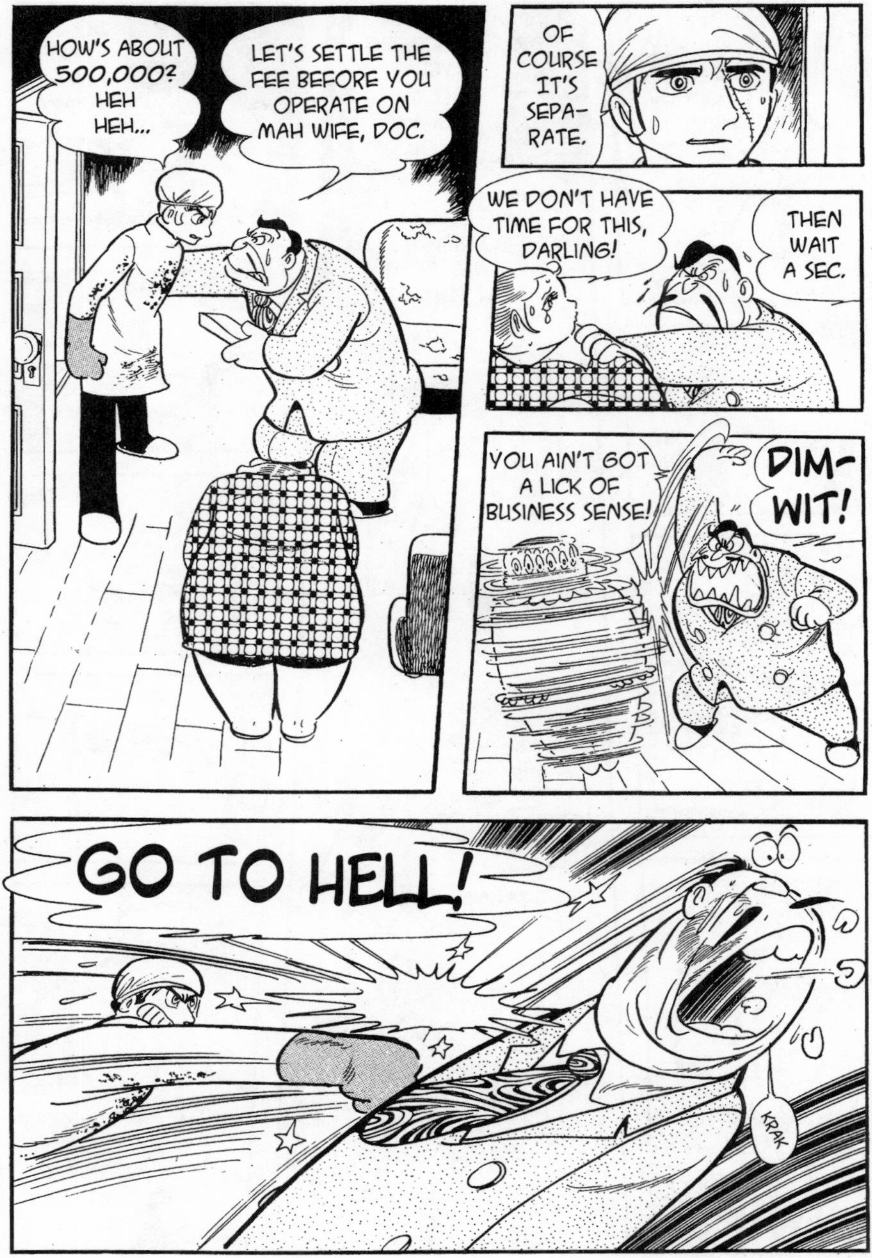
OF COURSE IT'S SEPA-RATE.
THEN WAIT A SEC.
WE DON'T HAVE TIME FOR THIS, DARLING!
DIM-WIT!
YOU AIN'T GOT A LICK OF BUSINESS SENSE!
LET'S SETTLE THE FEE BEFORE YOU OPERATE ON MAH WIFE, DOC.
HOW'S ABOUT 500,000? HEH HEH...
GO TO HELL!
KRAK

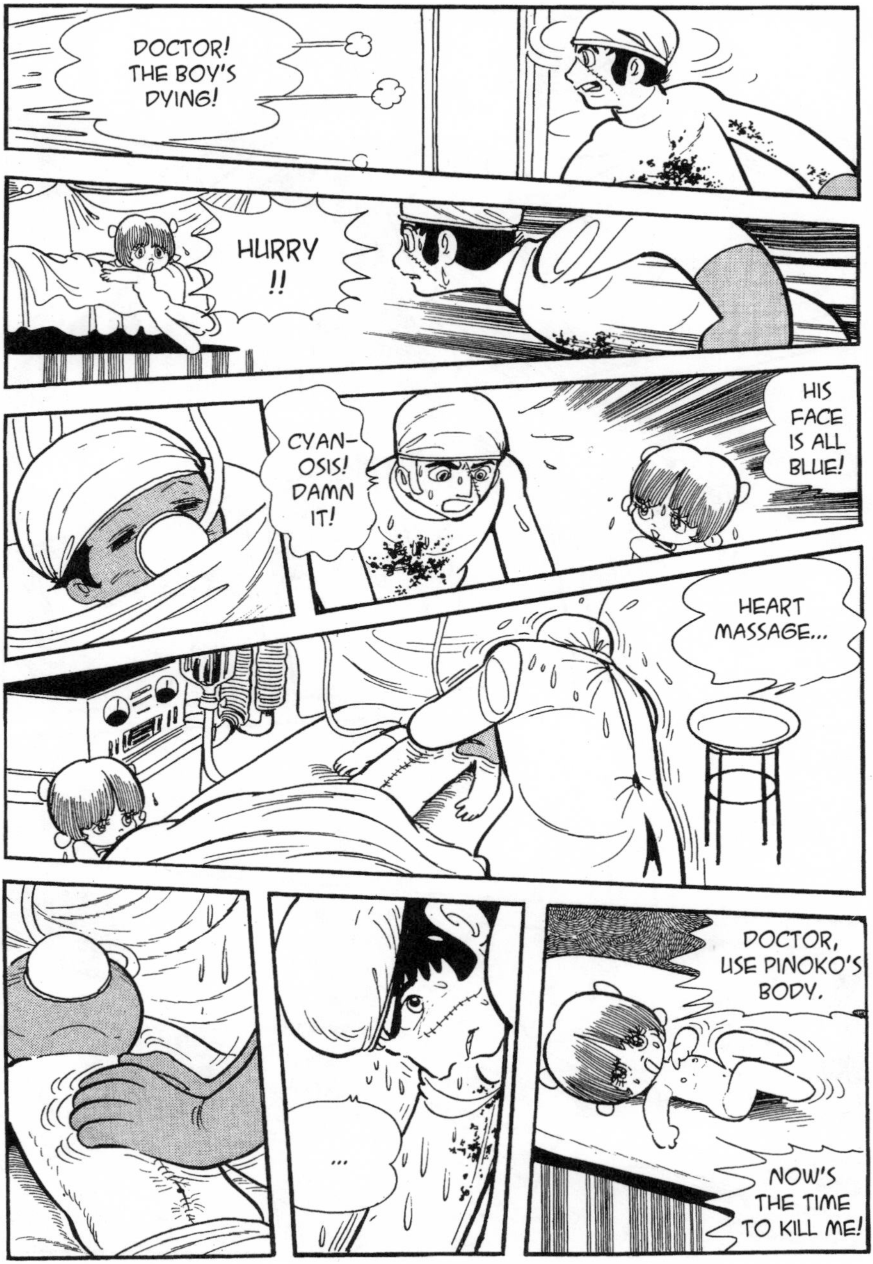

DOCTOR! THE BOY'S DYING!
HURRY !!
HIS FACE IS ALL BLUE!
CYAN-OSIS! DAMN IT!
HEART MASSAGE...
DOCTOR, USE PINOKO'S BODY.
NOW'S THE TIME TO KILL ME!
...

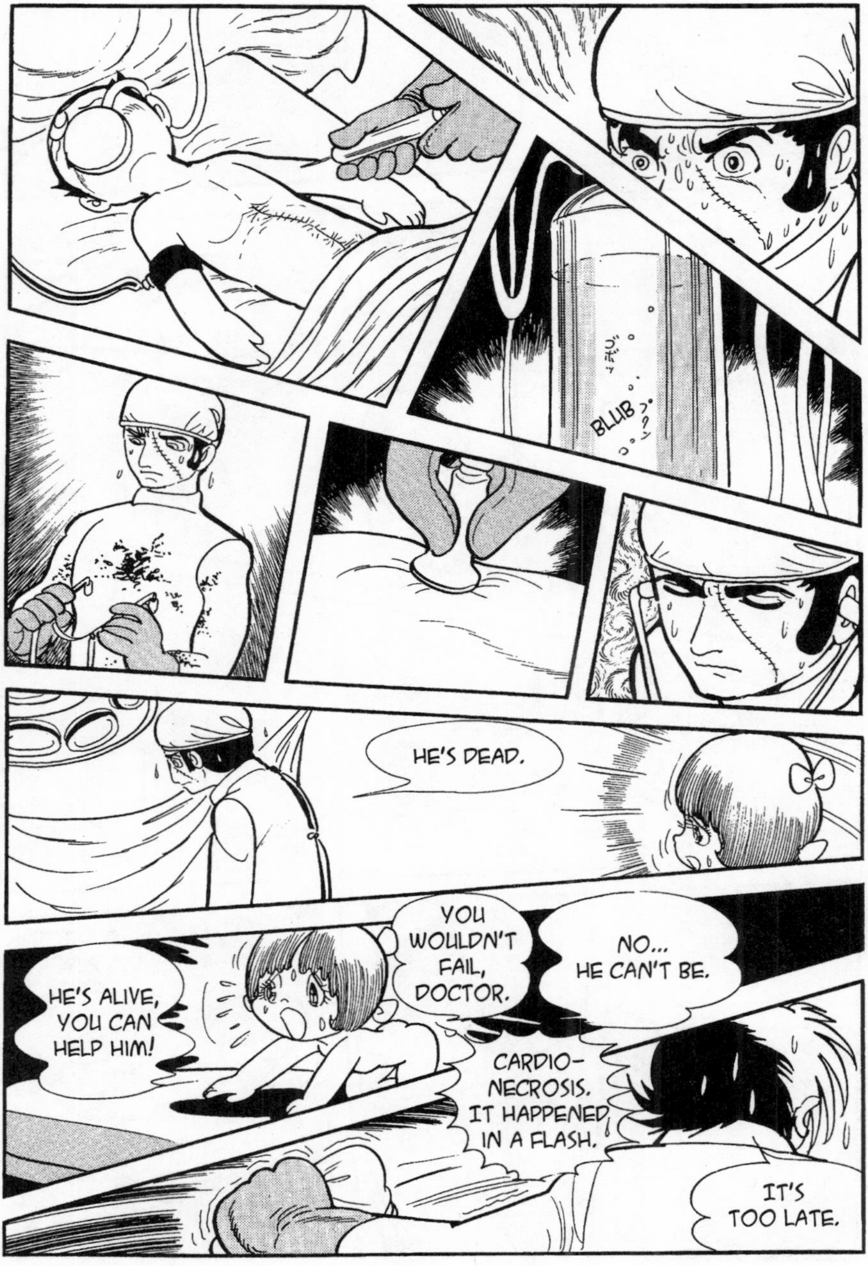
BLUB
HE'S DEAD.
NO... HE CAN'T BE.
YOU WOULDN'T FAIL, DOCTOR.
HE'S ALIVE, YOU CAN HELP HIM!
CARDIO-NECROSIS. IT HAPPENED IN A FLASH.
IT'S TOO LATE.

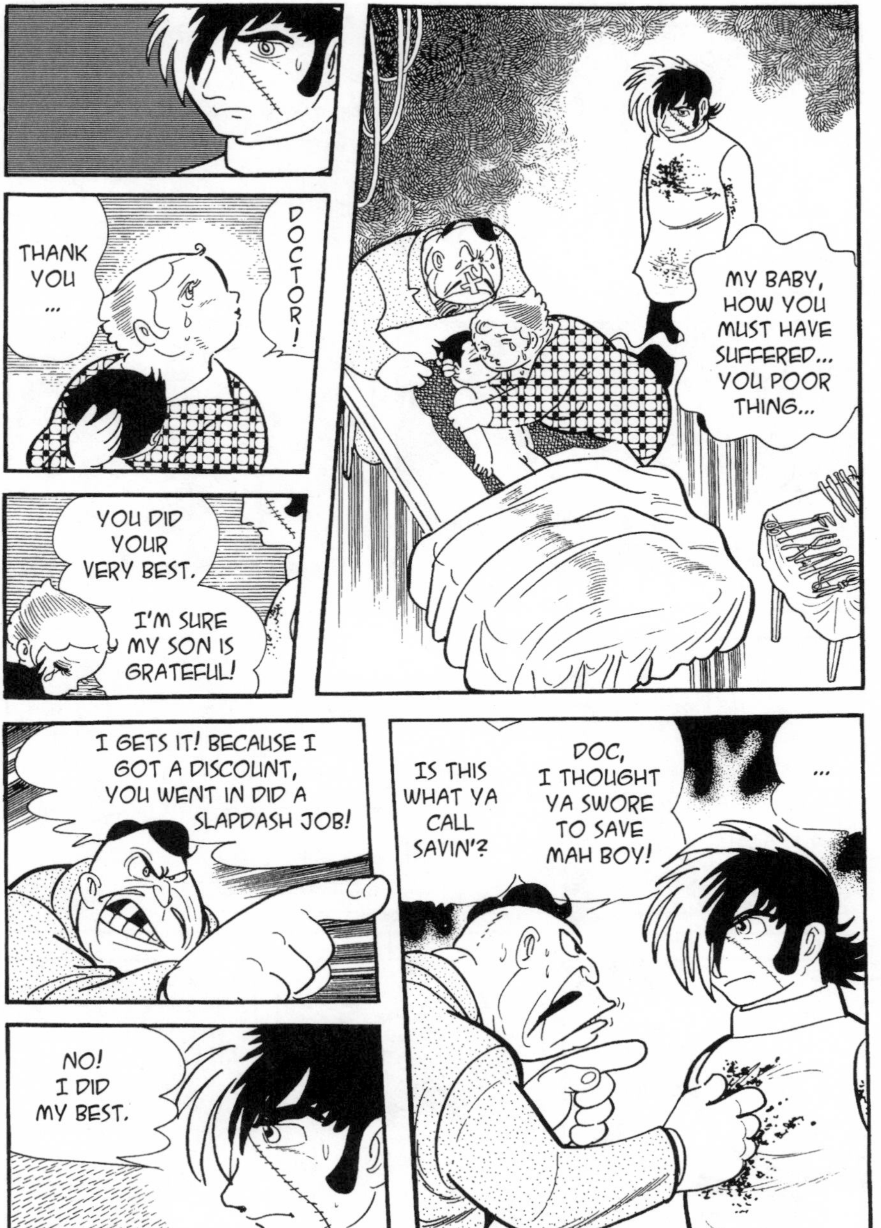
MY BABY, HOW YOU MUST HAVE SUFFERED... YOU POOR THING...
DOCTOR!
THANK YOU ...
YOU DID YOUR VERY BEST.
I'M SURE MY SON IS GRATEFUL!
...
DOC, I THOUGHT YA SWORE TO SAVE MAH BOY!
IS THIS WHAT YA CALL SAVIN'?
I GETS IT! BECAUSE I GOT A DISCOUNT, YOU WENT IN DID A SLAPDASH JOB!
NO! I DID MY BEST.

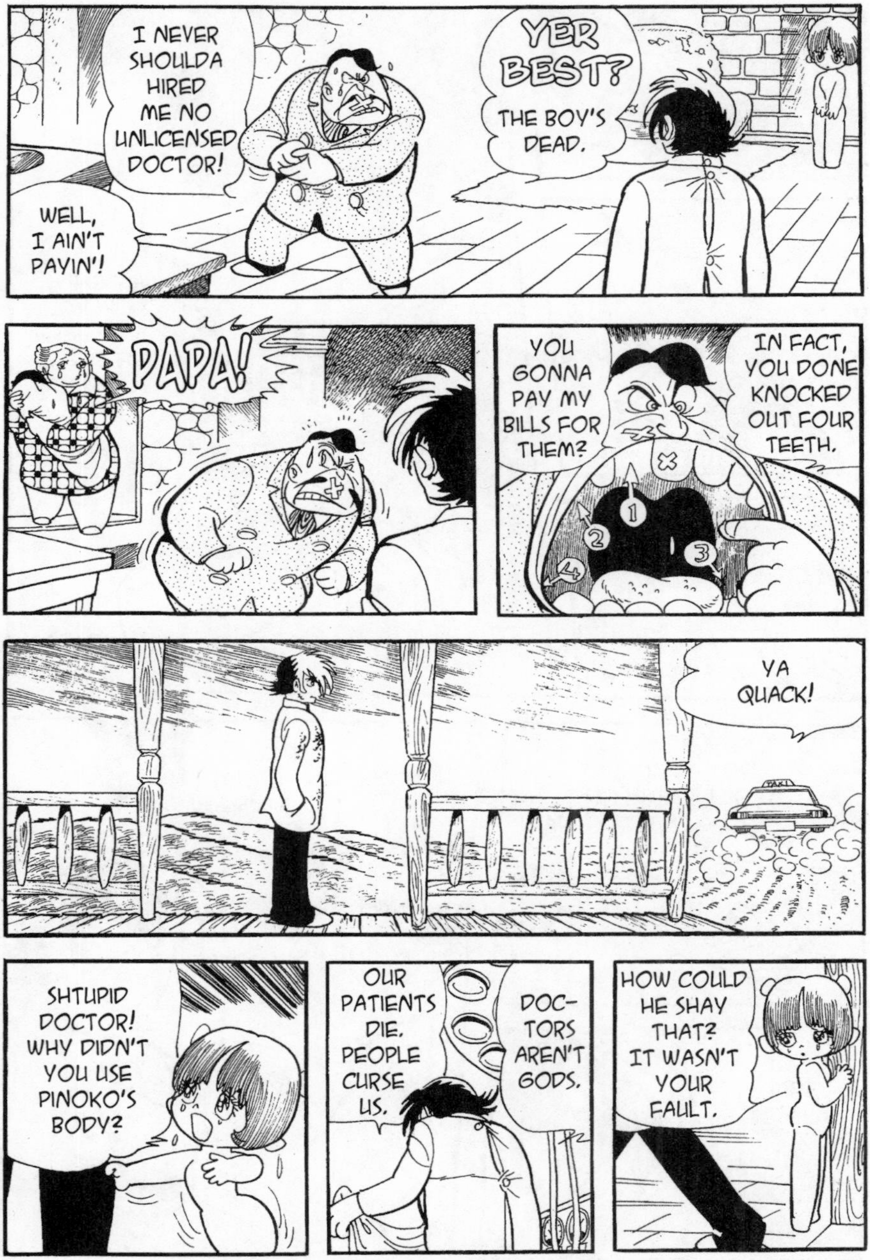
YER BEST?
THE BOY'S DEAD.
I NEVER SHOULDA HIRED ME NO UNLICENSED DOCTOR!
WELL, I AIN'T PAYIN'!
IN FACT, YOU DONE KNOCKED OUT FOUR TEETH.
YOU GONNA PAY MY BILLS FOR THEM?
PAPA!
YA QUACK!
TAXI
HOW COULD HE SHAY THAT? IT WASN'T YOUR FAULT.
DOC-TORS AREN'T GODS.
OUR PATIENTS DIE, PEOPLE CURSE US.
SHTUPID DOCTOR! WHY DIDN'T YOU USE PINOKO'S BODY?

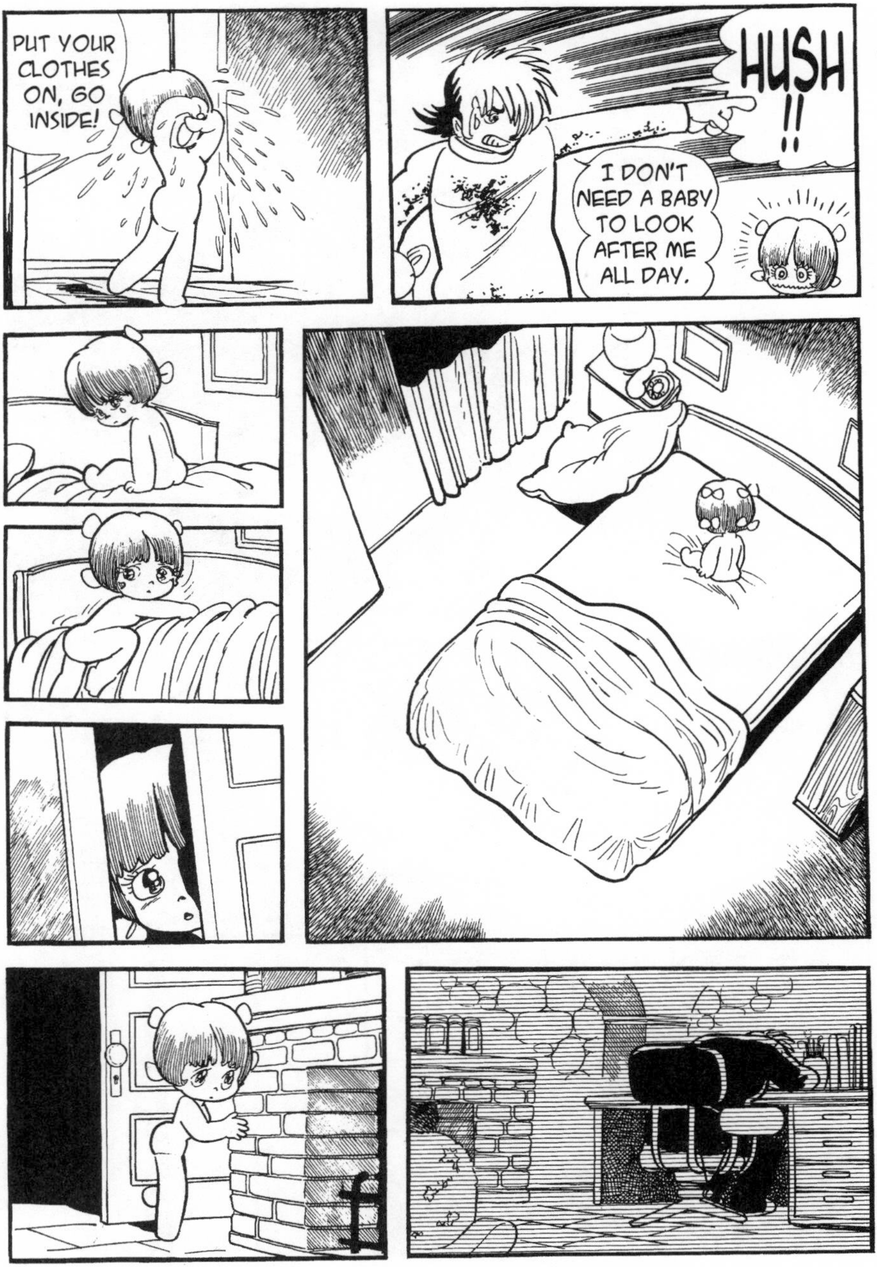
HUSH !!
I DON'T NEED A BABY TO LOOK AFTER ME ALL DAY.
PUT YOUR CLOTHES ON, GO INSIDE!

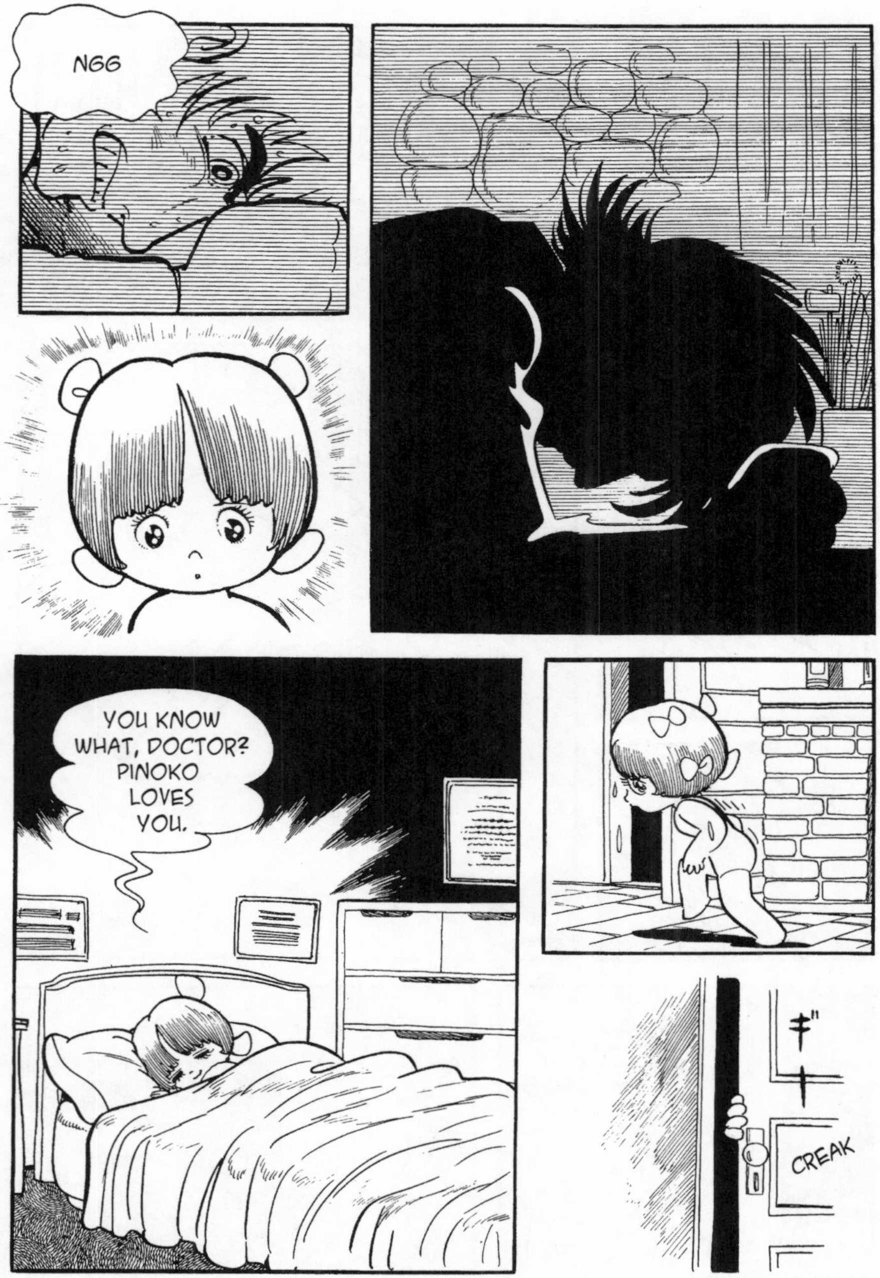
NGG
ギ
CREAK
YOU KNOW WHAT, DOCTOR? PINOKO LOVES YOU.

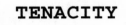

TENACITY

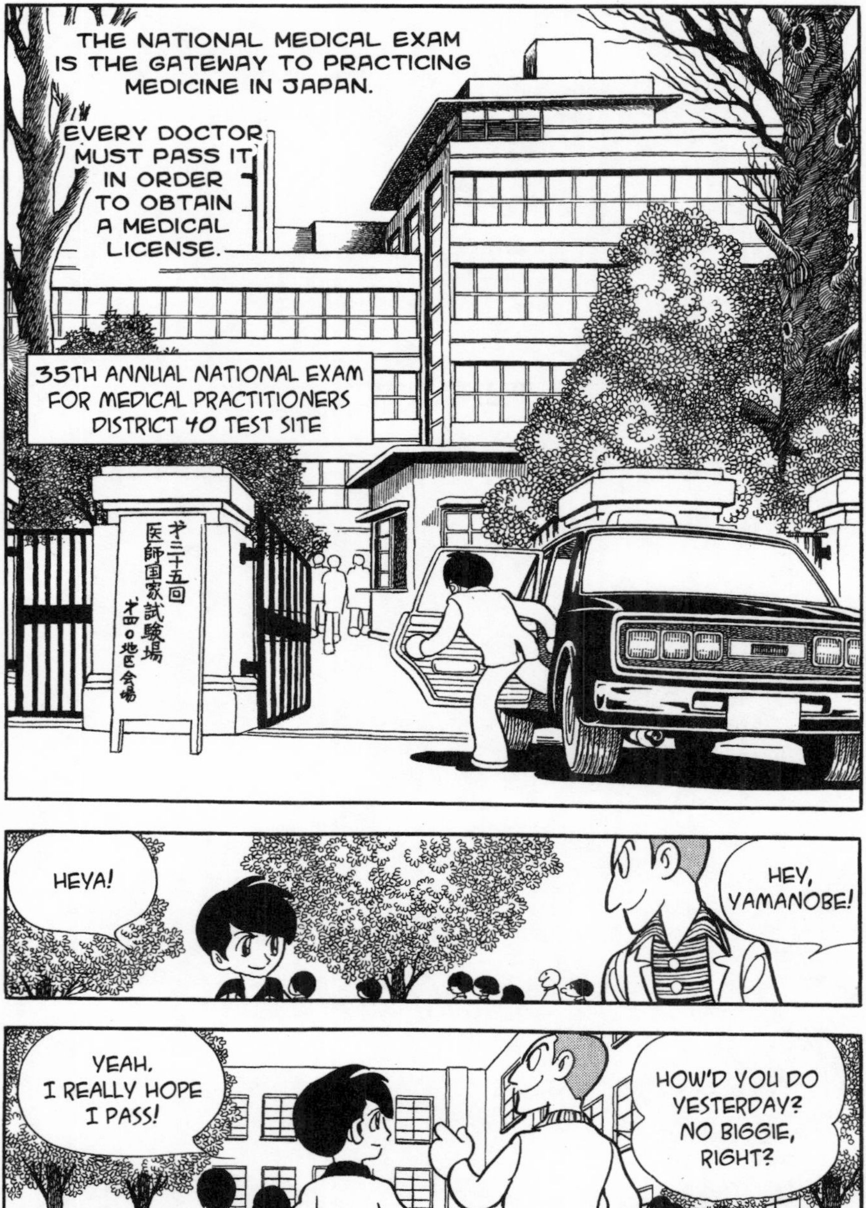
THE NATIONAL MEDICAL EXAM IS THE GATEWAY TO PRACTICING MEDICINE IN JAPAN.
EVERY DOCTOR MUST PASS IT IN ORDER TO OBTAIN A MEDICAL LICENSE.
35TH ANNUAL NATIONAL EXAM FOR MEDICAL PRACTITIONERS DISTRICT 40 TEST SITE
才三十五回 医師国家試験場 才四0地区会場
HEY, YAMANOBE!
HEYA!
HOW'D YOU DO YESTERDAY? NO BIGGIE, RIGHT?
YEAH, I REALLY HOPE I PASS!

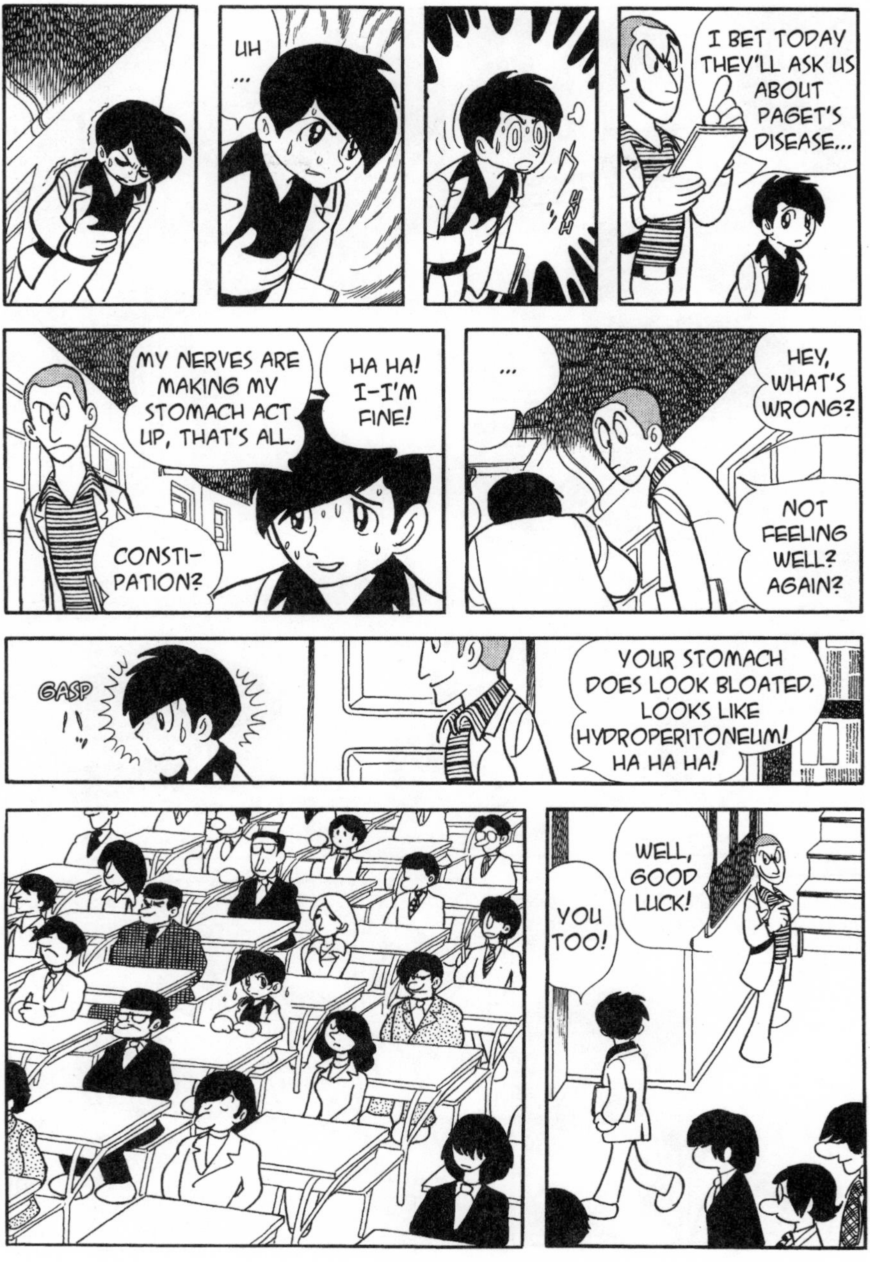
I BET TODAY THEY'LL ASK US ABOUT PAGET'S DISEASE...
UH ...
HEY, WHAT'S WRONG?
...
NOT FEELING WELL? AGAIN?
HA HA! I-I'M FINE!
MY NERVES ARE MAKING MY STOMACH ACT UP, THAT'S ALL.
CONSTI-PATION?
YOUR STOMACH DOES LOOK BLOATED. LOOKS LIKE HYDROPERITONEUM! HA HA HA!
GASP !!
WELL, GOOD LUCK!
YOU TOO!

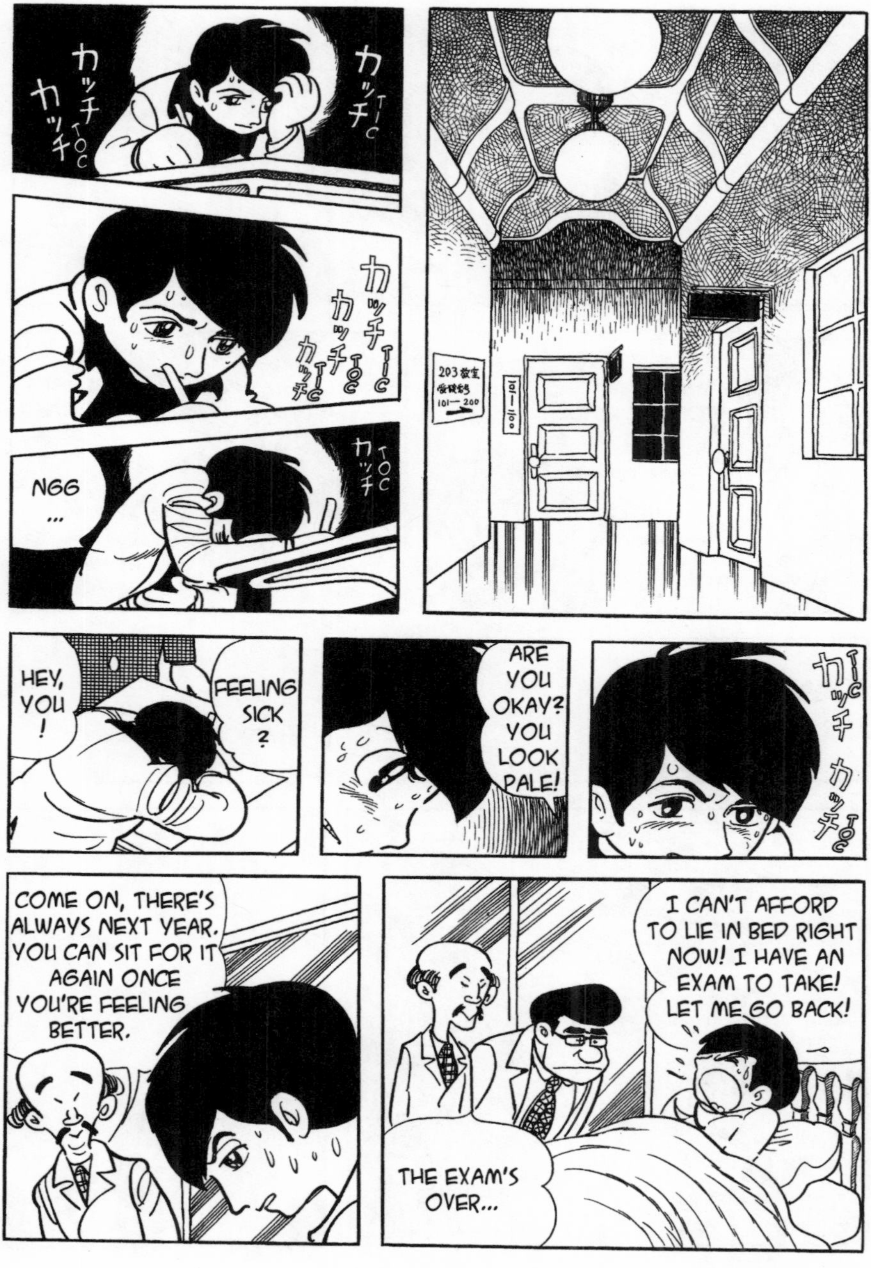
カッチ TIC
カッチ TOC カッチ
カッチ TIC
カッチ TOC
カッチ TIC
カッチ TOC
NGG ...
カッチ TIC
カッチ TOC
ARE YOU OKAY? YOU LOOK PALE!
FEELING SICK?
HEY, YOU!
I CAN'T AFFORD TO LIE IN BED RIGHT NOW! I HAVE AN EXAM TO TAKE! LET ME GO BACK!
THE EXAM'S OVER...
COME ON, THERE'S ALWAYS NEXT YEAR. YOU CAN SIT FOR IT AGAIN ONCE YOU'RE FEELING BETTER.

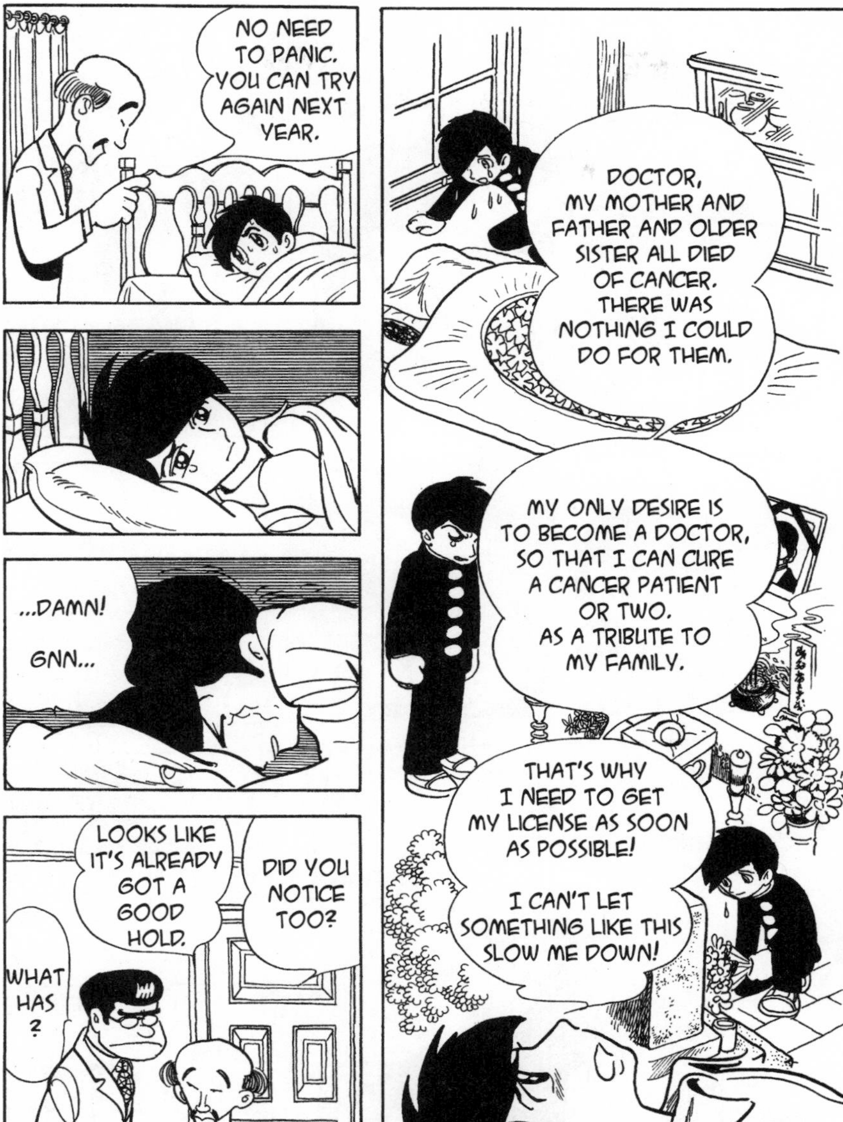
DOCTOR, MY MOTHER AND FATHER AND OLDER SISTER ALL DIED OF CANCER. THERE WAS NOTHING I COULD DO FOR THEM.
MY ONLY DESIRE IS TO BECOME A DOCTOR, SO THAT I CAN CURE A CANCER PATIENT OR TWO. AS A TRIBUTE TO MY FAMILY.
THAT'S WHY I NEED TO GET MY LICENSE AS SOON AS POSSIBLE!
I CAN'T LET SOMETHING LIKE THIS SLOW ME DOWN!
NO NEED TO PANIC. YOU CAN TRY AGAIN NEXT YEAR.
...DAMN!
GNN...
DID YOU NOTICE TOO?
LOOKS LIKE IT'S ALREADY GOT A GOOD HOLD.
WHAT HAS ?
CANCER, OF COURSE!

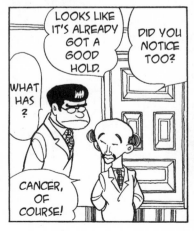

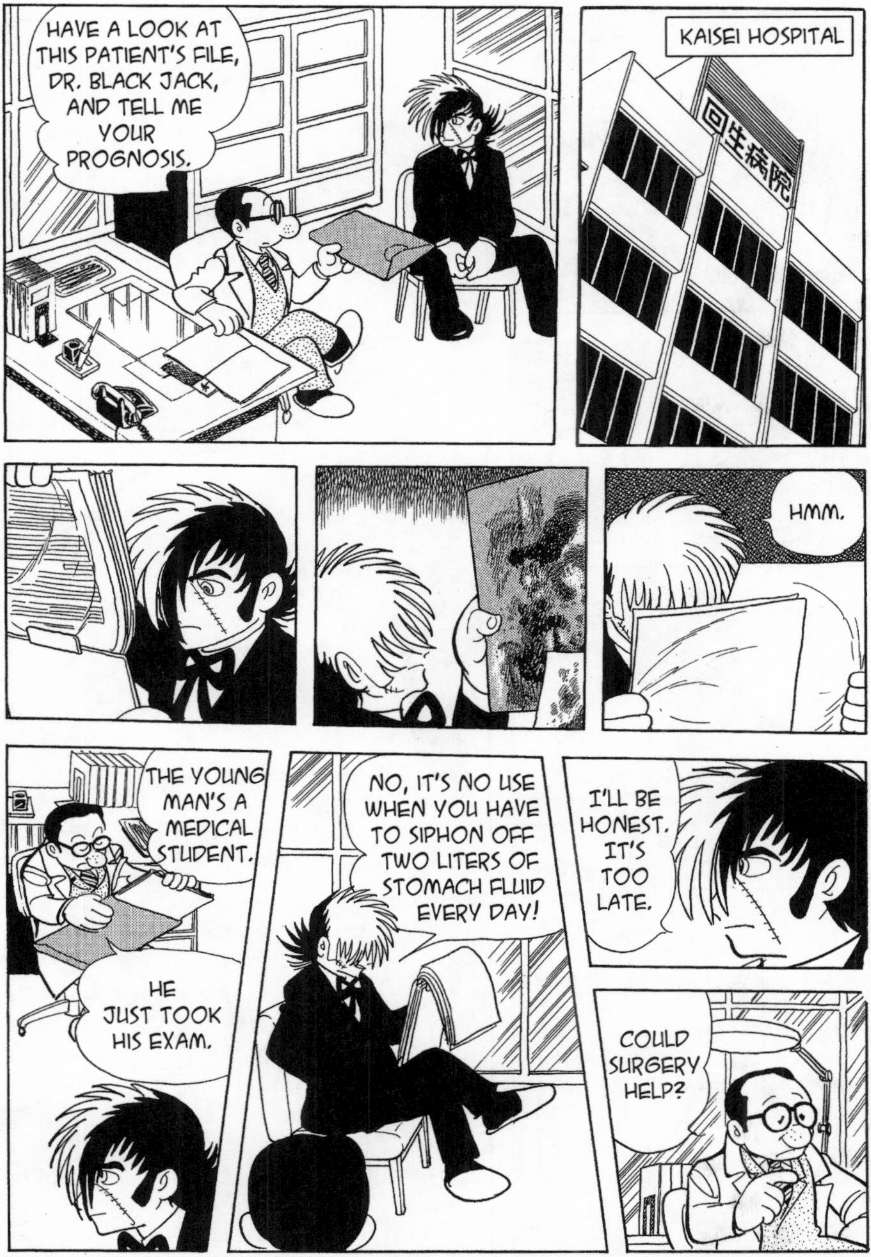
KAISEI HOSPITAL
回生病院
HAVE A LOOK AT THIS PATIENT'S FILE, DR. BLACK JACK, AND TELL ME YOUR PROGNOSIS.
HMM.
I'LL BE HONEST. IT'S TOO LATE.
COULD SURGERY HELP?
NO, IT'S NO USE WHEN YOU HAVE TO SIPHON OFF TWO LITERS OF STOMACH FLUID EVERY DAY!
THE YOUNG MAN'S A MEDICAL STUDENT.
HE JUST TOOK HIS EXAM.

NOTE: THOUGH SPELLED DIFFERENTLY, "KAISEI" IS A GENERAL HOSPITAL OF NOTE IN TEZUKA'S NATIVE KANSAI REGION.

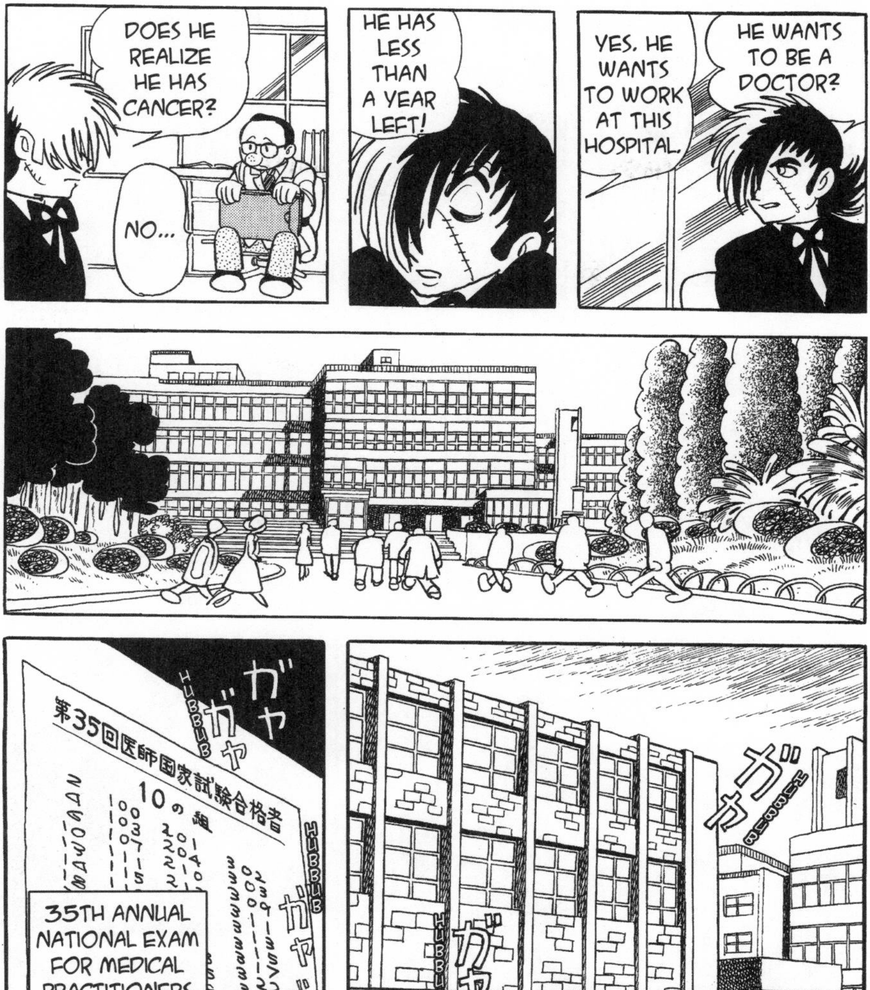
HE WANTS TO BE A DOCTOR?
YES. HE WANTS TO WORK AT THIS HOSPITAL.
HE HAS LESS THAN A YEAR LEFT!
DOES HE REALIZE HE HAS CANCER?
NO...
ガヤ
HUBBUB
ガヤ
HUBBUB
ガヤ
HUBBUB
ガヤ
HUBBUB
ガヤ
HUBBUB
ガヤガヤ
HUBBUB
ガヤガヤ
第35回医師国家試験合格者
10の組
35TH ANNUAL NATIONAL EXAM FOR MEDICAL PRACTITIONERS SUCCESSFUL CANDIDATES GROUP 10

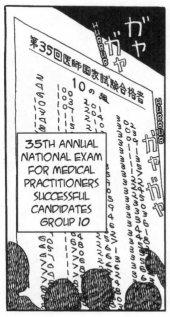

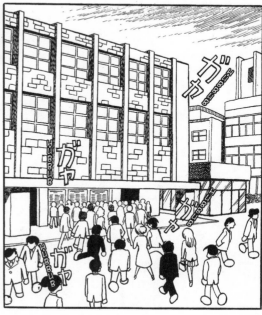

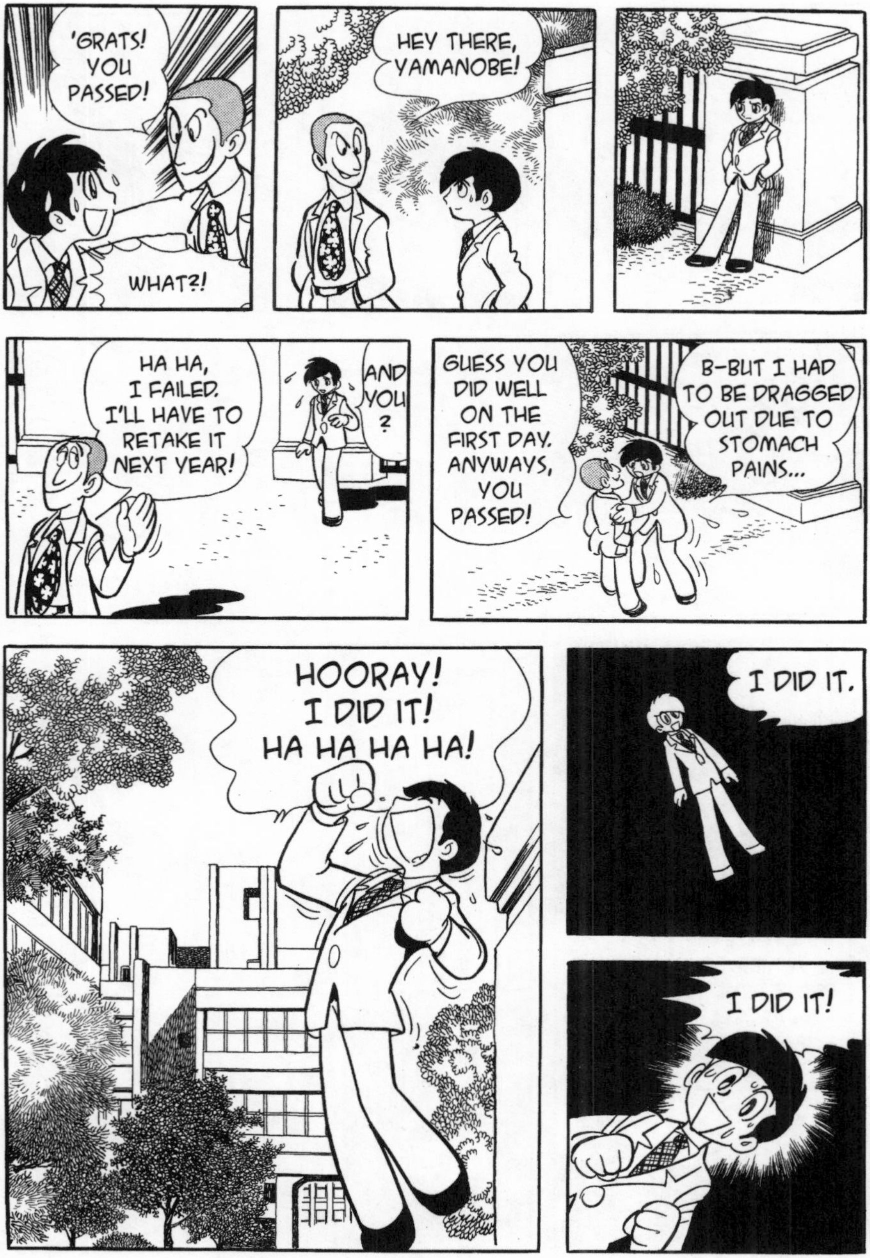
HEY THERE, YAMANOBE!
'GRATS! YOU PASSED!
WHAT?!
B-BUT I HAD TO BE DRAGGED OUT DUE TO STOMACH PAINS...
GUESS YOU DID WELL ON THE FIRST DAY. ANYWAYS, YOU PASSED!
AND YOU ?
HA HA, I FAILED. I'LL HAVE TO RETAKE IT NEXT YEAR!
I DID IT.
I DID IT!
HOORAY! I DID IT! HA HA HA HA!

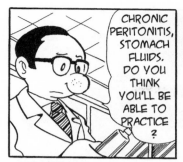

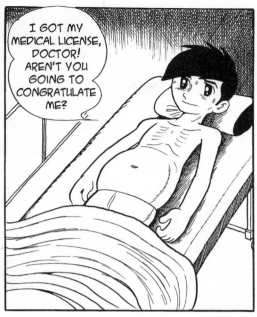

I GOT MY MEDICAL LICENSE, DOCTOR! AREN'T YOU GOING TO CONGRATULATE ME?
CHRONIC PERITONITIS, STOMACH FLUIDS. DO YOU THINK YOU'LL BE ABLE TO PRACTICE?
I WILL! I HAVE TO!
I'LL BE BLUNT. YOU CAN'T.
IN YOUR CONDITION, YOU WON'T BE ABLE TO CURE A SINGLE PATIENT.
TIME TO THROW IN THE TOWEL.
HOW CAN YOU SAY THAT WHEN I'VE JUST GOTTEN MY LICENSE?!
AS THE OLD SAYING GOES, PHYSICIAN, HEAL THY-SELF!
YOU'RE GRAVELY ILL. YOU THINK A DOCTOR IN YOUR CONDI-TION...
CAN EARN HIS WARDS' TRUST?

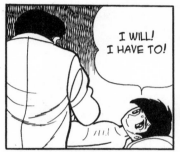

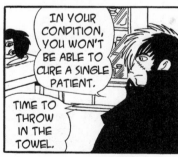

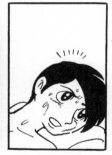

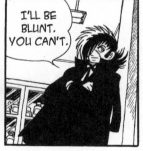

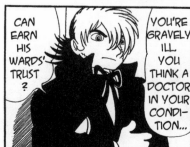

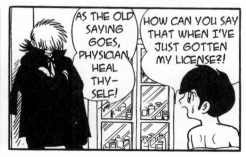

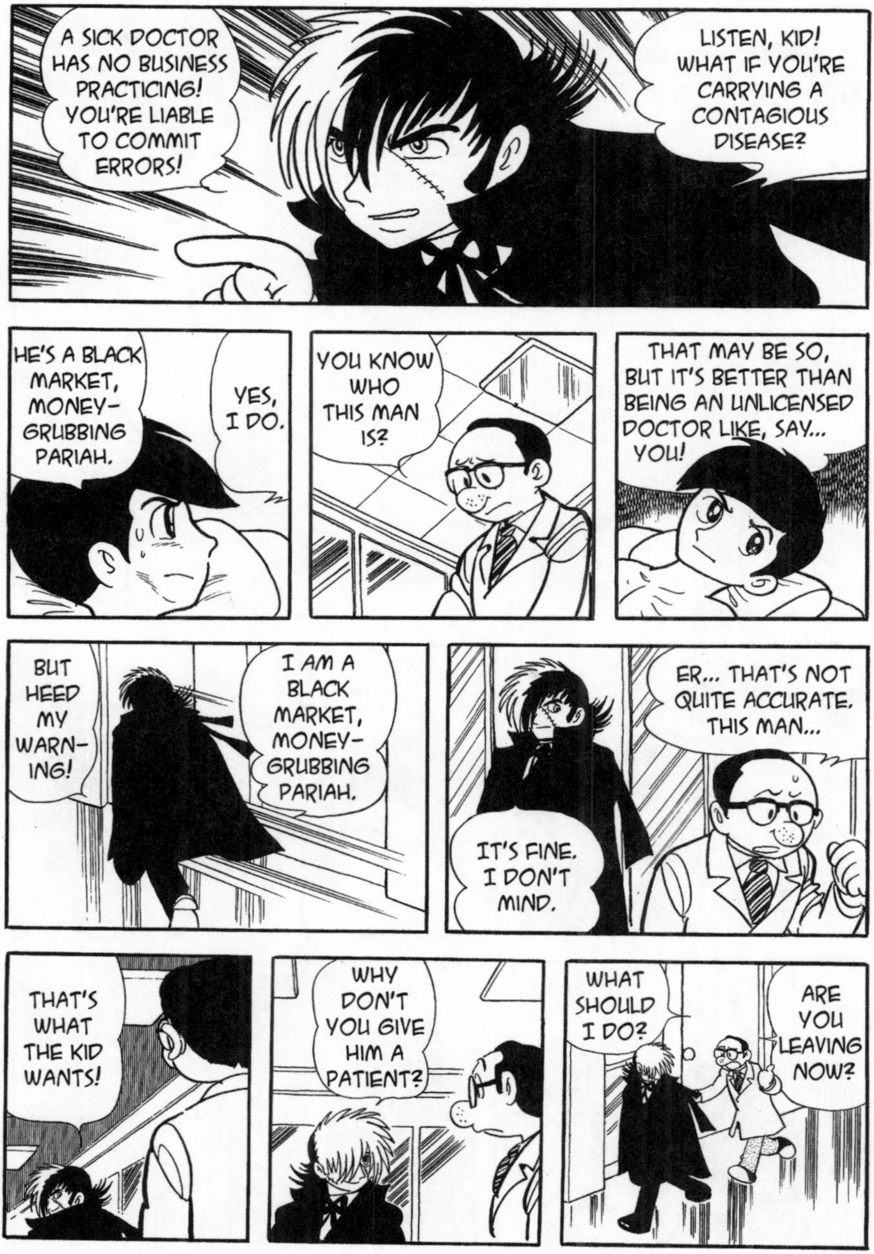
LISTEN, KID! WHAT IF YOU'RE CARRYING A CONTAGIOUS DISEASE?
A SICK DOCTOR HAS NO BUSINESS PRACTICING! YOU'RE LIABLE TO COMMIT ERRORS!
THAT MAY BE SO, BUT IT'S BETTER THAN BEING AN UNLICENSED DOCTOR LIKE, SAY... YOU!
YOU KNOW WHO THIS MAN IS?
YES, I DO.
HE'S A BLACK MARKET, MONEY-GRUBBING PARIAH.
ER... THAT'S NOT QUITE ACCURATE. THIS MAN...
IT'S FINE. I DON'T MIND.
I AM A BLACK MARKET, MONEY-GRUBBING PARIAH.
BUT HEED MY WARN-ING!
ARE YOU LEAVING NOW?
WHAT SHOULD I DO?
WHY DON'T YOU GIVE HIM A PATIENT?
THAT'S WHAT THE KID WANTS!

YOUR PATIENT IS INSIDE THIS ROOM.
WHAT IS THIS ?!
OOPS! SORRY.
HOW'S THE PAIN?
THIS IS DR. YAMANOBE. HE'LL BE YOUR DOCTOR FROM NOW ON.
PLEASED TO MEET YOU, DOCTOR.
AH... UH... PLEASED TO MEET YOU.
W-WELL, LET ME EXAMINE YOU!

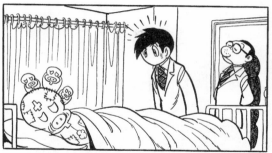

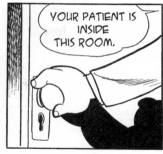

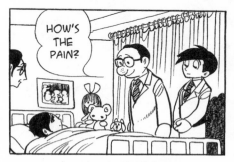

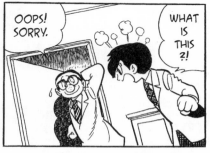

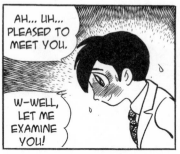

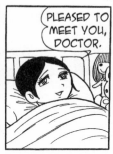

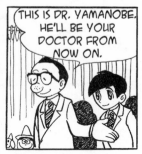

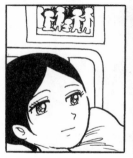

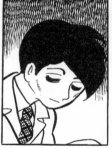

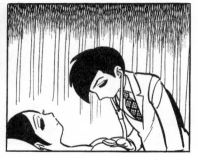

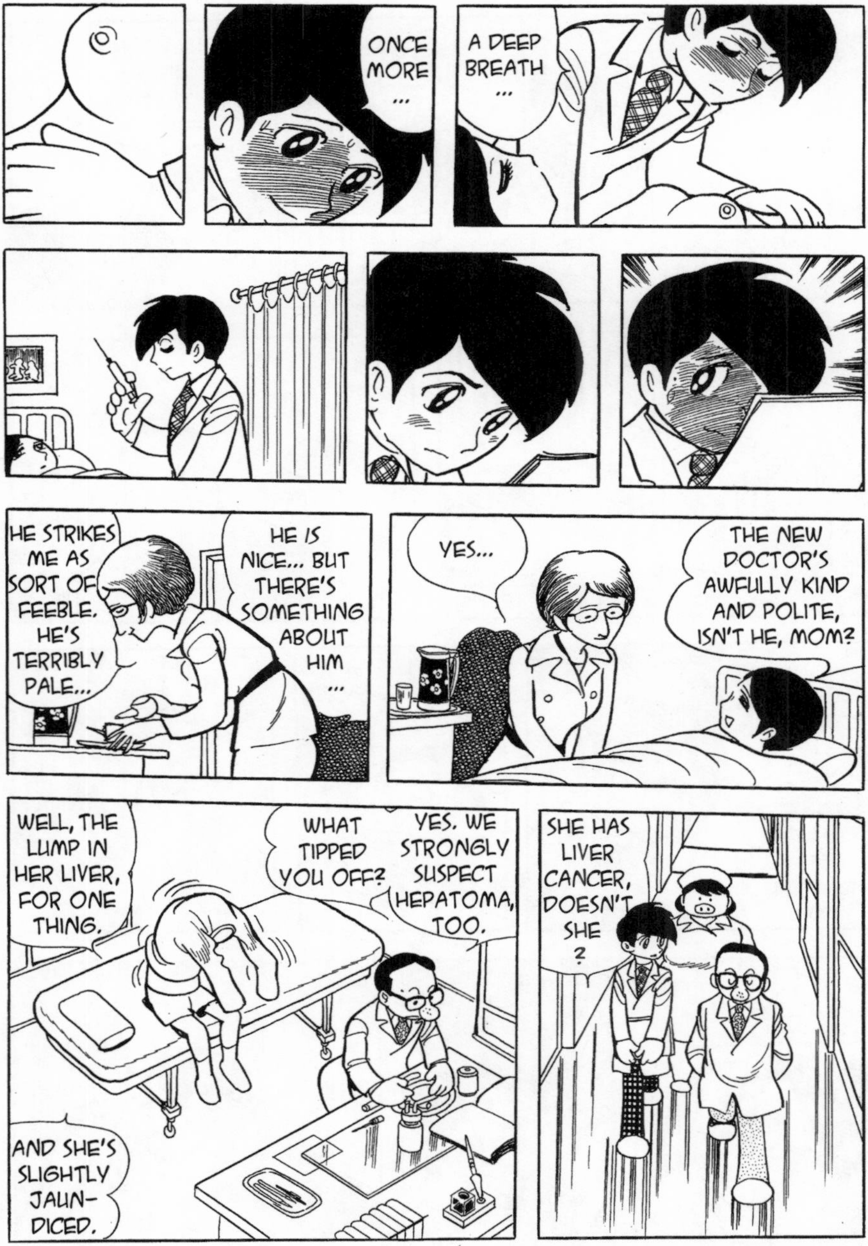
A DEEP BREATH ...
ONCE MORE ...
THE NEW DOCTOR'S AWFULLY KIND AND POLITE, ISN'T HE, MOM?
YES...
HE IS NICE... BUT THERE'S SOMETHING ABOUT HIM ...
HE STRIKES ME AS SORT OF FEEBLE. HE'S TERRIBLY PALE...
SHE HAS LIVER CANCER, DOESN'T SHE ?
YES. WE STRONGLY SUSPECT HEPATOMA, TOO.
WHAT TIPPED YOU OFF?
WELL, THE LUMP IN HER LIVER, FOR ONE THING.
AND SHE'S SLIGHTLY JAUN-DICED.

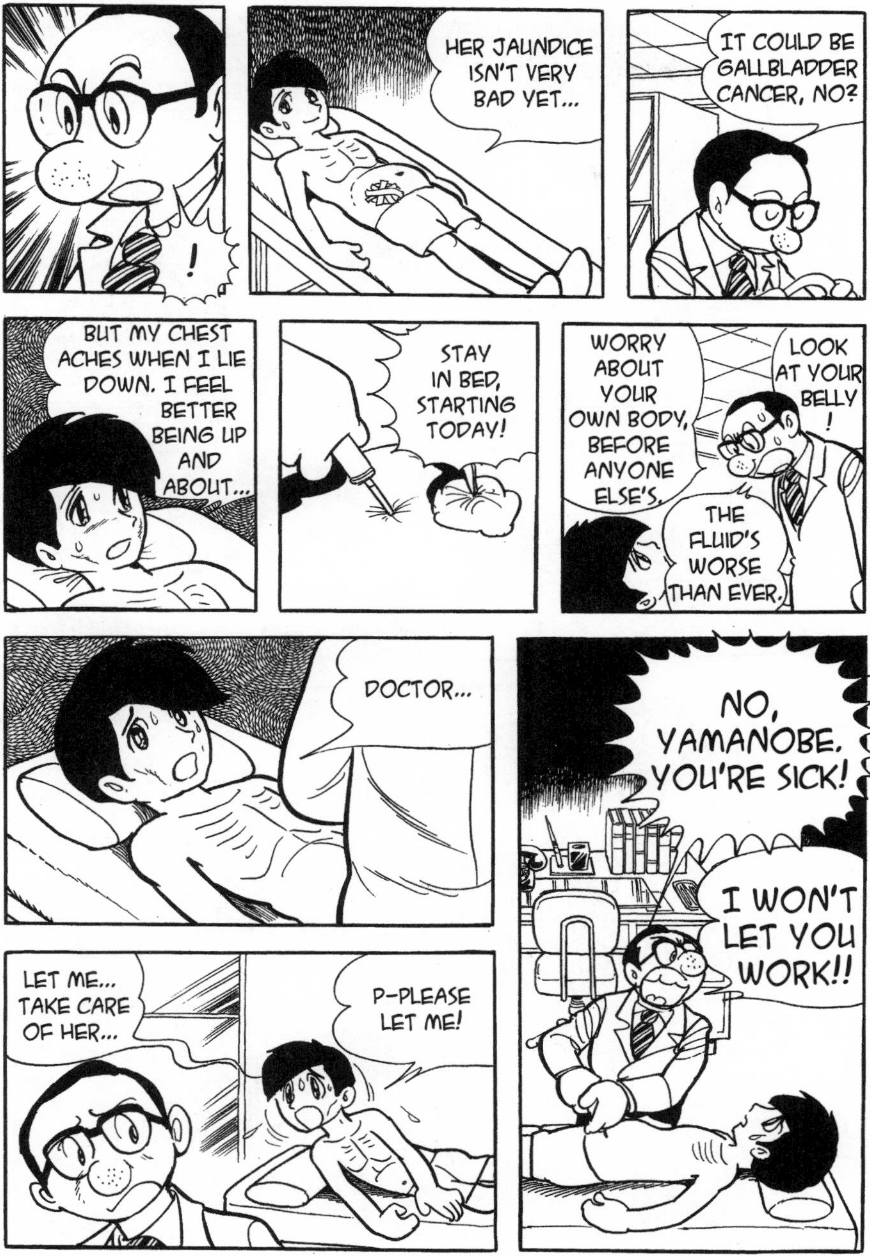
IT COULD BE GALLBLADDER CANCER, NO?
HER JAUNDICE ISN'T VERY BAD YET...
!
LOOK AT YOUR BELLY!
WORRY ABOUT YOUR OWN BODY, BEFORE ANYONE ELSE'S.
THE FLUID'S WORSE THAN EVER.
STAY IN BED, STARTING TODAY!
BUT MY CHEST ACHES WHEN I LIE DOWN. I FEEL BETTER BEING UP AND ABOUT...
NO, YAMANOBE. YOU'RE SICK!
I WON'T LET YOU WORK!!
DOCTOR...
P-PLEASE LET ME!
LET ME... TAKE CARE OF HER...

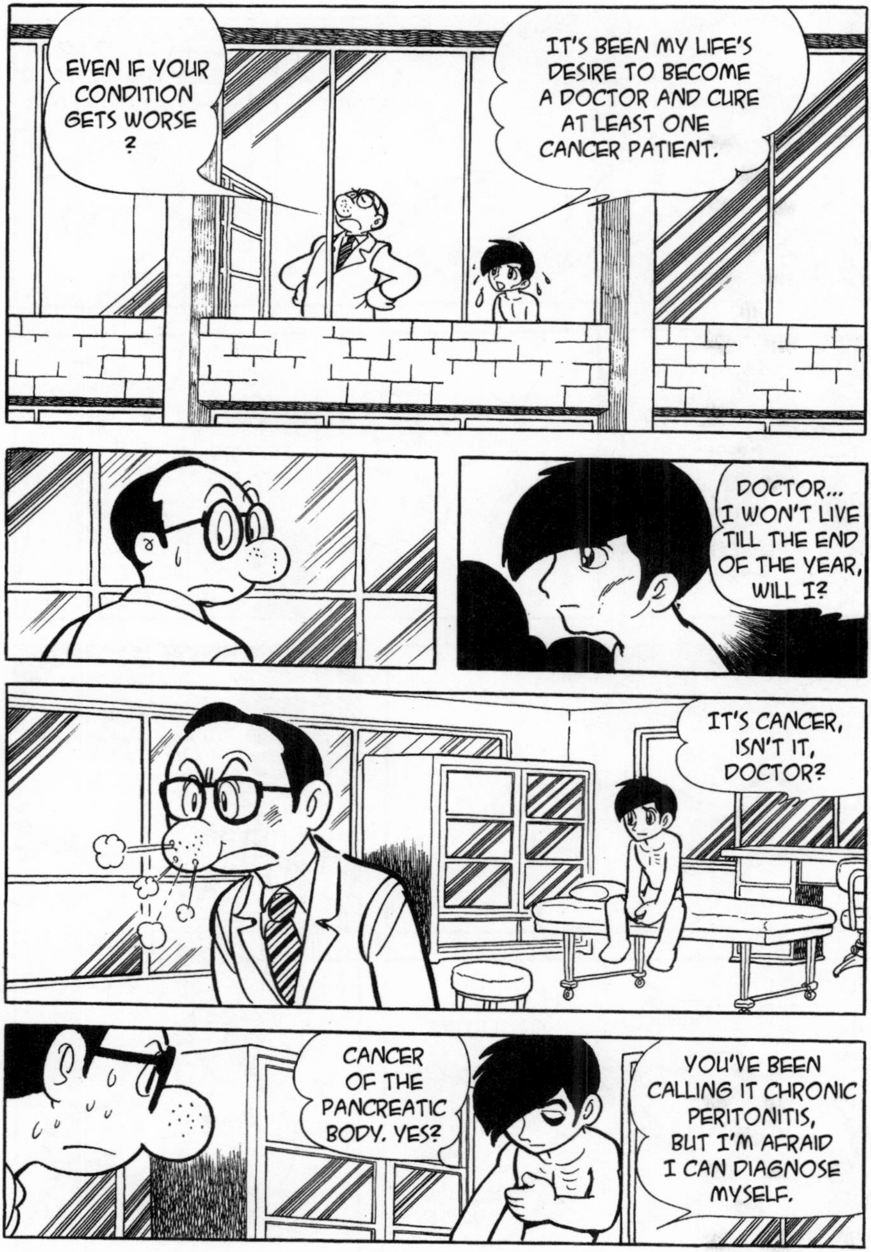
IT'S BEEN MY LIFE'S DESIRE TO BECOME A DOCTOR AND CURE AT LEAST ONE CANCER PATIENT.
EVEN IF YOUR CONDITION GETS WORSE ?
DOCTOR... I WON'T LIVE TILL THE END OF THE YEAR, WILL I?
IT'S CANCER, ISN'T IT, DOCTOR?
YOU'VE BEEN CALLING IT CHRONIC PERITONITIS, BUT I'M AFRAID I CAN DIAGNOSE MYSELF.
CANCER OF THE PANCREATIC BODY. YES?

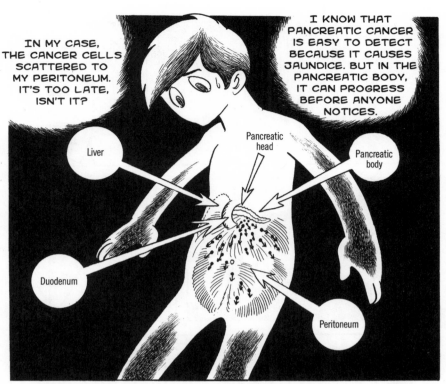

I KNOW THAT PANCREATIC CANCER IS EASY TO DETECT BECAUSE IT CAUSES JAUNDICE. BUT IN THE PANCREATIC BODY, IT CAN PROGRESS BEFORE ANYONE NOTICES.
IN MY CASE, THE CANCER CELLS SCATTERED TO MY PERITONEUM. IT'S TOO LATE, ISN'T IT?
Pancreatic body
Pancreatic head
Liver
Duodenum
Peritoneum
YOU KNEW?
CANCER KILLED MY ENTIRE FAMILY, AND NOW IT'S KILLING ME!
BEFORE I GO, JUST ONCE, I WANT TO CURE A CANCER PATIENT WHO STILL HAS A CHANCE!

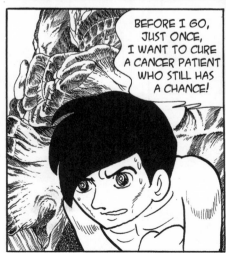

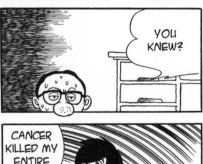

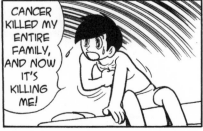

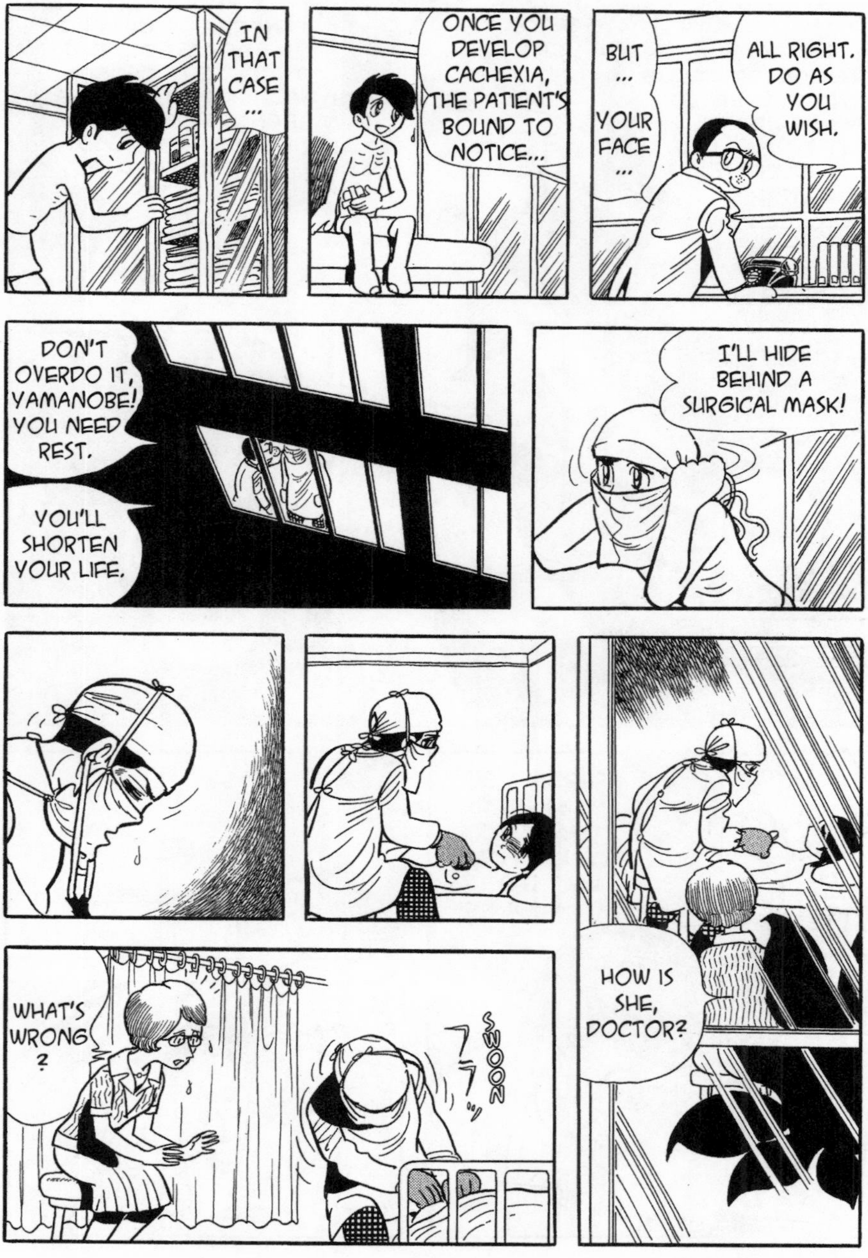
ALL RIGHT. DO AS YOU WISH.
BUT ... YOUR FACE ...
ONCE YOU DEVELOP CACHEXIA, THE PATIENT'S BOUND TO NOTICE...
IN THAT CASE ...
I'LL HIDE BEHIND A SURGICAL MASK!
DON'T OVERDO IT, YAMANOBE! YOU NEED REST.
YOU'LL SHORTEN YOUR LIFE.
HOW IS SHE, DOCTOR?
SWOON
WHAT'S WRONG?

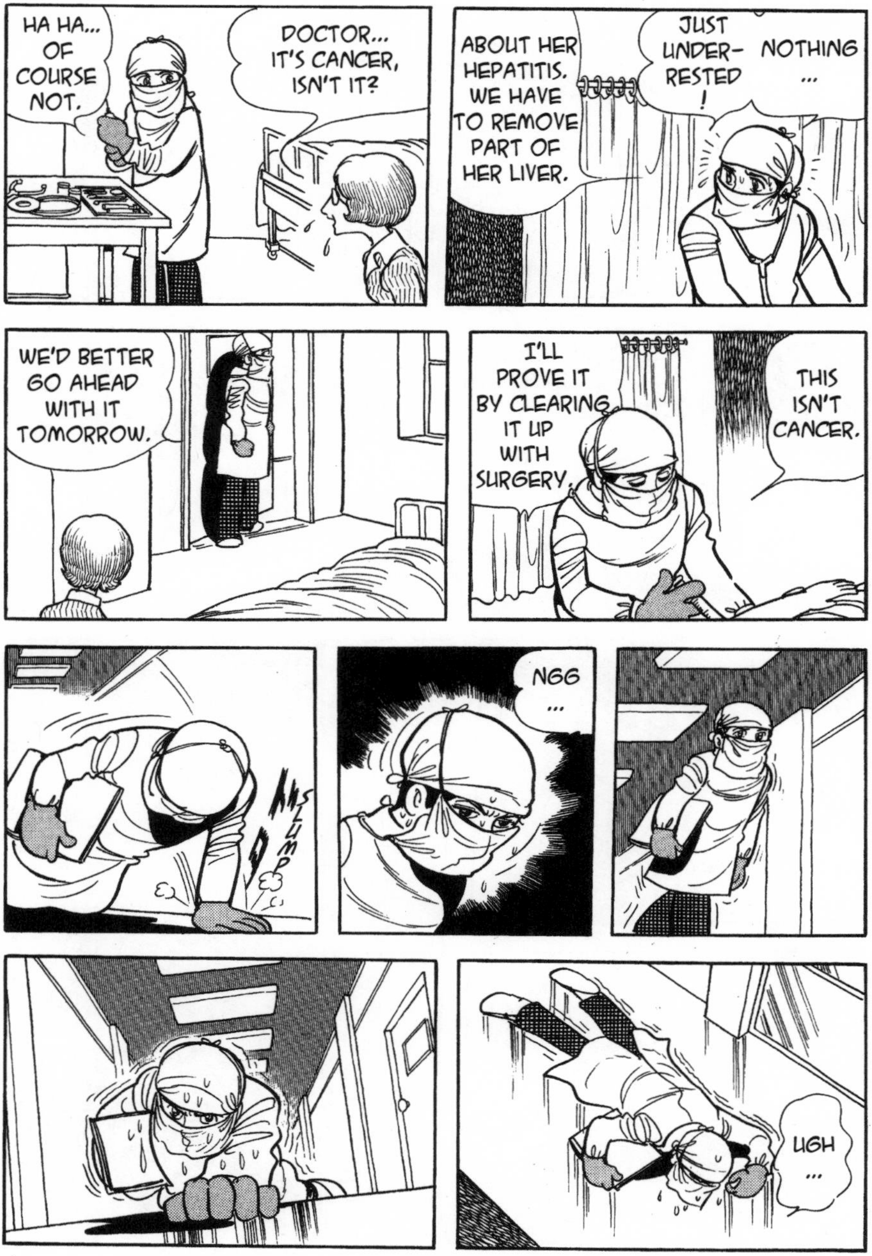
NOTHING ...
JUST UNDER-RESTED!
ABOUT HER HEPATITIS. WE HAVE TO REMOVE PART OF HER LIVER.
DOCTOR... IT'S CANCER, ISN'T IT?
HA HA... OF COURSE NOT.
THIS ISN'T CANCER.
I'LL PROVE IT BY CLEARING IT UP WITH SURGERY.
WE'D BETTER GO AHEAD WITH IT TOMORROW.
NGG ...
SLUMP
UGH ...

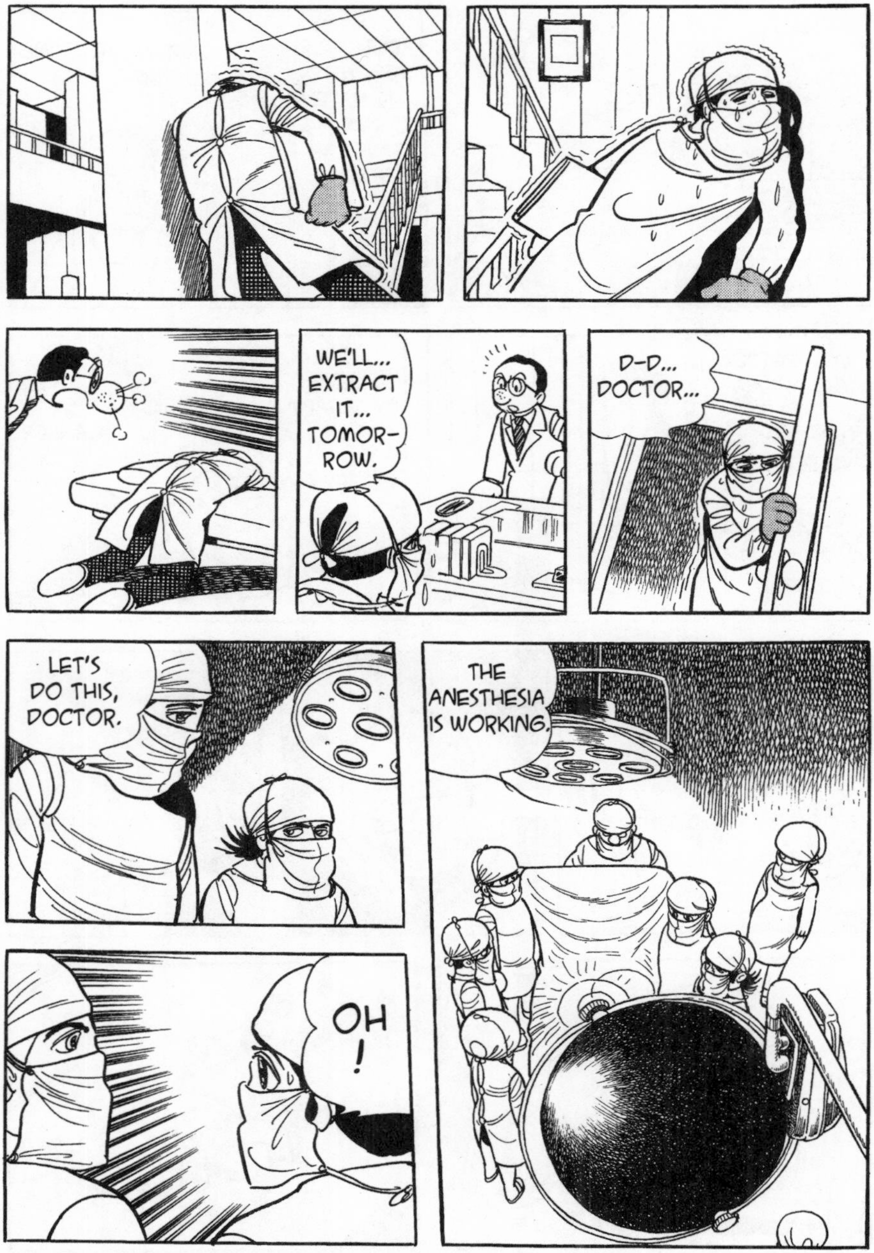
D-D... DOCTOR...
WE'LL... EXTRACT IT... TOMORROW.
THE ANESTHESIA IS WORKING.
LET'S DO THIS, DOCTOR.
OH!

WHY, DOCTOR BLACK JACK, IT'S YOU!
I WAS ASKED TO COME IN AND ASSIST YOU.
I DON'T WANT YOUR HELP!
HEY, THE ANESTHETIC'S WORKING. BETTER GET TO IT.
I... I KNOW.
INCISE UPPER ABDOMEN AT MIDLINE.
HERE!
COME ON, THE LIVER! THAT'S NOT WHERE.
INTESTINAL CLAMP!
...

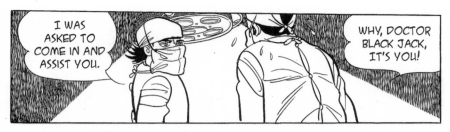

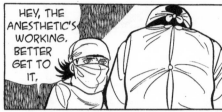

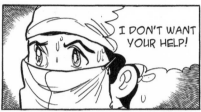

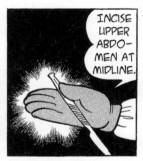

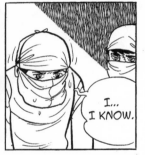

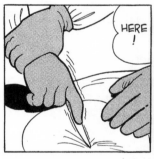

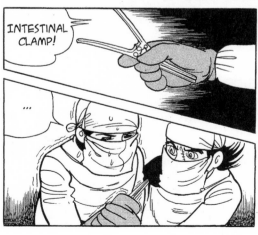

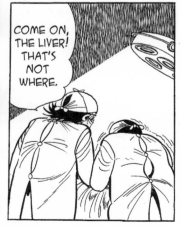

GOOD. SEVER WITH ELECTRIC SCALPEL.
YES. THAT PART.
ポタリ
PLOP
WELL DONE! YOU DID IT... YOU GOT THE WHOLE TUMOR. YOU'VE SAVED HER!
グラ
WOBBLE
THUD

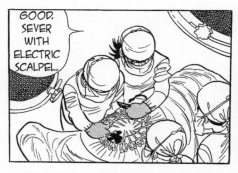

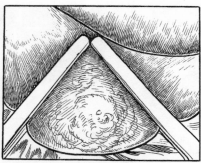

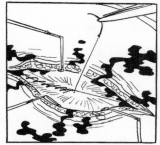

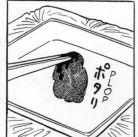

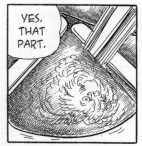

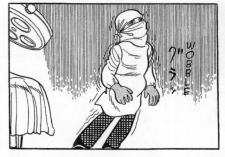

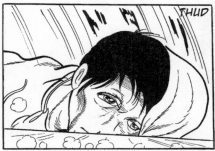

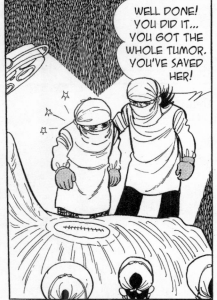

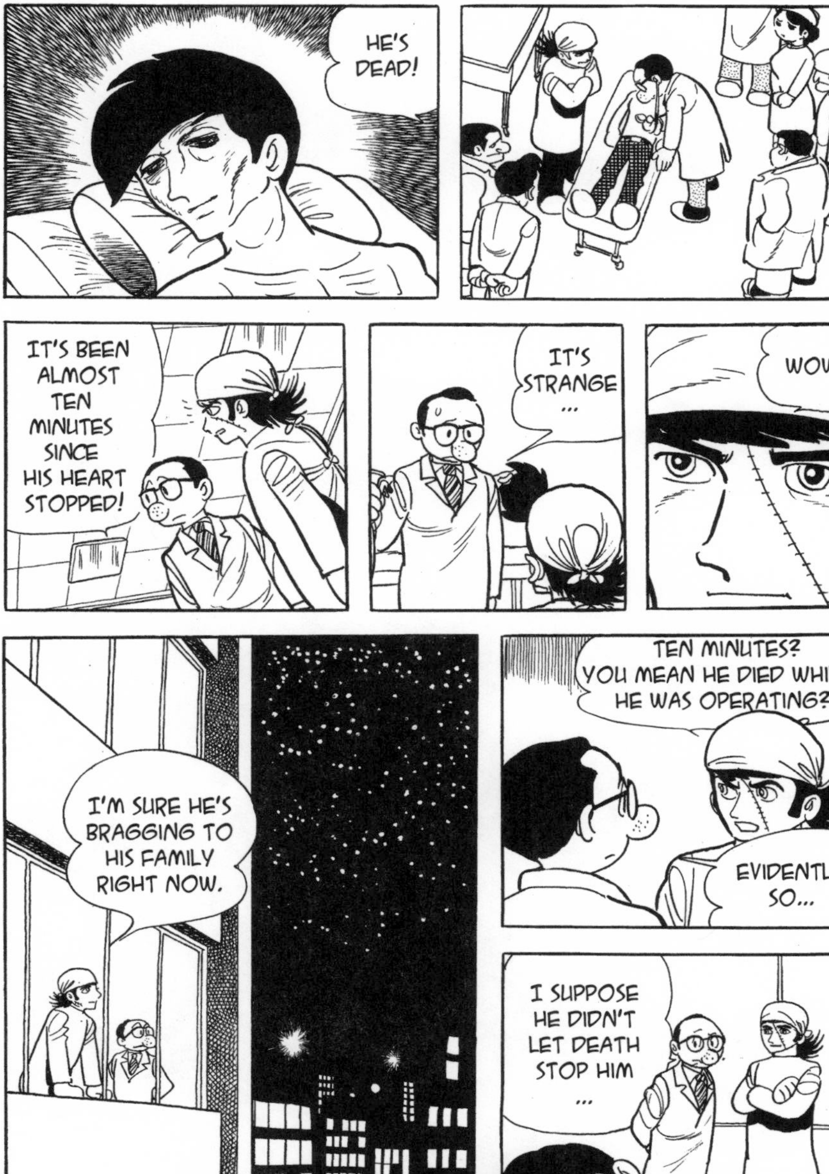
HE'S DEAD!
WOW.
IT'S STRANGE ...
IT'S BEEN ALMOST TEN MINUTES SINCE HIS HEART STOPPED!
TEN MINUTES? YOU MEAN HE DIED WHILE HE WAS OPERATING?!
EVIDENTLY SO...
I SUPPOSE HE DIDN'T LET DEATH STOP HIM ...
I'M SURE HE'S BRAGGING TO HIS FAMILY RIGHT NOW.

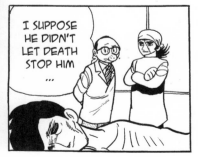

AN ODD RELATIONSHIP

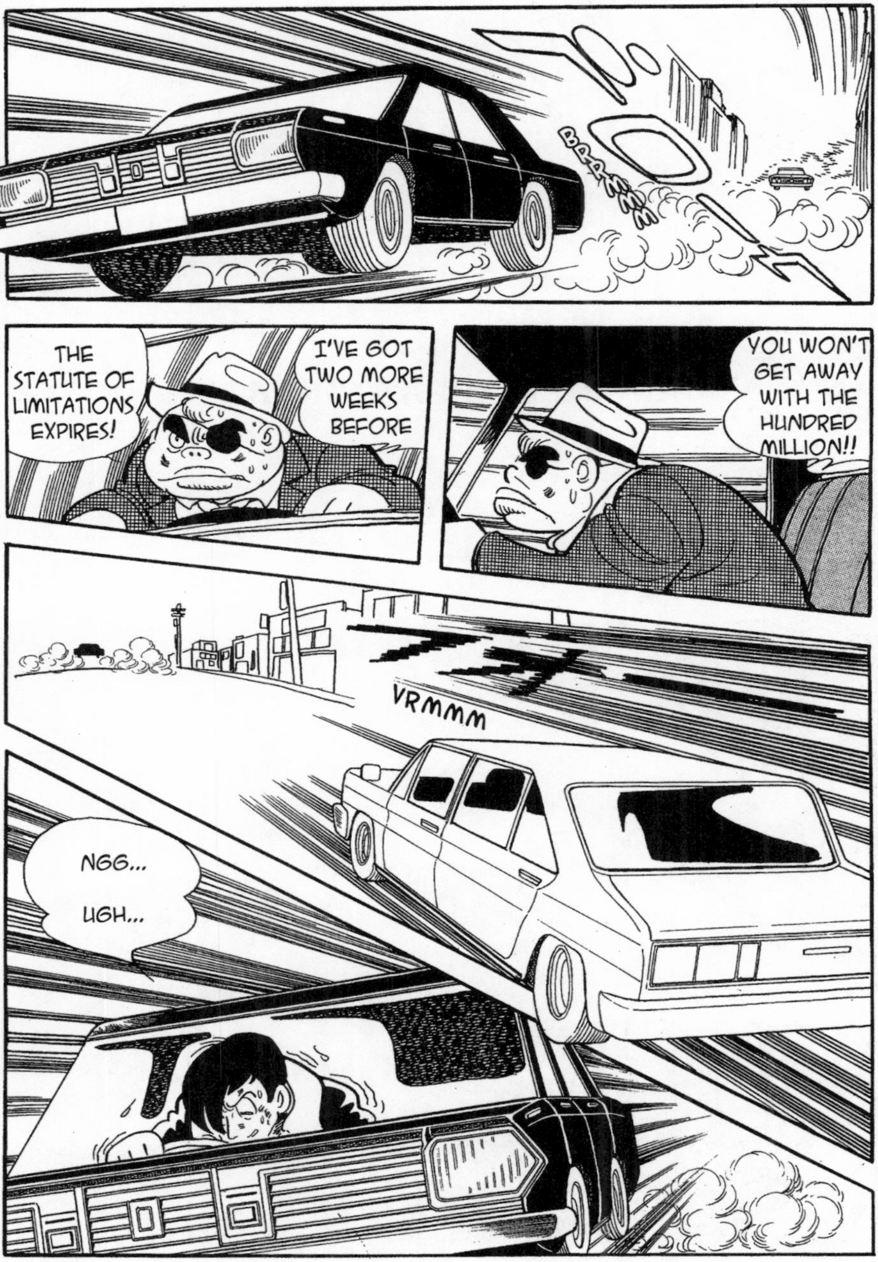
BRRAMMM
YOU WON'T GET AWAY WITH THE HUNDRED MILLION!!
I'VE GOT TWO MORE WEEKS BEFORE
THE STATUTE OF LIMITATIONS EXPIRES!
VRMMM
NGG...
UGH...

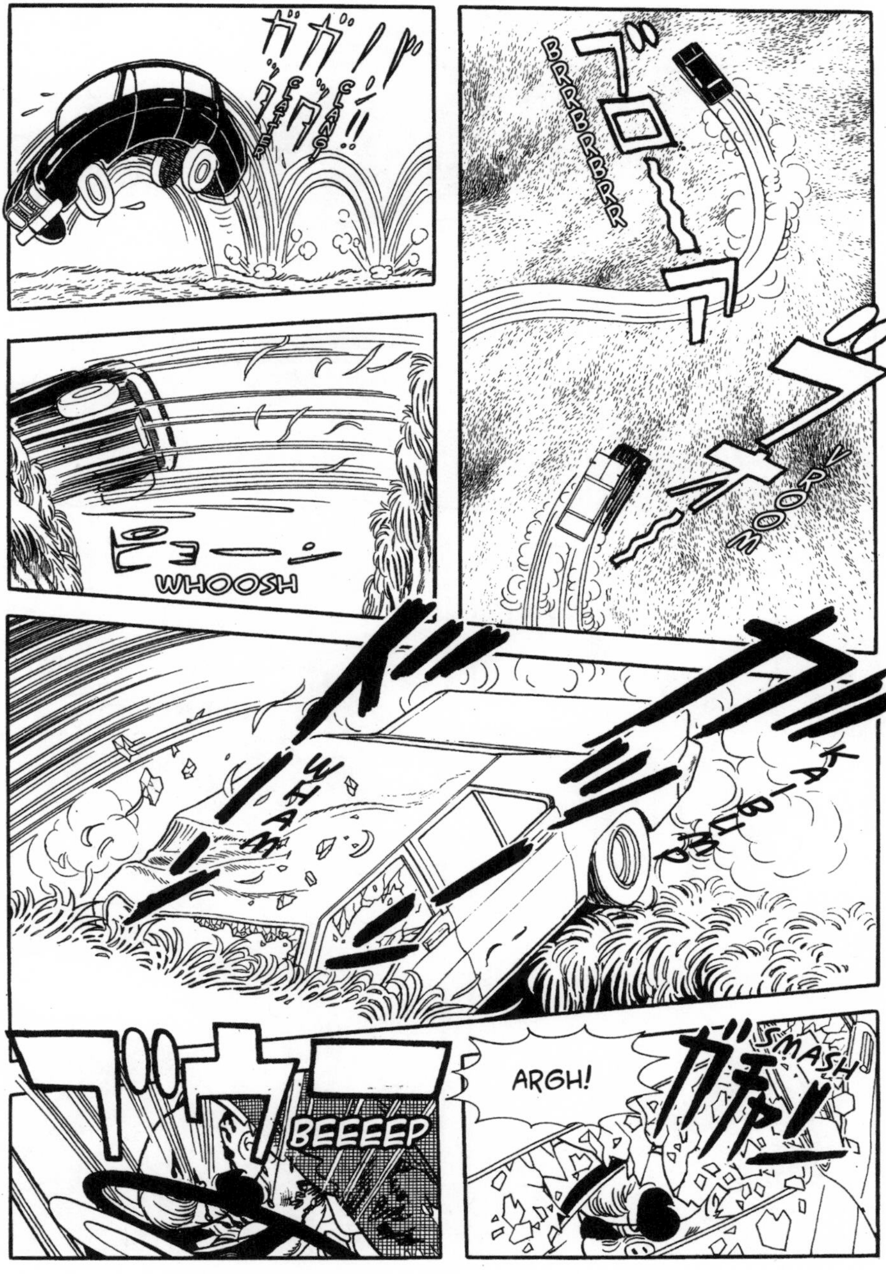
BRRRBRBRRR
VROOM
CLANG!!
CLATTER
WHOOSH
KA-BUMP
WHAM
ARGH!
SMASH
BEEEEP

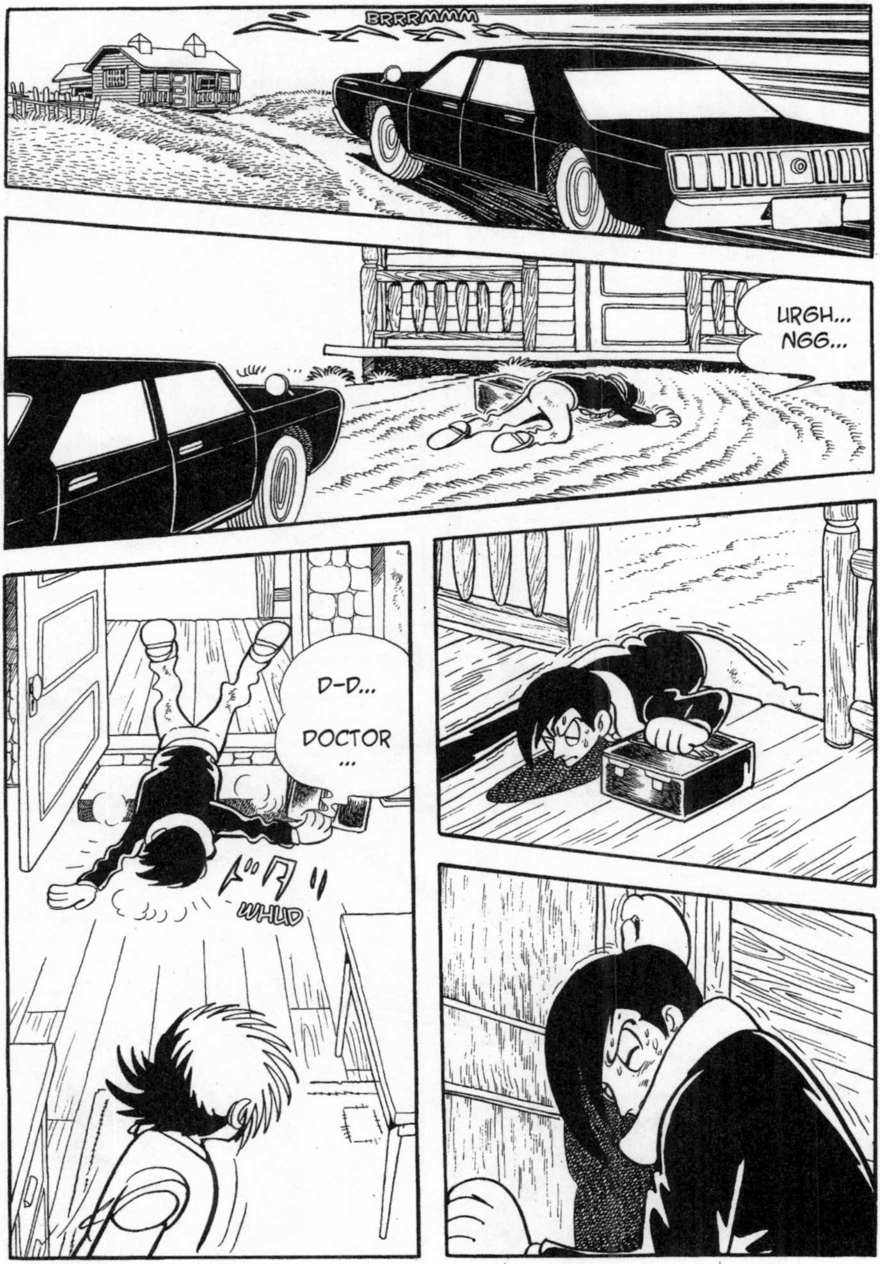
BRRRMMM
URGH... NGG...
D-D... DOCTOR ...
WHUD

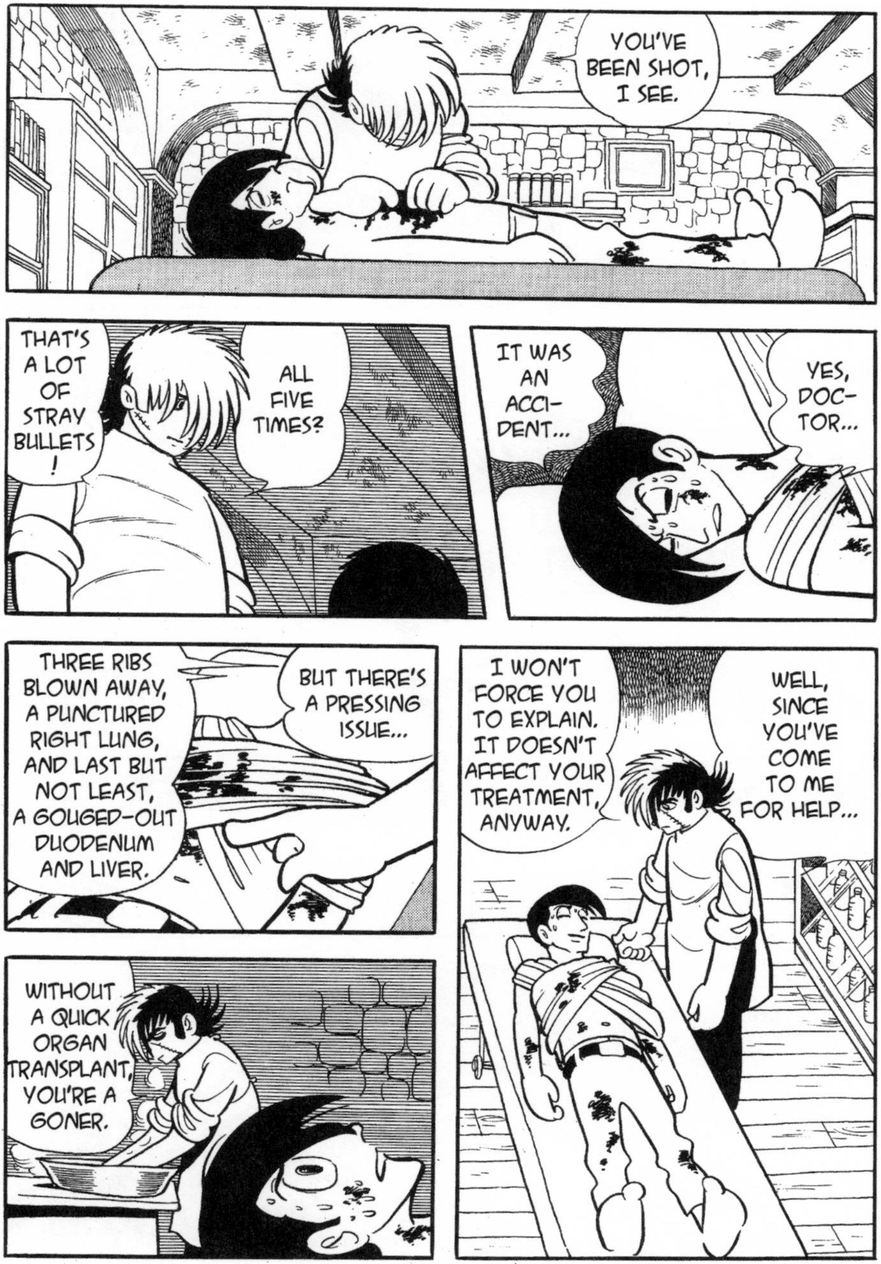
YOU'VE BEEN SHOT, I SEE.
YES, DOCTOR...
IT WAS AN ACCIDENT...
ALL FIVE TIMES?
THAT'S A LOT OF STRAY BULLETS!
WELL, SINCE YOU'VE COME TO ME FOR HELP...
I WON'T FORCE YOU TO EXPLAIN. IT DOESN'T AFFECT YOUR TREATMENT, ANYWAY.
BUT THERE'S A PRESSING ISSUE...
THREE RIBS BLOWN AWAY, A PUNCTURED RIGHT LUNG, AND LAST BUT NOT LEAST, A GOUGED-OUT DUODENUM AND LIVER.
WITHOUT A QUICK ORGAN TRANSPLANT, YOU'RE A GONER.

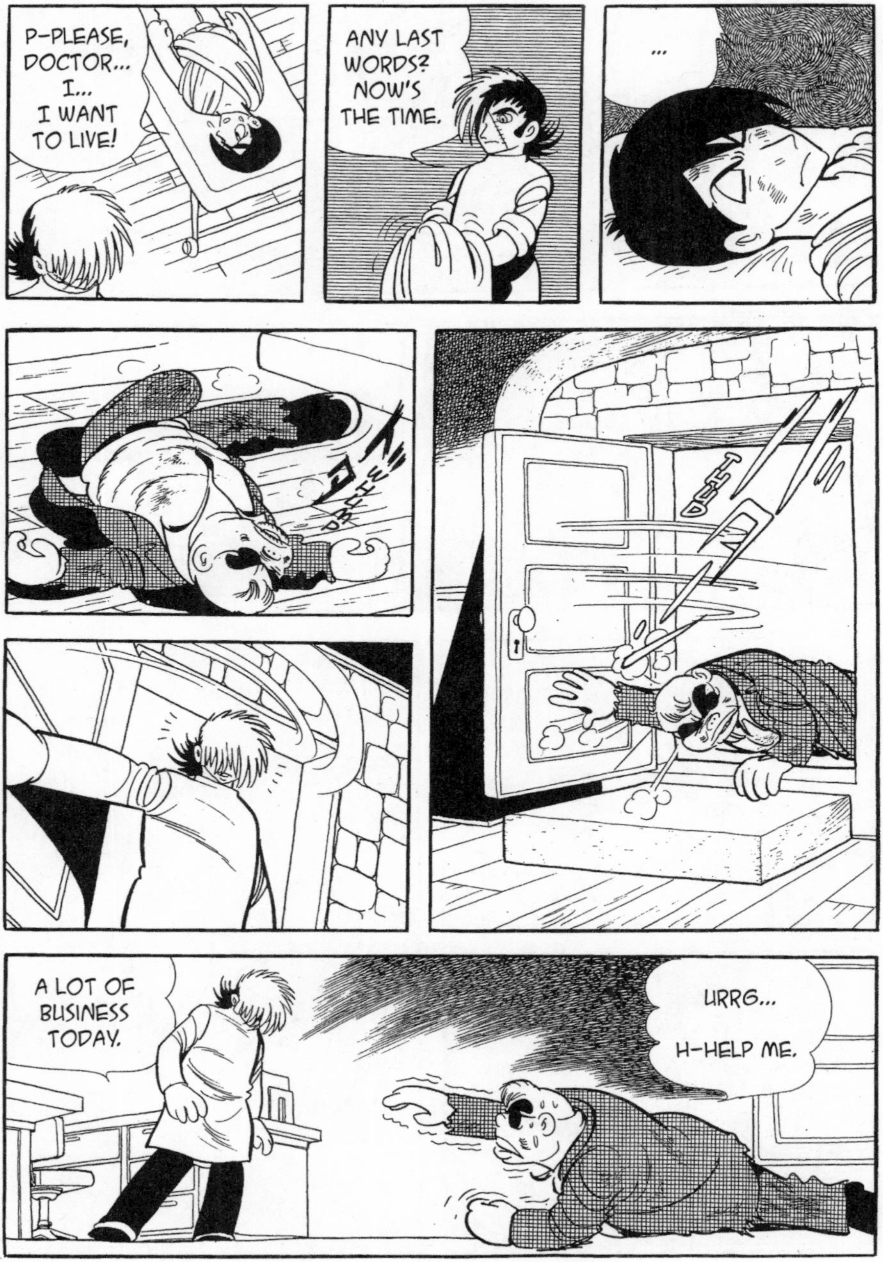
...
ANY LAST WORDS? NOW'S THE TIME.
P-PLEASE, DOCTOR... I... I WANT TO LIVE!
THUD
WHUMP
URRG... H-HELP ME.
A LOT OF BUSINESS TODAY.

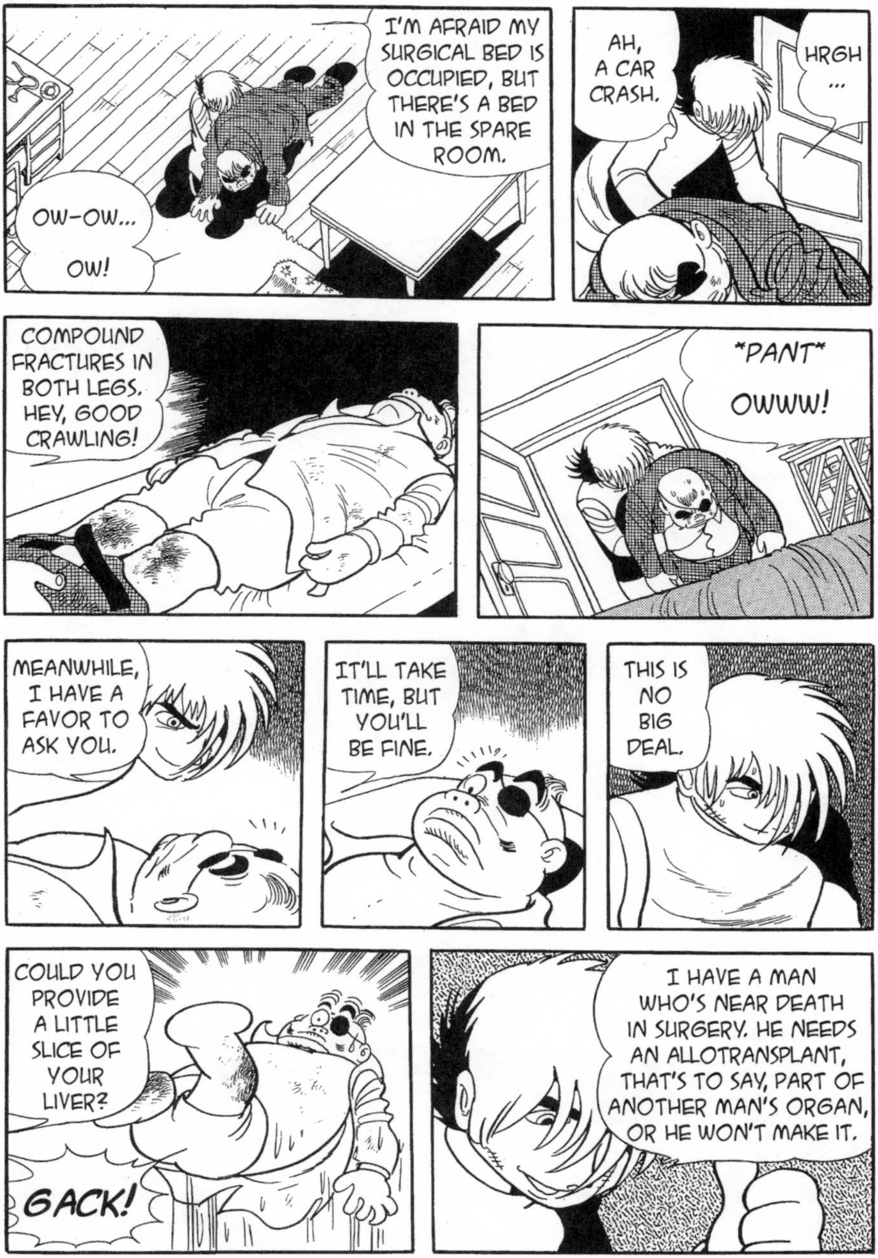
HRGH ...
AH, A CAR CRASH.
I'M AFRAID MY SURGICAL BED IS OCCUPIED, BUT THERE'S A BED IN THE SPARE ROOM.
OW-OW... OW!
PANT OWWW!
COMPOUND FRACTURES IN BOTH LEGS. HEY, GOOD CRAWLING!
THIS IS NO BIG DEAL.
IT'LL TAKE TIME, BUT YOU'LL BE FINE.
MEANWHILE, I HAVE A FAVOR TO ASK YOU.
I HAVE A MAN WHO'S NEAR DEATH IN SURGERY. HE NEEDS AN ALLOTRANSPLANT, THAT'S TO SAY, PART OF ANOTHER MAN'S ORGAN, OR HE WON'T MAKE IT.
COULD YOU PROVIDE A LITTLE SLICE OF YOUR LIVER?
GACK!

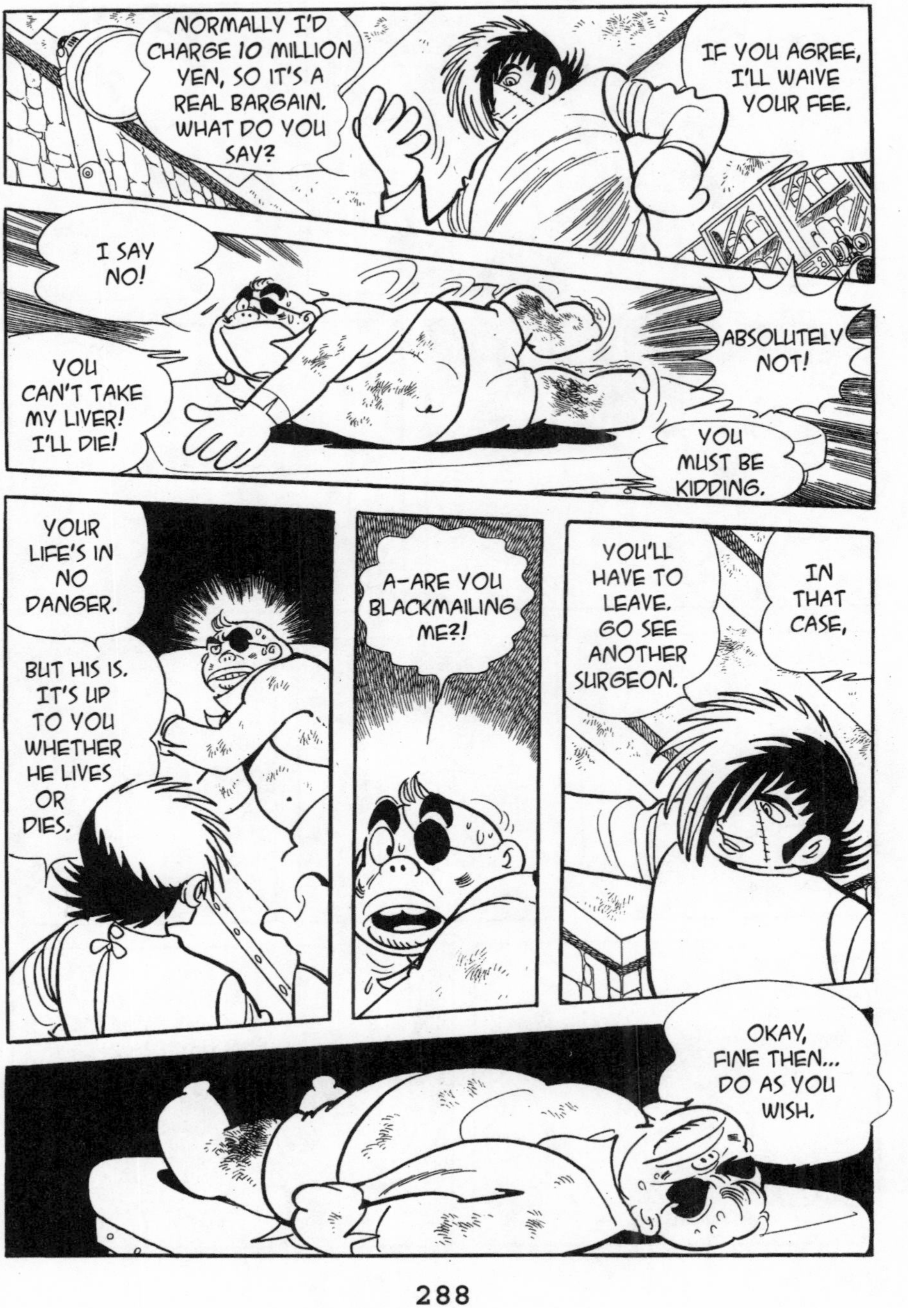
IF YOU AGREE, I'LL WAIVE YOUR FEE.
NORMALLY I'D CHARGE 10 MILLION YEN, SO IT'S A REAL BARGAIN. WHAT DO YOU SAY?
I SAY NO!
ABSOLUTELY NOT!
YOU MUST BE KIDDING.
YOU CAN'T TAKE MY LIVER! I'LL DIE!
IN THAT CASE,
YOU'LL HAVE TO LEAVE. GO SEE ANOTHER SURGEON.
A-ARE YOU BLACKMAILING ME?!
YOUR LIFE'S IN NO DANGER.
BUT HIS IS. IT'S UP TO YOU WHETHER HE LIVES OR DIES.
OKAY, FINE THEN... DO AS YOU WISH.

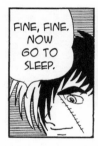

GOOD ...
I'LL PUT YOU UNDER RIGHT NOW.
I'M A SPECIAL INVESTIGATIONS OFFICER OF THE TOKYO METROPOLITAN POLICE. I'LL HAVE YOU PROSECUTED FOR THIS, YOU KNOW!
FINE, FINE. NOW GO TO SLEEP.
A VERY KIND MAN HAS COME FORTH TO BE YOUR DONOR.
PINOKO!
AYE AYE!
AND THE DOUBLE-HEADER BEGINS!
ARE YOU SERIOUS? TWO AT ONCE? AND, UH, YOUR ASSISTANT IS A CHILD...
SHE'S 20 AND A GIFTED DOCTOR!

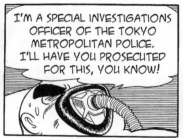

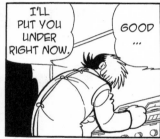

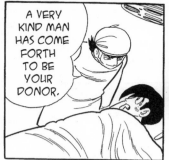

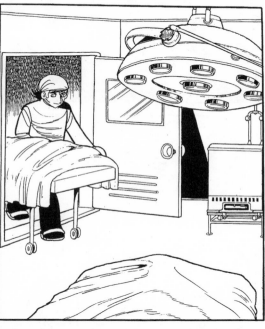

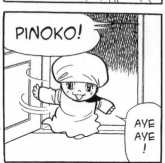

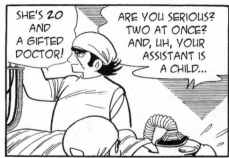

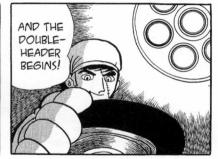

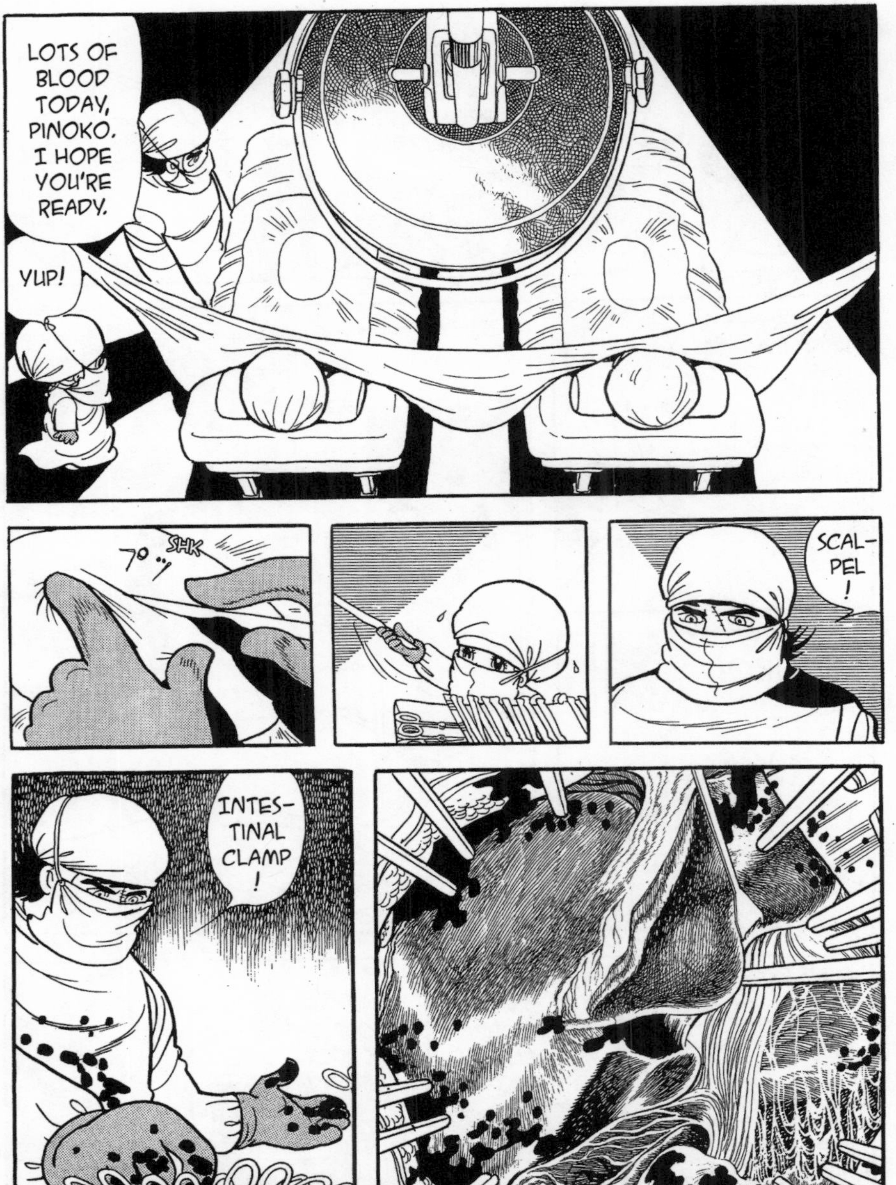
LOTS OF BLOOD TODAY, PINOKO. I HOPE YOU'RE READY.
YUP!
SCAL-PEL!
SHK
INTES-TINAL CLAMP!

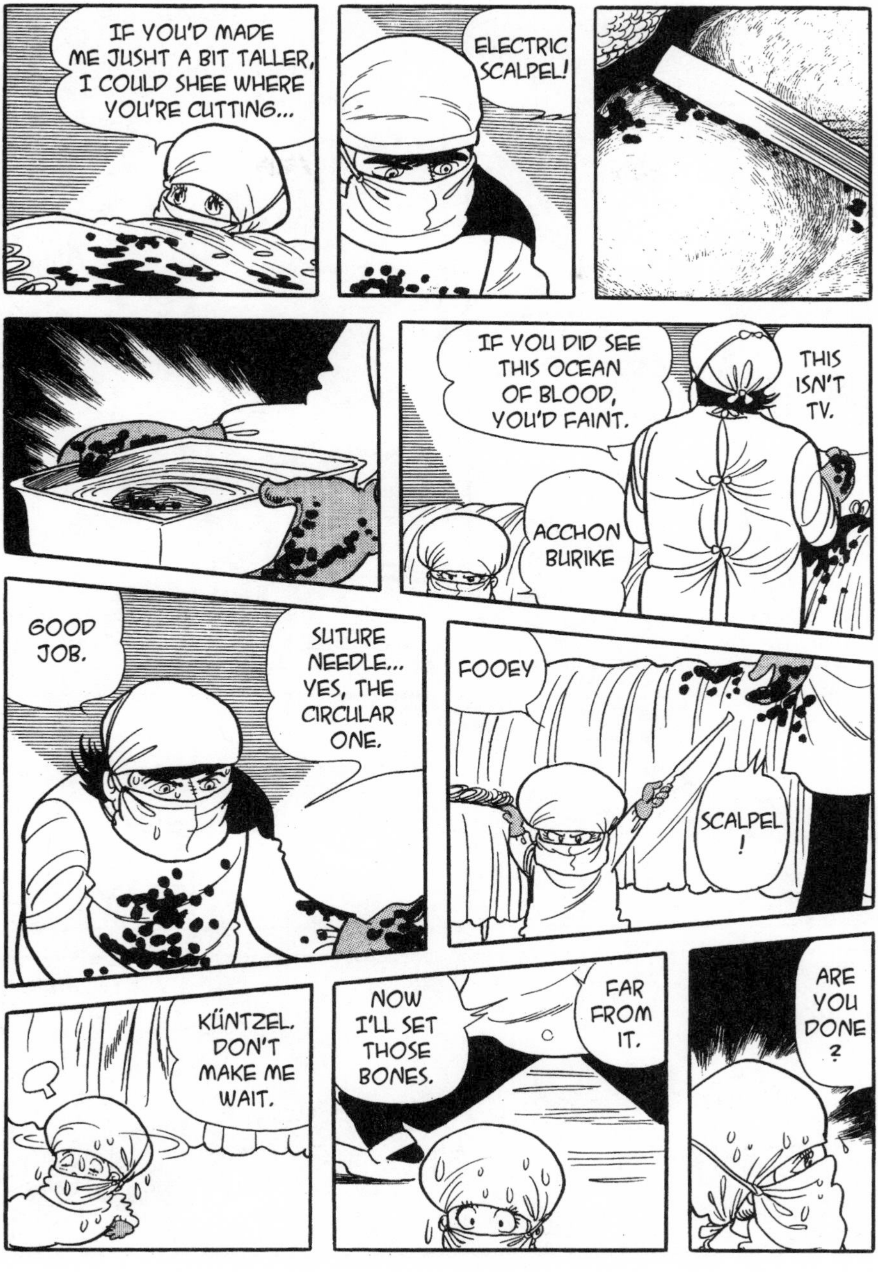
ELECTRIC SCALPEL!
IF YOU'D MADE ME JUSHT A BIT TALLER, I COULD SHEE WHERE YOU'RE CUTTING...
THIS ISN'T TV.
IF YOU DID SEE THIS OCEAN OF BLOOD, YOU'D FAINT.
ACCHON BURIKE
FOOEY
SCALPEL!
SUTURE NEEDLE... YES, THE CIRCULAR ONE.
GOOD JOB.
ARE YOU DONE?
FAR FROM IT.
NOW I'LL SET THOSE BONES.
KÜNTZEL. DON'T MAKE ME WAIT.

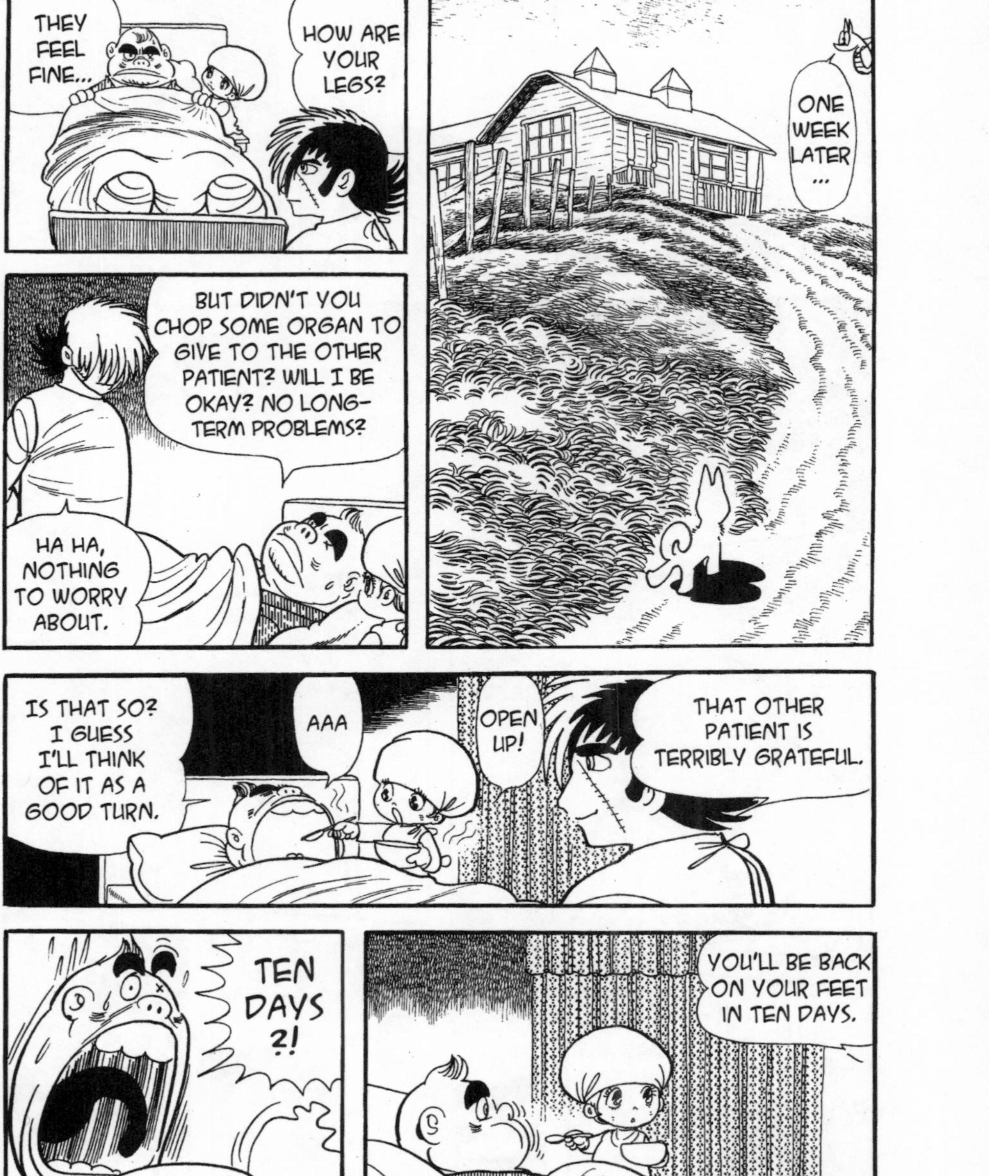
ONE WEEK LATER ...
HOW ARE YOUR LEGS?
THEY FEEL FINE...
BUT DIDN'T YOU CHOP SOME ORGAN TO GIVE TO THE OTHER PATIENT? WILL I BE OKAY? NO LONG-TERM PROBLEMS?
HA HA, NOTHING TO WORRY ABOUT.
THAT OTHER PATIENT IS TERRIBLY GRATEFUL.
OPEN UP!
AAA
IS THAT SO? I GUESS I'LL THINK OF IT AS A GOOD TURN.
YOU'LL BE BACK ON YOUR FEET IN TEN DAYS.
TEN DAYS ?!

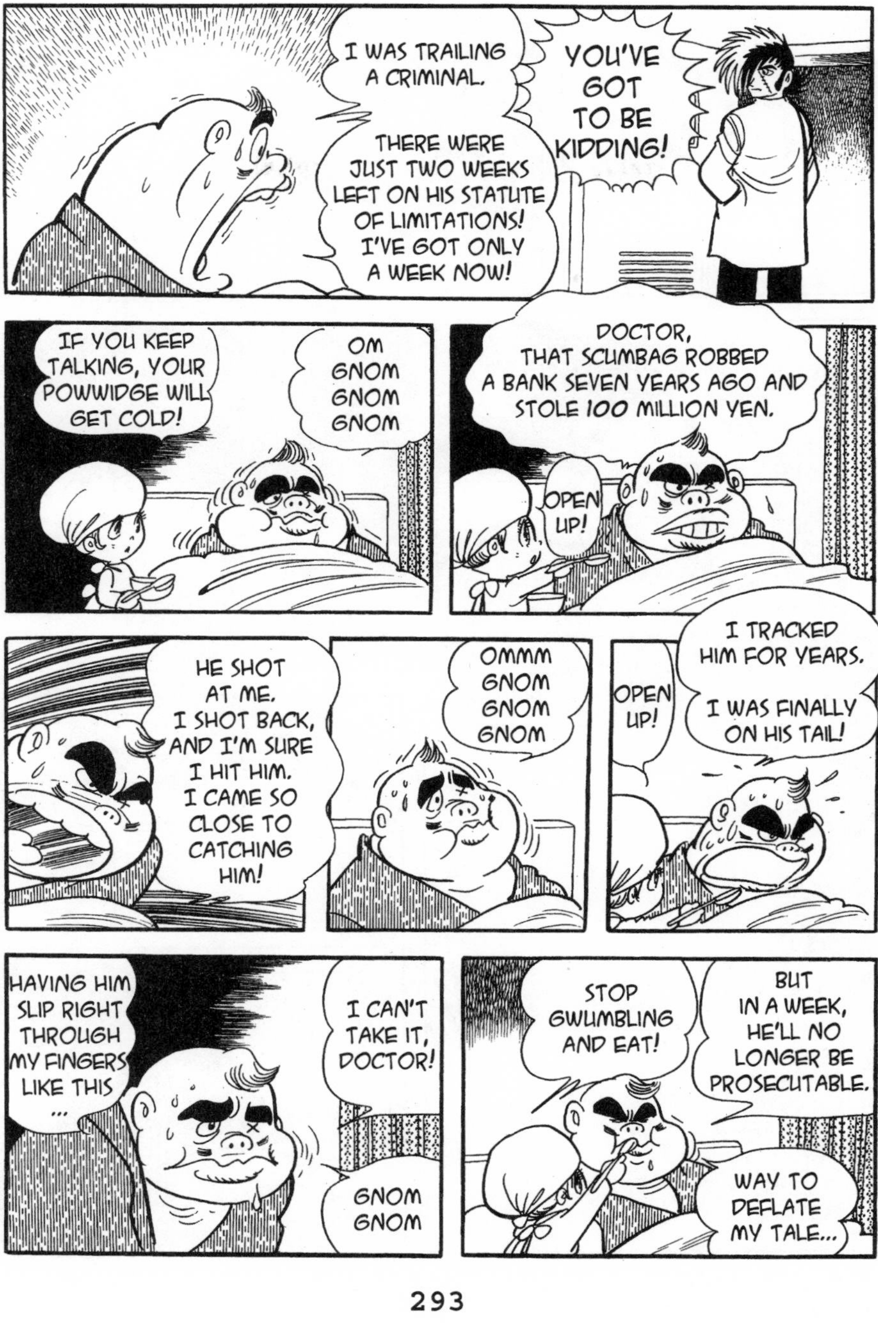
YOU'VE GOT TO BE KIDDING!
I WAS TRAILING A CRIMINAL.
THERE WERE JUST TWO WEEKS LEFT ON HIS STATUTE OF LIMITATIONS! I'VE GOT ONLY A WEEK NOW!
DOCTOR, THAT SCUMBAG ROBBED A BANK SEVEN YEARS AGO AND STOLE 100 MILLION YEN.
OPEN UP!
OM GNOM GNOM GNOM
IF YOU KEEP TALKING, YOUR POWWIDGE WILL GET COLD!
I TRACKED HIM FOR YEARS.
I WAS FINALLY ON HIS TAIL!
OPEN UP!
OMMM GNOM GNOM GNOM
HE SHOT AT ME. I SHOT BACK, AND I'M SURE I HIT HIM. I CAME SO CLOSE TO CATCHING HIM!
BUT IN A WEEK, HE'LL NO LONGER BE PROSECUTABLE.
STOP GWUMBLING AND EAT!
WAY TO DEFLATE MY TALE...
I CAN'T TAKE IT, DOCTOR!
HAVING HIM SLIP RIGHT THROUGH MY FINGERS LIKE THIS ...
GNOM GNOM

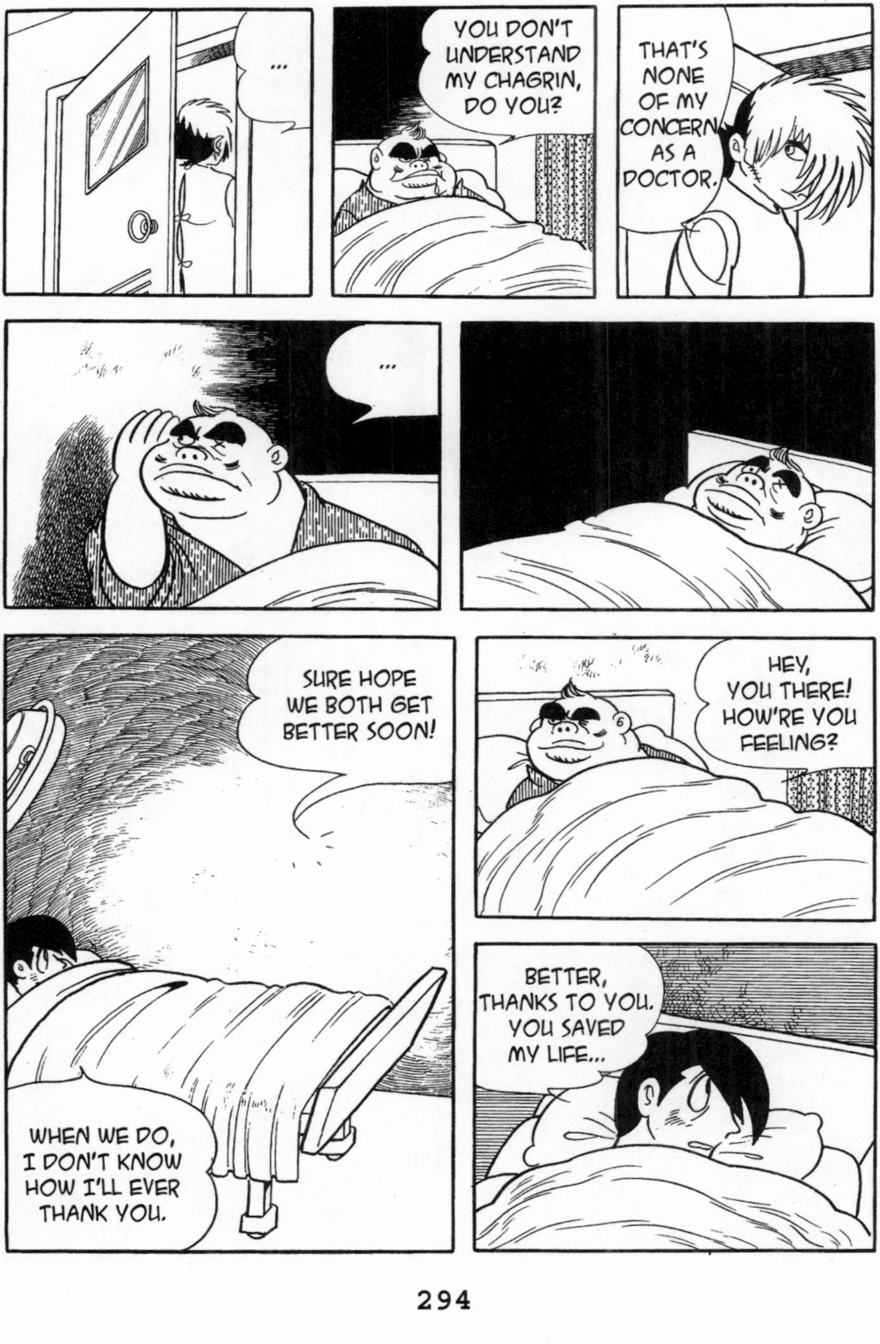
THAT'S NONE OF MY CONCERN AS A DOCTOR.
YOU DON'T UNDERSTAND MY CHAGRIN, DO YOU?
...
...
HEY, YOU THERE! HOW'RE YOU FEELING?
BETTER, THANKS TO YOU. YOU SAVED MY LIFE...
SURE HOPE WE BOTH GET BETTER SOON!
WHEN WE DO, I DON'T KNOW HOW I'LL EVER THANK YOU.

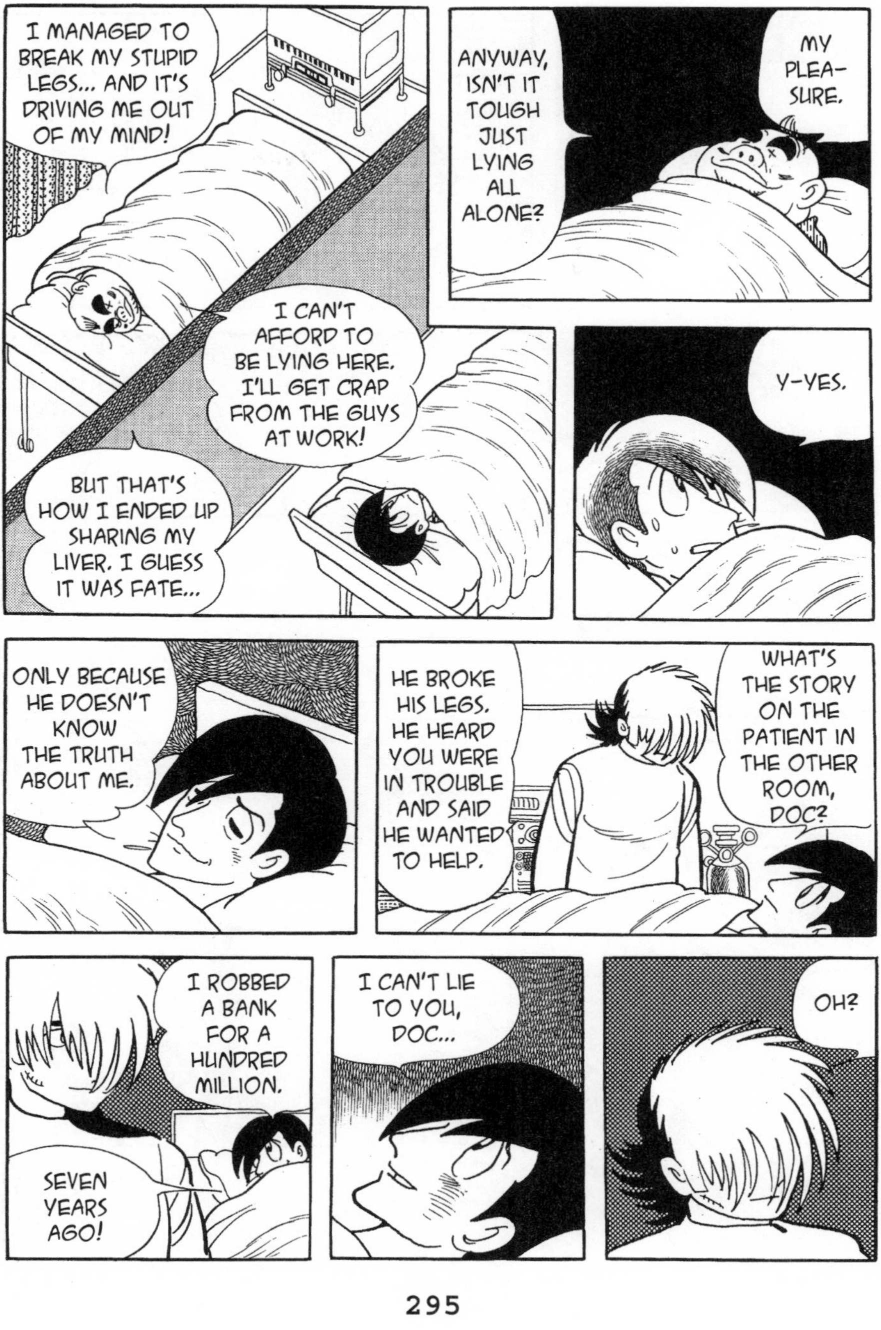
MY PLEASURE.
ANYWAY, ISN'T IT TOUGH JUST LYING ALL ALONE?
I MANAGED TO BREAK MY STUPID LEGS... AND IT'S DRIVING ME OUT OF MY MIND!
Y-YES.
I CAN'T AFFORD TO BE LYING HERE. I'LL GET CRAP FROM THE GUYS AT WORK!
BUT THAT'S HOW I ENDED UP SHARING MY LIVER. I GUESS IT WAS FATE...
WHAT'S THE STORY ON THE PATIENT IN THE OTHER ROOM, DOC?
HE BROKE HIS LEGS. HE HEARD YOU WERE IN TROUBLE AND SAID HE WANTED TO HELP.
ONLY BECAUSE HE DOESN'T KNOW THE TRUTH ABOUT ME.
OH?
I CAN'T LIE TO YOU, DOC...
I ROBBED A BANK FOR A HUNDRED MILLION.
SEVEN YEARS AGO!

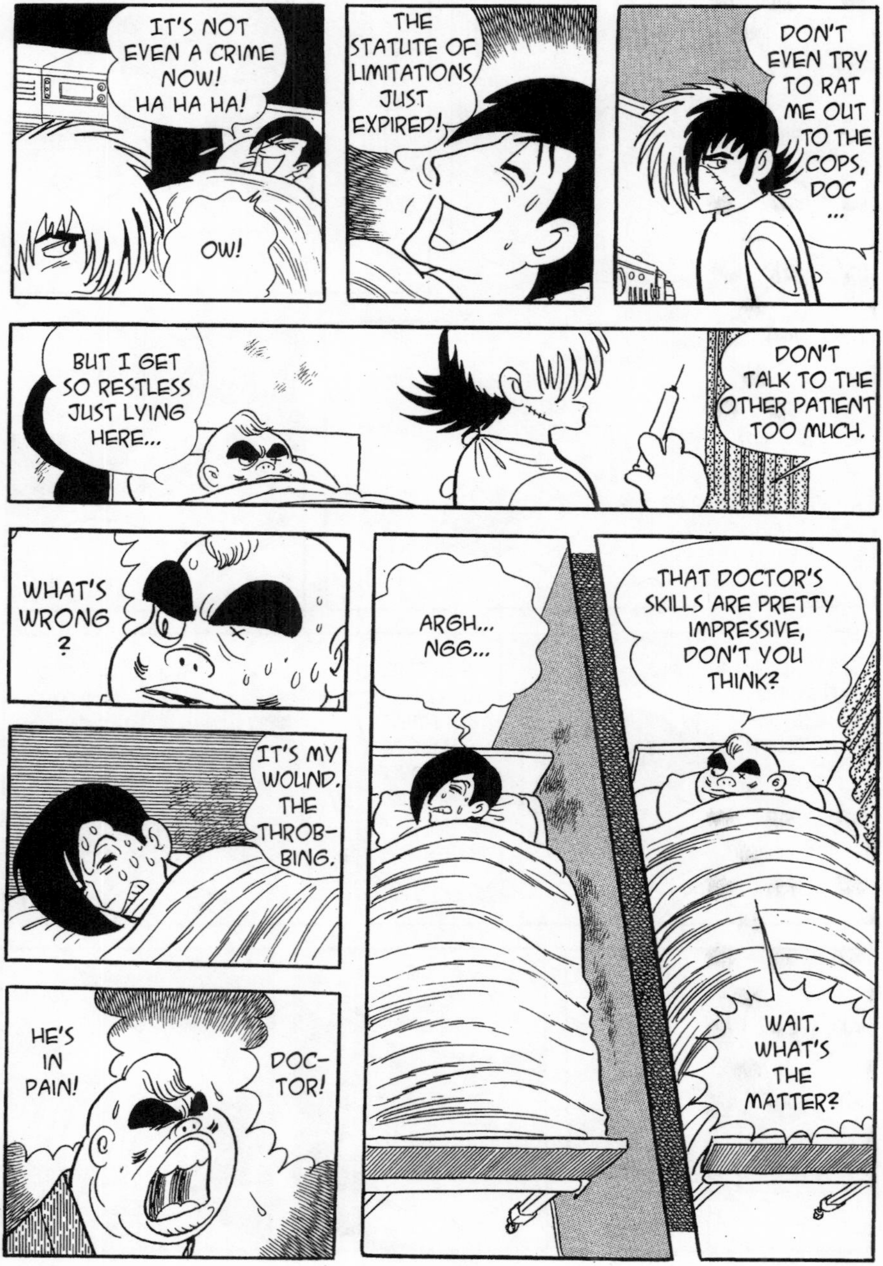
DON'T EVEN TRY TO RAT ME OUT TO THE COPS, DOC ...
THE STATUTE OF LIMITATIONS JUST EXPIRED!
IT'S NOT EVEN A CRIME NOW! HA HA HA!
OW!
DON'T TALK TO THE OTHER PATIENT TOO MUCH.
BUT I GET SO RESTLESS JUST LYING HERE...
THAT DOCTOR'S SKILLS ARE PRETTY IMPRESSIVE, DON'T YOU THINK?
WAIT. WHAT'S THE MATTER?
ARGH... NGG...
WHAT'S WRONG?
IT'S MY WOUND. THE THROB-BING.
DOC-TOR!
HE'S IN PAIN!

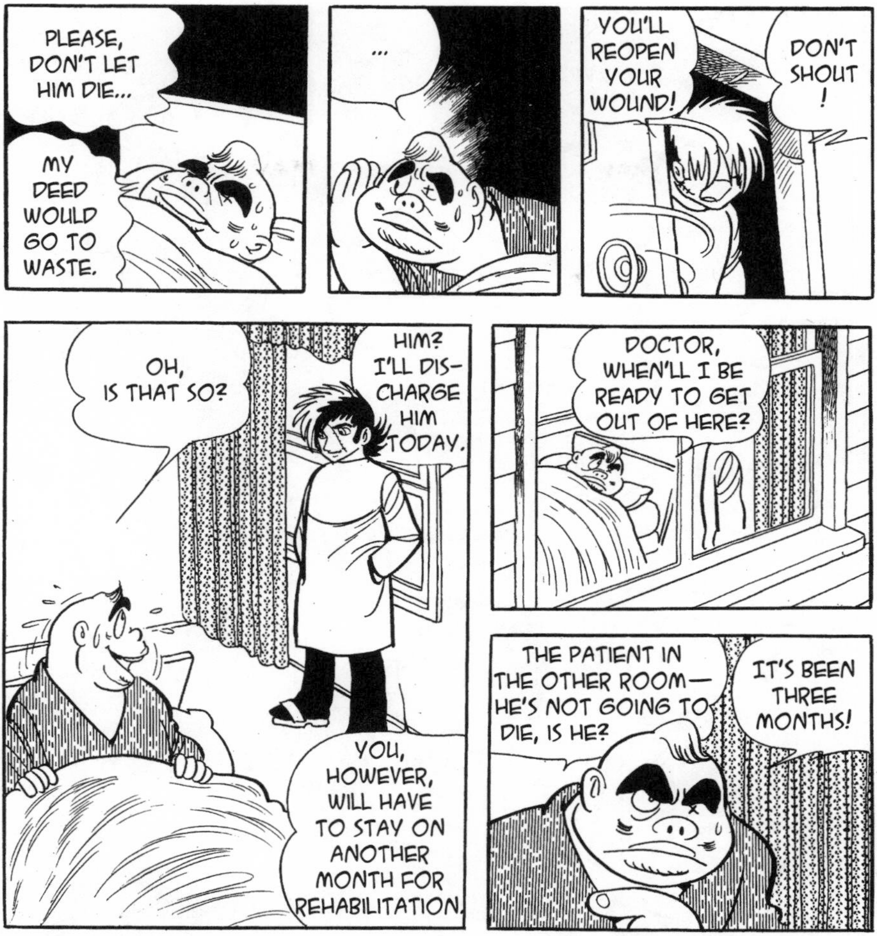
DON'T SHOUT!
YOU'LL REOPEN YOUR WOUND!
...
PLEASE, DON'T LET HIM DIE...
MY DEED WOULD GO TO WASTE.
DOCTOR, WHEN'LL I BE READY TO GET OUT OF HERE?
IT'S BEEN THREE MONTHS!
THE PATIENT IN THE OTHER ROOM— HE'S NOT GOING TO DIE, IS HE?
HIM? I'LL DISCHARGE HIM TODAY.
OH, IS THAT SO?
YOU, HOWEVER, WILL HAVE TO STAY ON ANOTHER MONTH FOR REHABILITATION.
THANKS TO YOU, I GET TO GO HOME TODAY!
I'D DO ANYTHING IN MY POWER TO THANK YOU...
JUST NAME IT!
AH. I'M SO HAPPY FOR YOU.

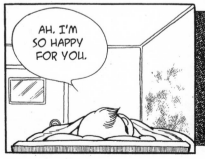

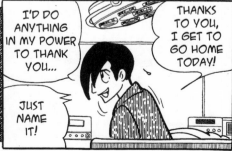

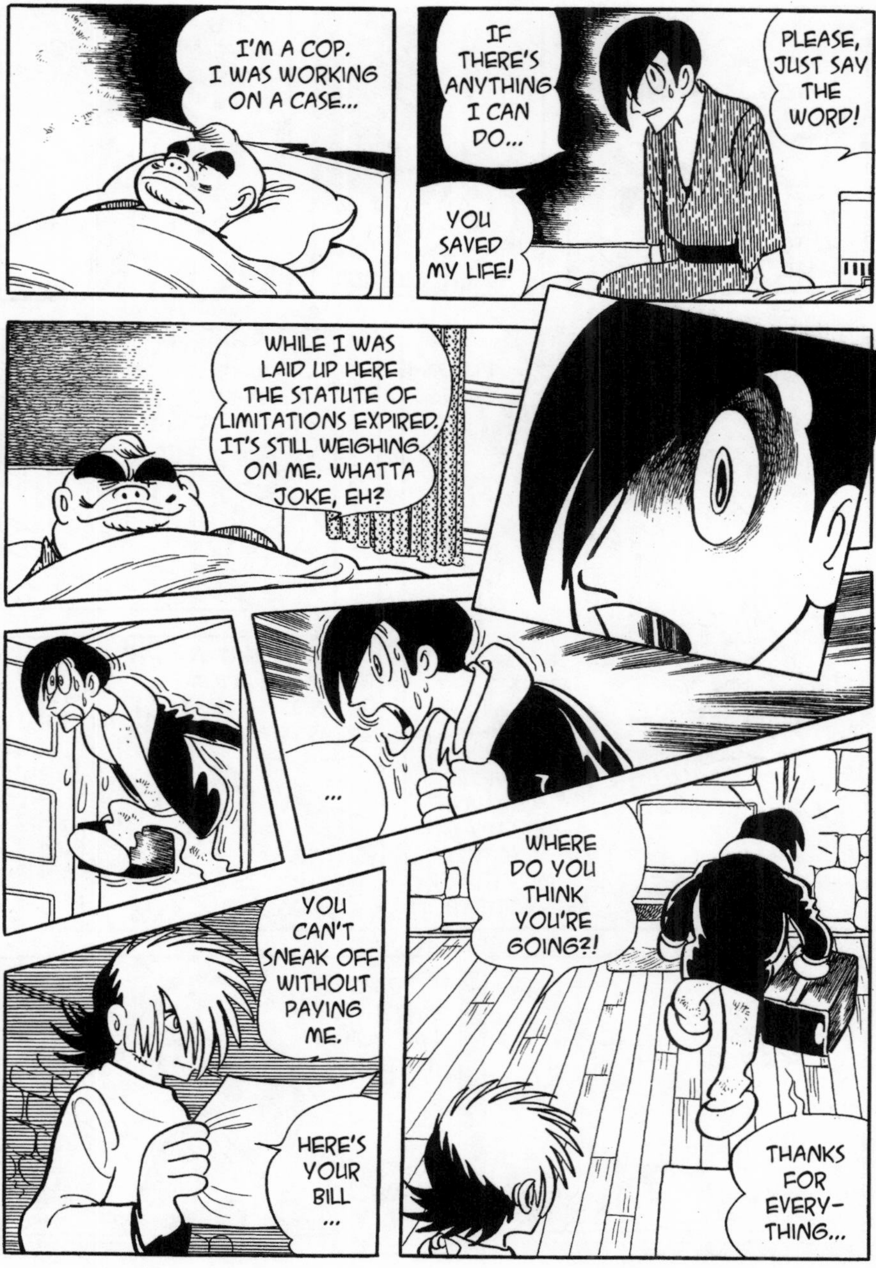
PLEASE, JUST SAY THE WORD!
IF THERE'S ANYTHING I CAN DO...
YOU SAVED MY LIFE!
I'M A COP. I WAS WORKING ON A CASE...
WHILE I WAS LAID UP HERE THE STATUTE OF LIMITATIONS EXPIRED. IT'S STILL WEIGHING ON ME. WHATTA JOKE, EH?
...
WHERE DO YOU THINK YOU'RE GOING?!
THANKS FOR EVERY-THING...
YOU CAN'T SNEAK OFF WITHOUT PAYING ME.
HERE'S YOUR BILL ...

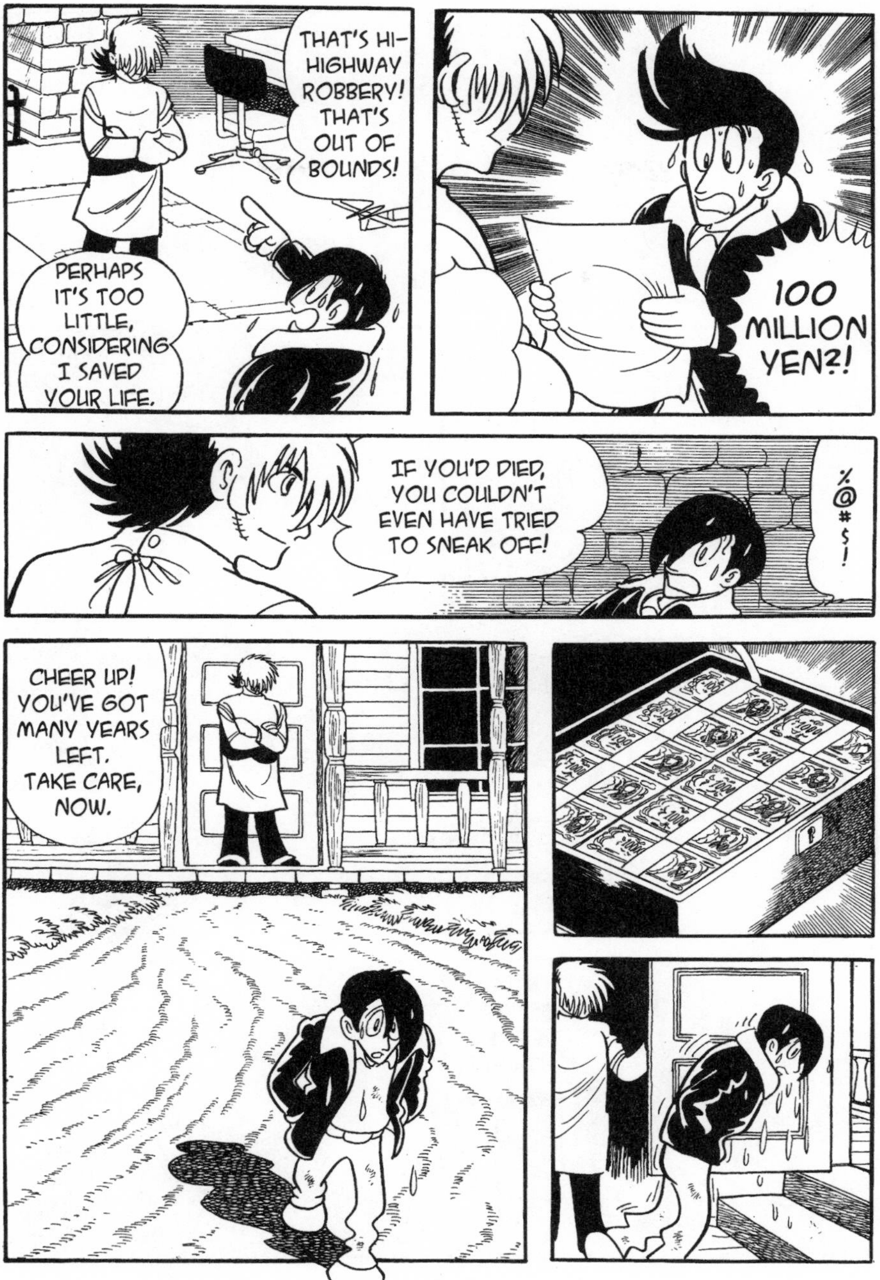
100 MILLION YEN?!
THAT'S HI-HIGHWAY ROBBERY! THAT'S OUT OF BOUNDS!
PERHAPS IT'S TOO LITTLE, CONSIDERING I SAVED YOUR LIFE.
%@#$!
IF YOU'D DIED, YOU COULDN'T EVEN HAVE TRIED TO SNEAK OFF!
CHEER UP! YOU'VE GOT MANY YEARS LEFT. TAKE CARE, NOW.

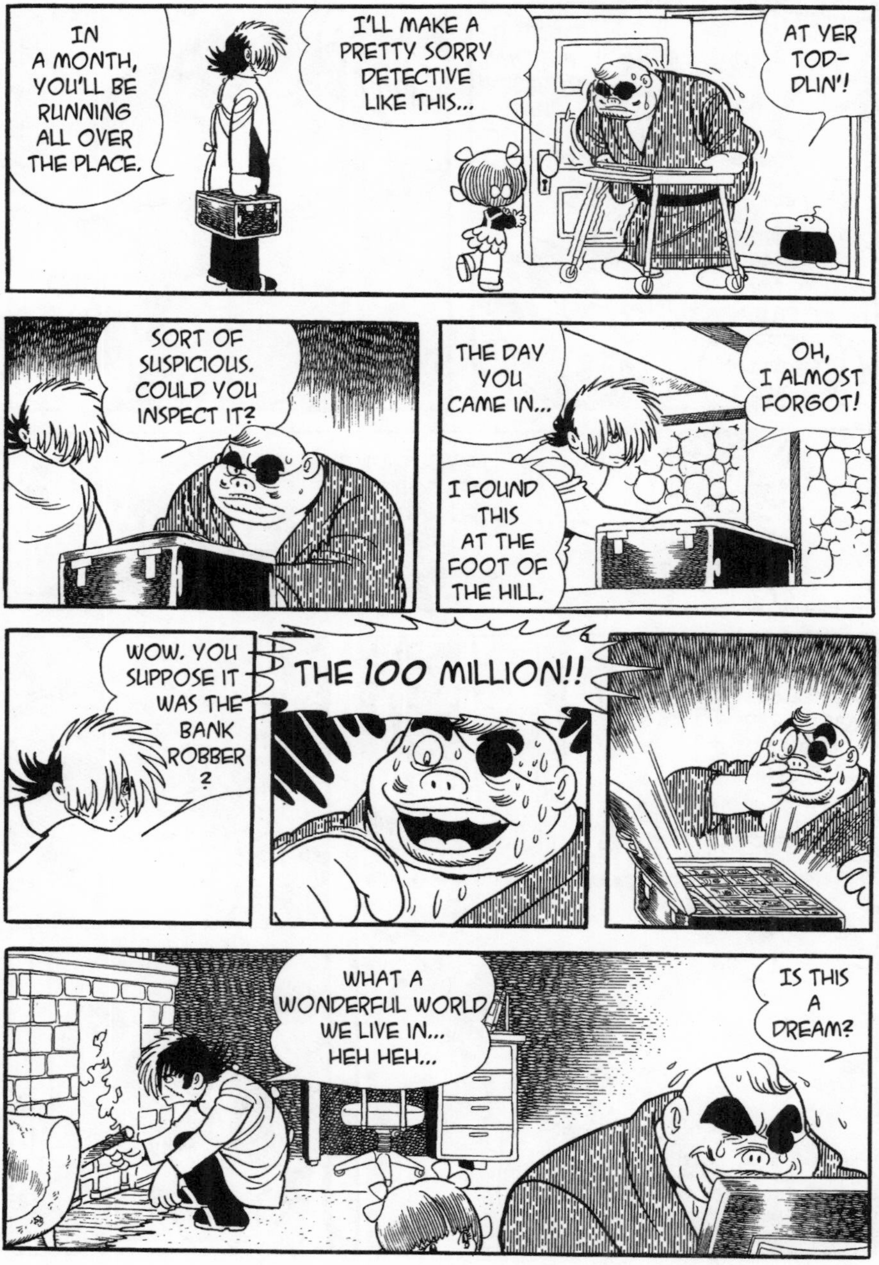
AT YER TOD-DLIN'!
I'LL MAKE A PRETTY SORRY DETECTIVE LIKE THIS...
IN A MONTH, YOU'LL BE RUNNING ALL OVER THE PLACE.
OH, I ALMOST FORGOT!
THE DAY YOU CAME IN...
I FOUND THIS AT THE FOOT OF THE HILL.
SORT OF SUSPICIOUS. COULD YOU INSPECT IT?
THE 100 MILLION!!
WOW. YOU SUPPOSE IT WAS THE BANK ROBBER?
IS THIS A DREAM?
WHAT A WONDERFUL WORLD WE LIVE IN... HEH HEH...

BABY BLUES

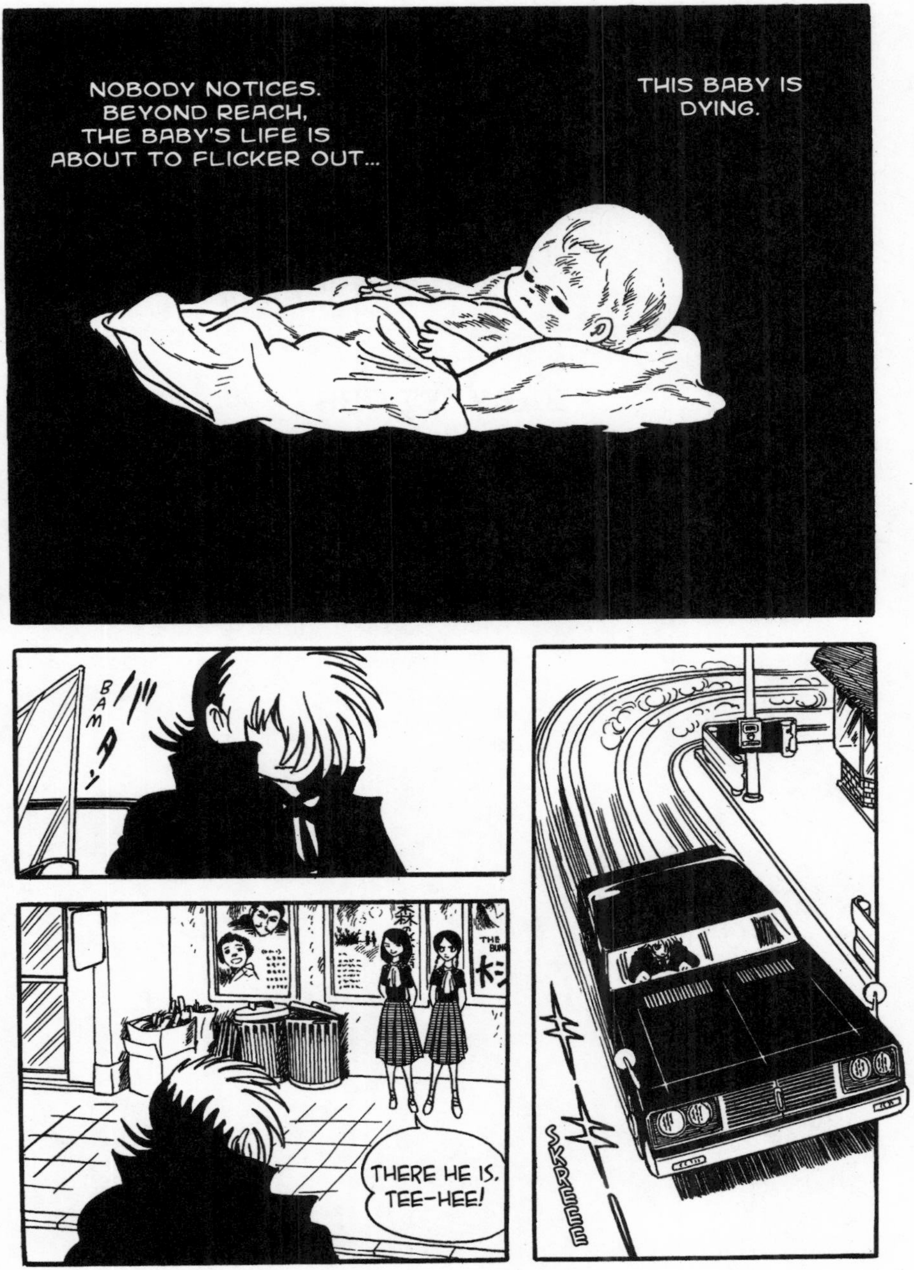

THIS BABY IS DYING.
NOBODY NOTICES. BEYOND REACH, THE BABY'S LIFE IS ABOUT TO FLICKER OUT...
SKREEEE
BAM
THERE HE IS, TEE-HEE!

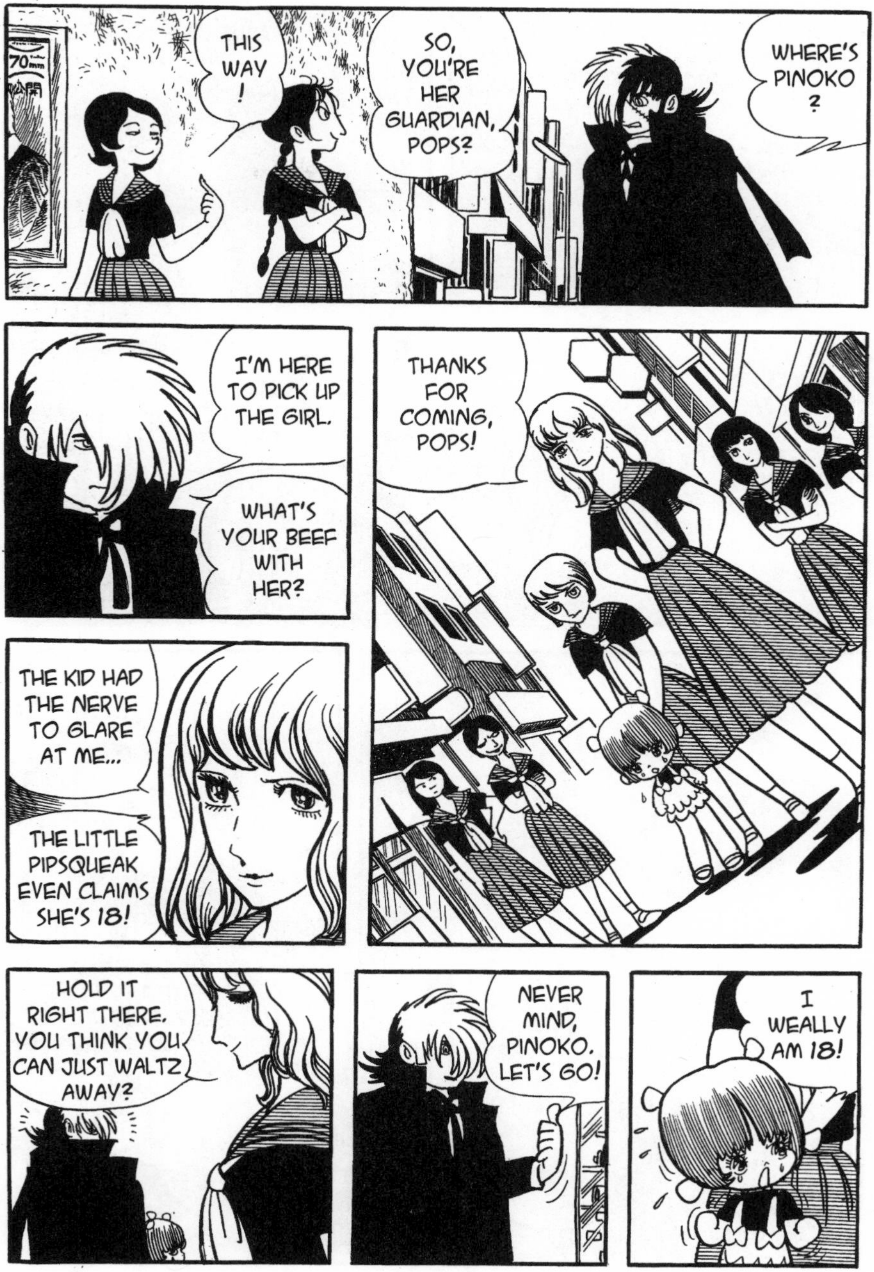
WHERE'S PINOKO?
SO, YOU'RE HER GUARDIAN, POPS?
THIS WAY!
THANKS FOR COMING, POPS!
I'M HERE TO PICK UP THE GIRL.
WHAT'S YOUR BEEF WITH HER?
THE KID HAD THE NERVE TO GLARE AT ME...
THE LITTLE PIPSQUEAK EVEN CLAIMS SHE'S 18!
I WEALLY AM 18!
NEVER MIND, PINOKO. LET'S GO!
HOLD IT RIGHT THERE. YOU THINK YOU CAN JUST WALTZ AWAY?

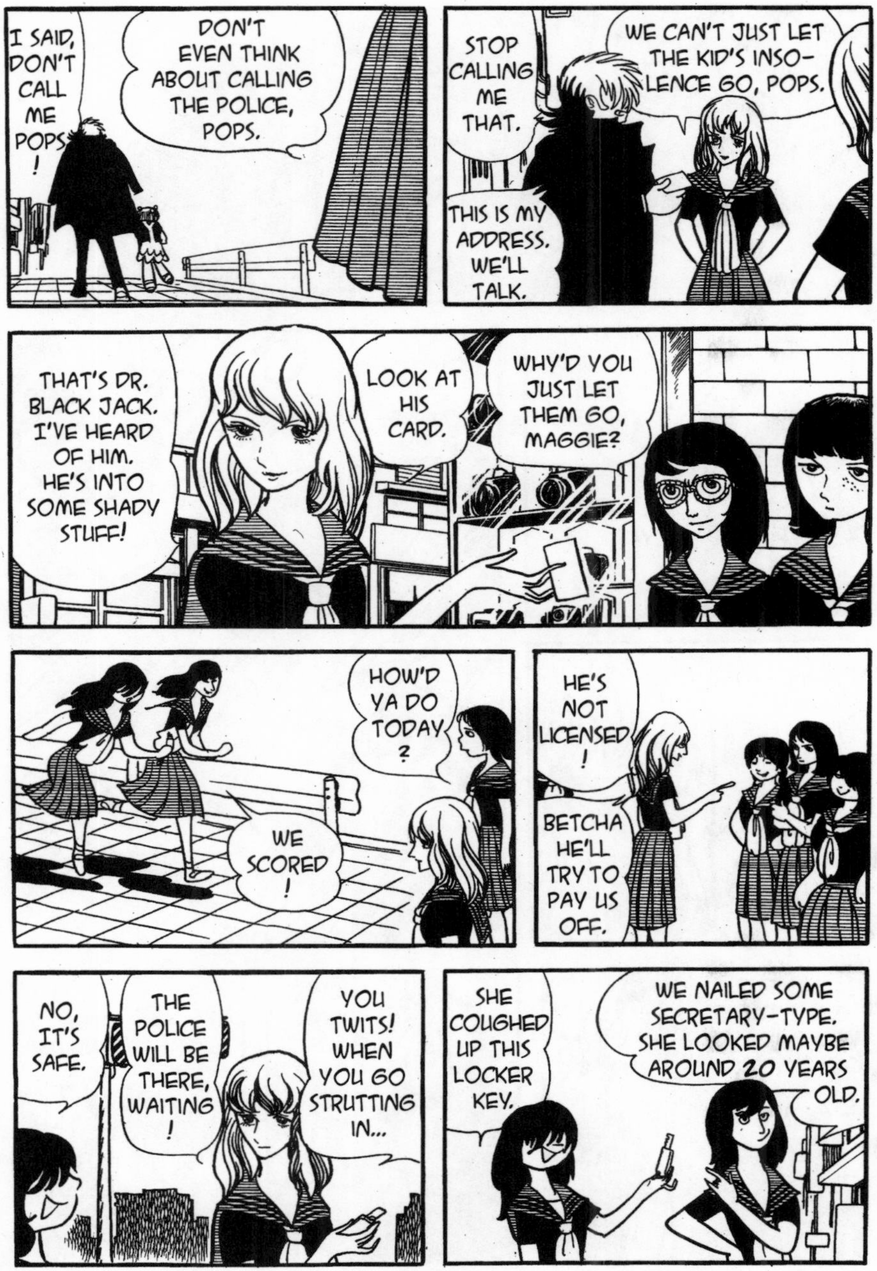
WE CAN'T JUST LET THE KID'S INSO-LENCE GO, POPS.
STOP CALLING ME THAT.
THIS IS MY ADDRESS. WE'LL TALK.
DON'T EVEN THINK ABOUT CALLING THE POLICE, POPS.
I SAID, DON'T CALL ME POPS!
WHY'D YOU JUST LET THEM GO, MAGGIE?
LOOK AT HIS CARD.
THAT'S DR. BLACK JACK. I'VE HEARD OF HIM. HE'S INTO SOME SHADY STUFF!
HE'S NOT LICENSED!
BETCHA HE'LL TRY TO PAY US OFF.
HOW'D YA DO TODAY?
WE SCORED!
WE NAILED SOME SECRETARY-TYPE. SHE LOOKED MAYBE AROUND 20 YEARS OLD.
SHE COUGHED UP THIS LOCKER KEY.
YOU TWITS! WHEN YOU GO STRUTTING IN...
THE POLICE WILL BE THERE, WAITING!
NO, IT'S SAFE.

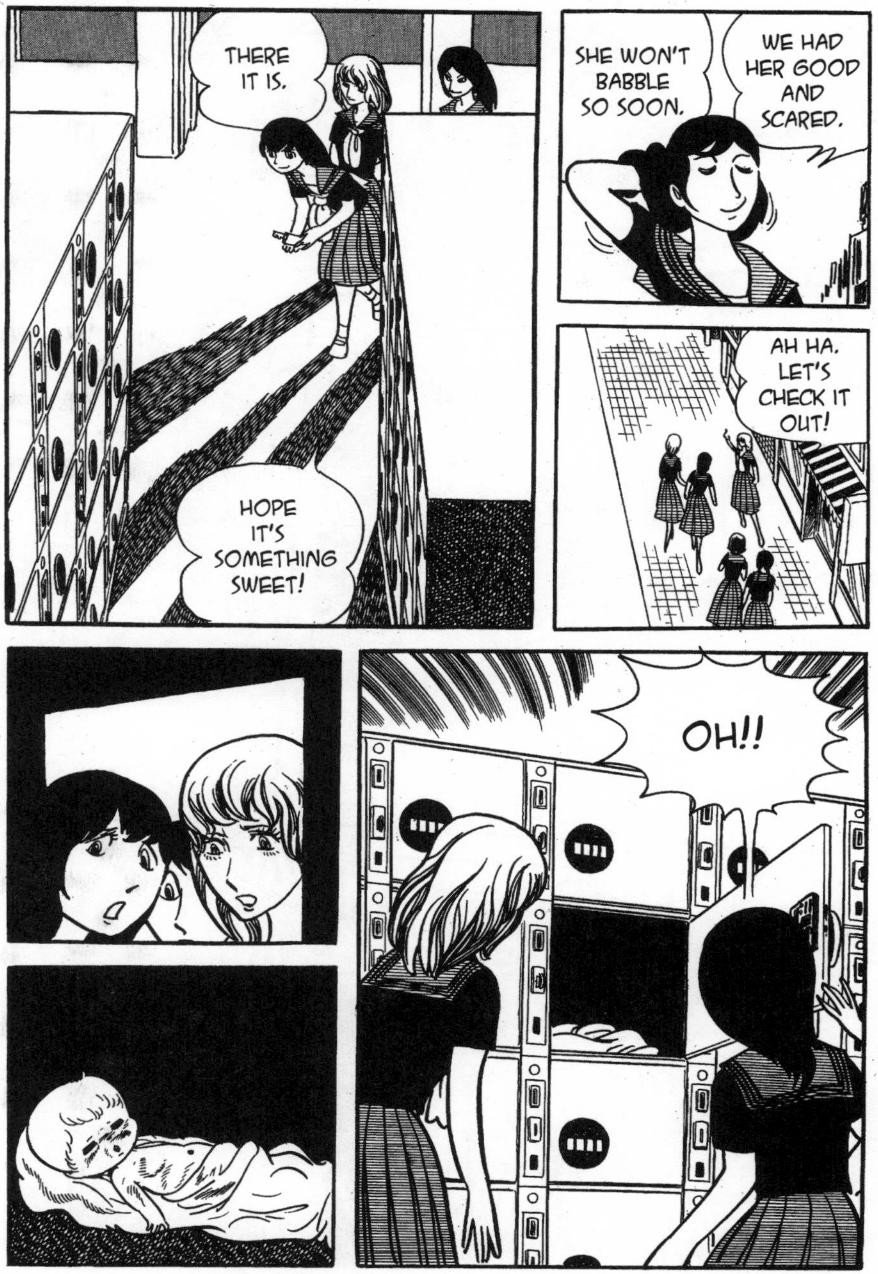
WE HAD HER GOOD AND SCARED.
SHE WON'T BABBLE SO SOON.
AH HA. LET'S CHECK IT OUT!
THERE IT IS.
HOPE IT'S SOMETHING SWEET!
OH!!

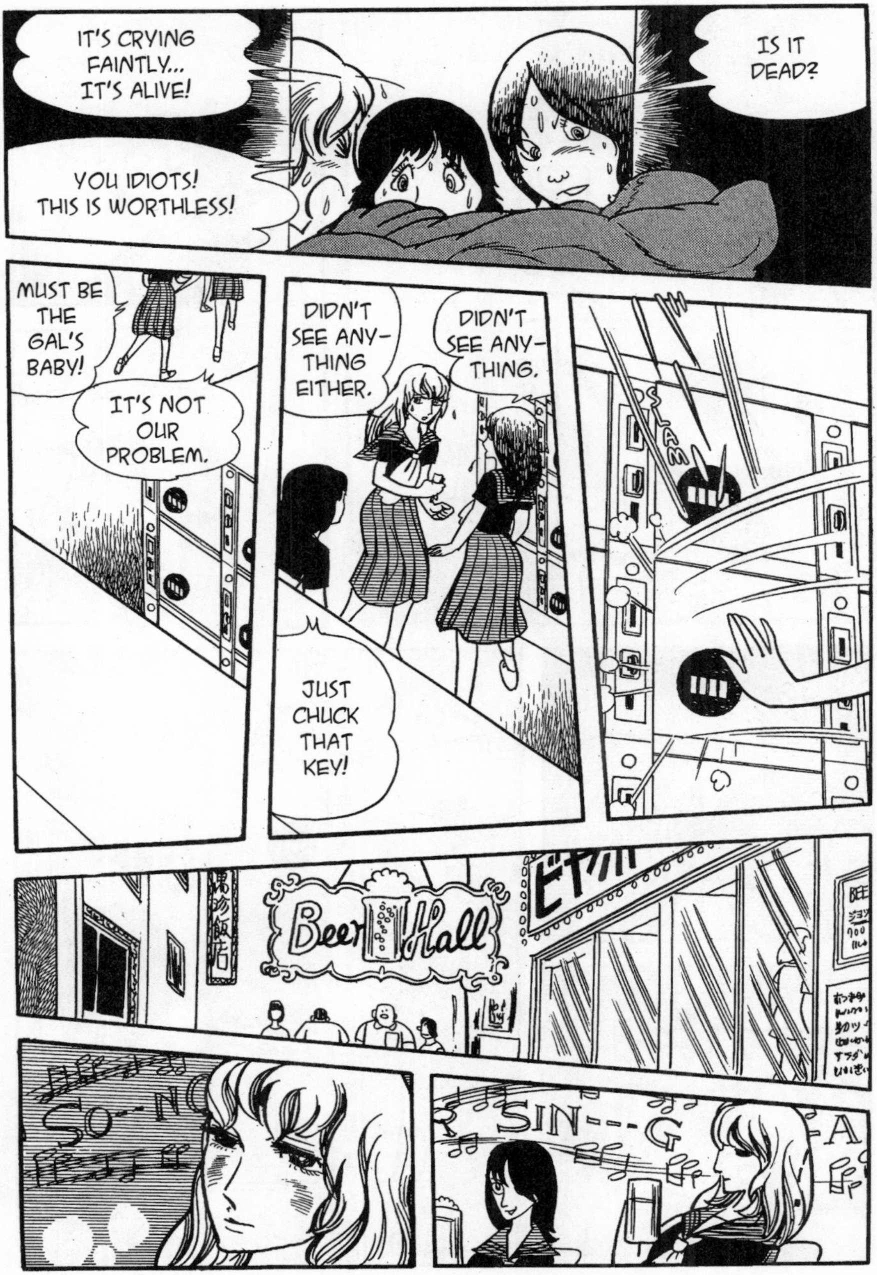

IS IT DEAD?
IT'S CRYING FAINTLY... IT'S ALIVE!
YOU IDIOTS! THIS IS WORTHLESS!
SLAM
DIDN'T SEE ANY-THING.
DIDN'T SEE ANY-THING EITHER.
JUST CHUCK THAT KEY!
MUST BE THE GAL'S BABY!
IT'S NOT OUR PROBLEM.
Beer Hall
SIN---G
SO--N

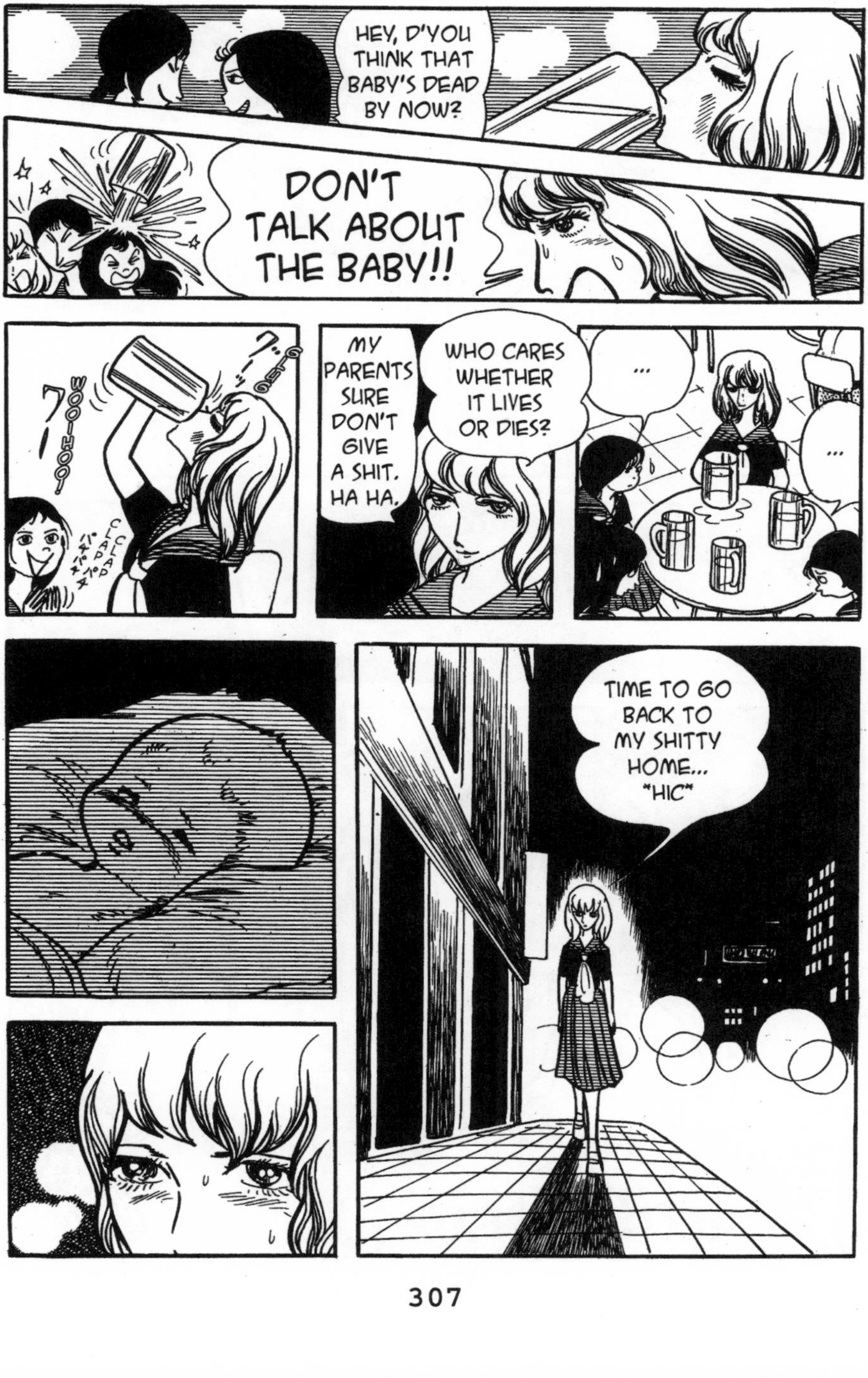
HEY, D'YOU THINK THAT BABY'S DEAD BY NOW?
DON'T TALK ABOUT THE BABY!!
...
...
WHO CARES WHETHER IT LIVES OR DIES?
MY PARENTS SURE DON'T GIVE A SHIT. HA HA.
WOO-HOO!
CLAP CLAP
TIME TO GO BACK TO MY SHITTY HOME... *HIC*

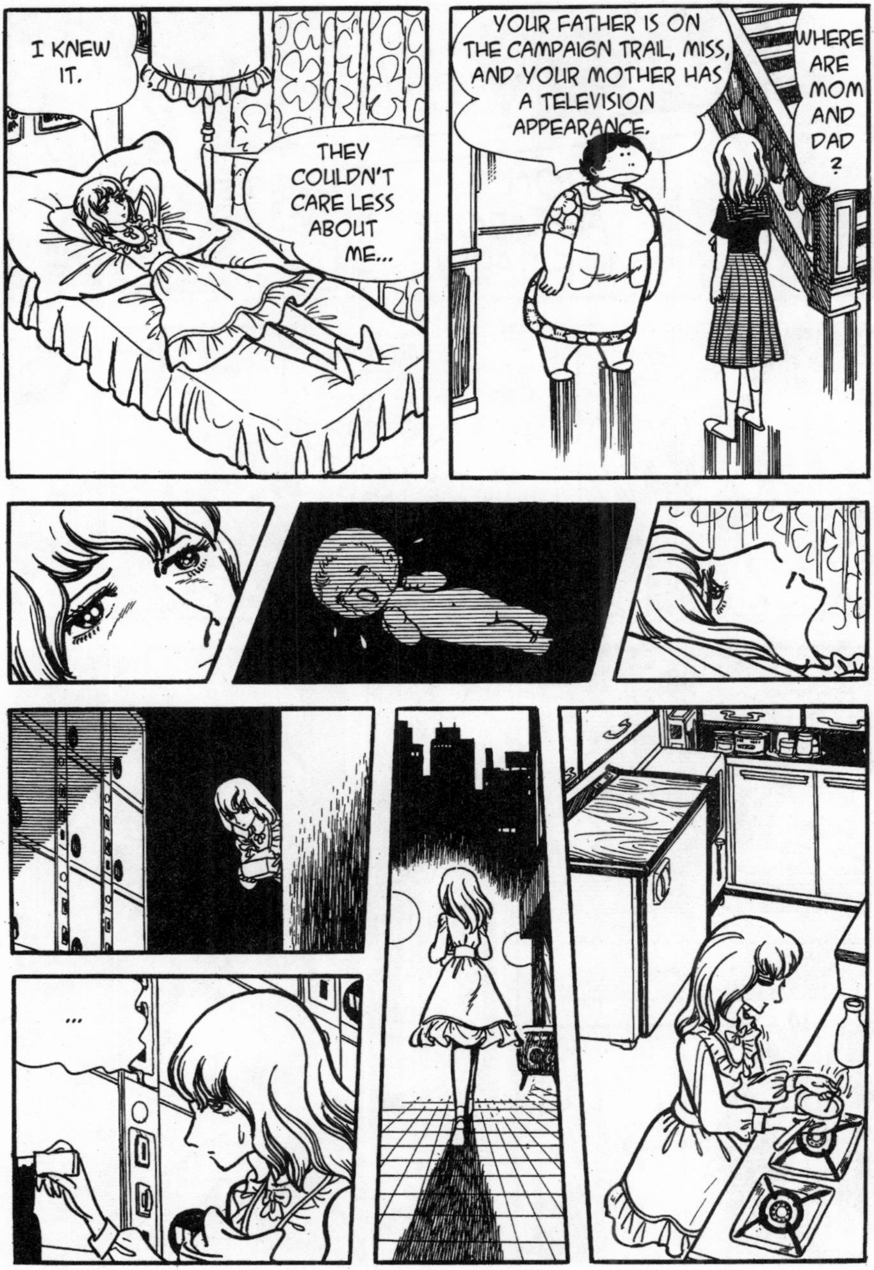
WHERE ARE MOM AND DAD?
YOUR FATHER IS ON THE CAMPAIGN TRAIL, MISS, AND YOUR MOTHER HAS A TELEVISION APPEARANCE.
I KNEW IT.
THEY COULDN'T CARE LESS ABOUT ME...
...

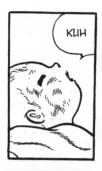
KUH

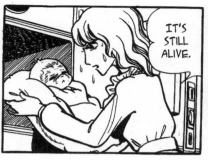
IT'S STILL ALIVE.

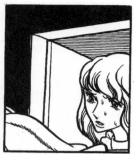

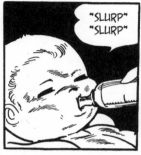
"SLURP" "SLURP"

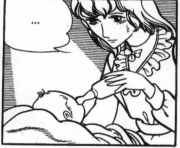
...

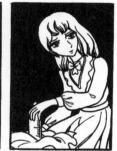

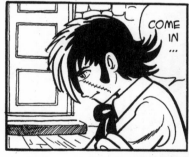
COME IN ...

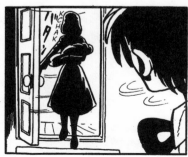

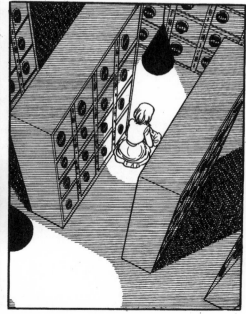

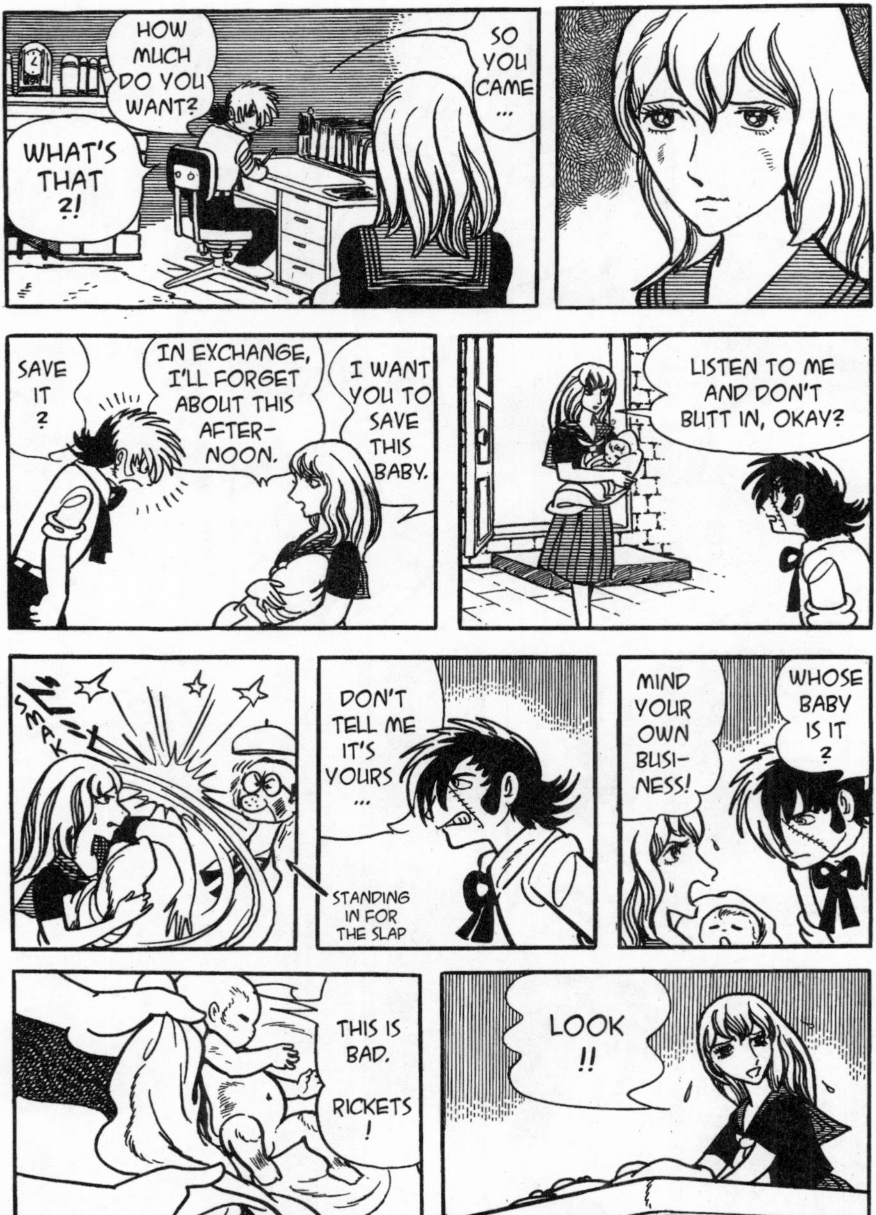
SO YOU CAME ...
HOW MUCH DO YOU WANT?
WHAT'S THAT ?!
LISTEN TO ME AND DON'T BUTT IN, OKAY?
I WANT YOU TO SAVE THIS BABY.
IN EXCHANGE, I'LL FORGET ABOUT THIS AFTERNOON.
SAVE IT ?
WHOSE BABY IS IT ?
MIND YOUR OWN BUSI-NESS!
DON'T TELL ME IT'S YOURS ...
SMAK
STANDING IN FOR THE SLAP
LOOK !!
THIS IS BAD.
RICKETS !

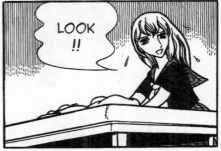

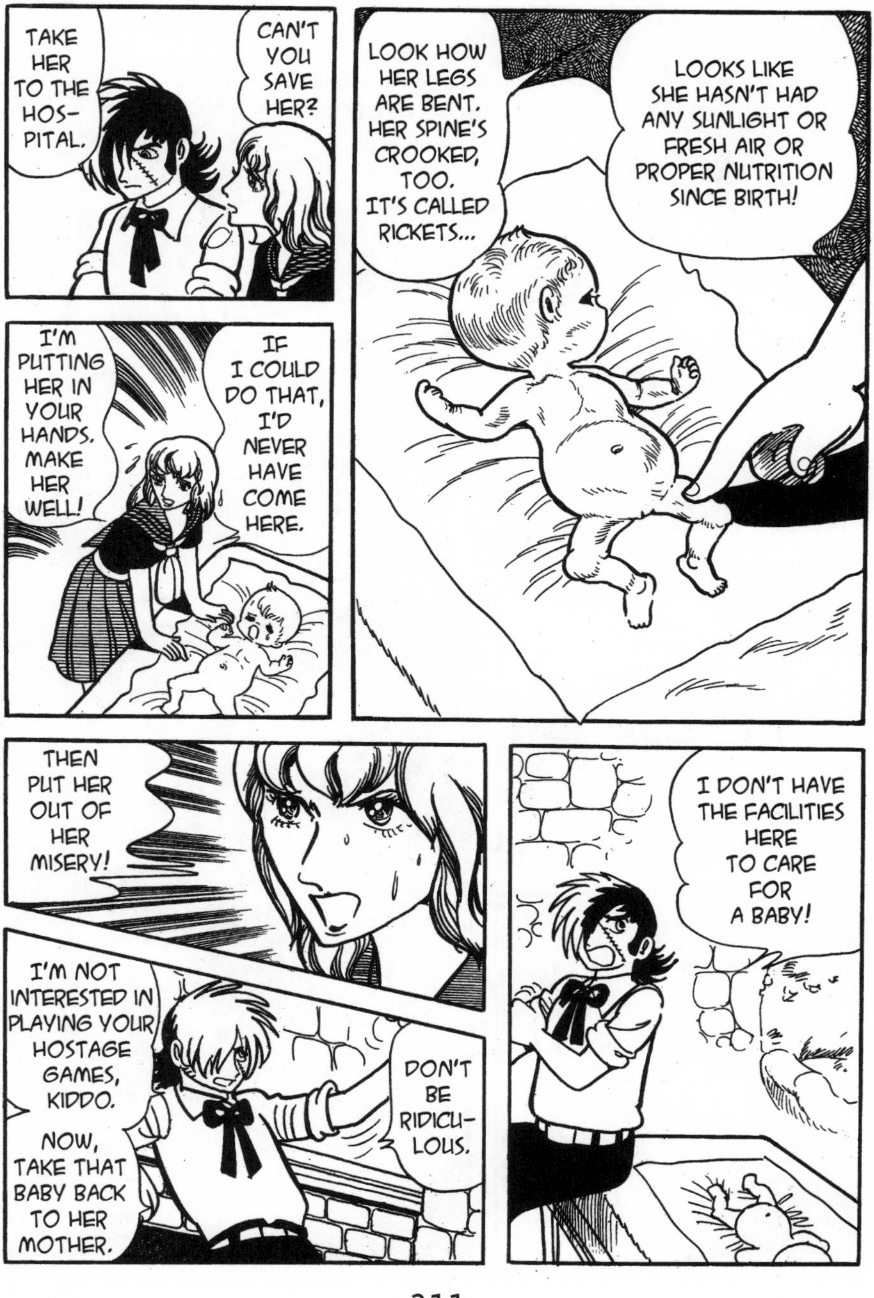
LOOKS LIKE SHE HASN'T HAD ANY SUNLIGHT OR FRESH AIR OR PROPER NUTRITION SINCE BIRTH!
LOOK HOW HER LEGS ARE BENT. HER SPINE'S CROOKED, TOO. IT'S CALLED RICKETS...
CAN'T YOU SAVE HER?
TAKE HER TO THE HOS-PITAL.
IF I COULD DO THAT, I'D NEVER HAVE COME HERE.
I'M PUTTING HER IN YOUR HANDS. MAKE HER WELL!
I DON'T HAVE THE FACILITIES HERE TO CARE FOR A BABY!
THEN PUT HER OUT OF HER MISERY!
DON'T BE RIDICU-LOUS.
I'M NOT INTERESTED IN PLAYING YOUR HOSTAGE GAMES, KIDDO.
NOW, TAKE THAT BABY BACK TO HER MOTHER.

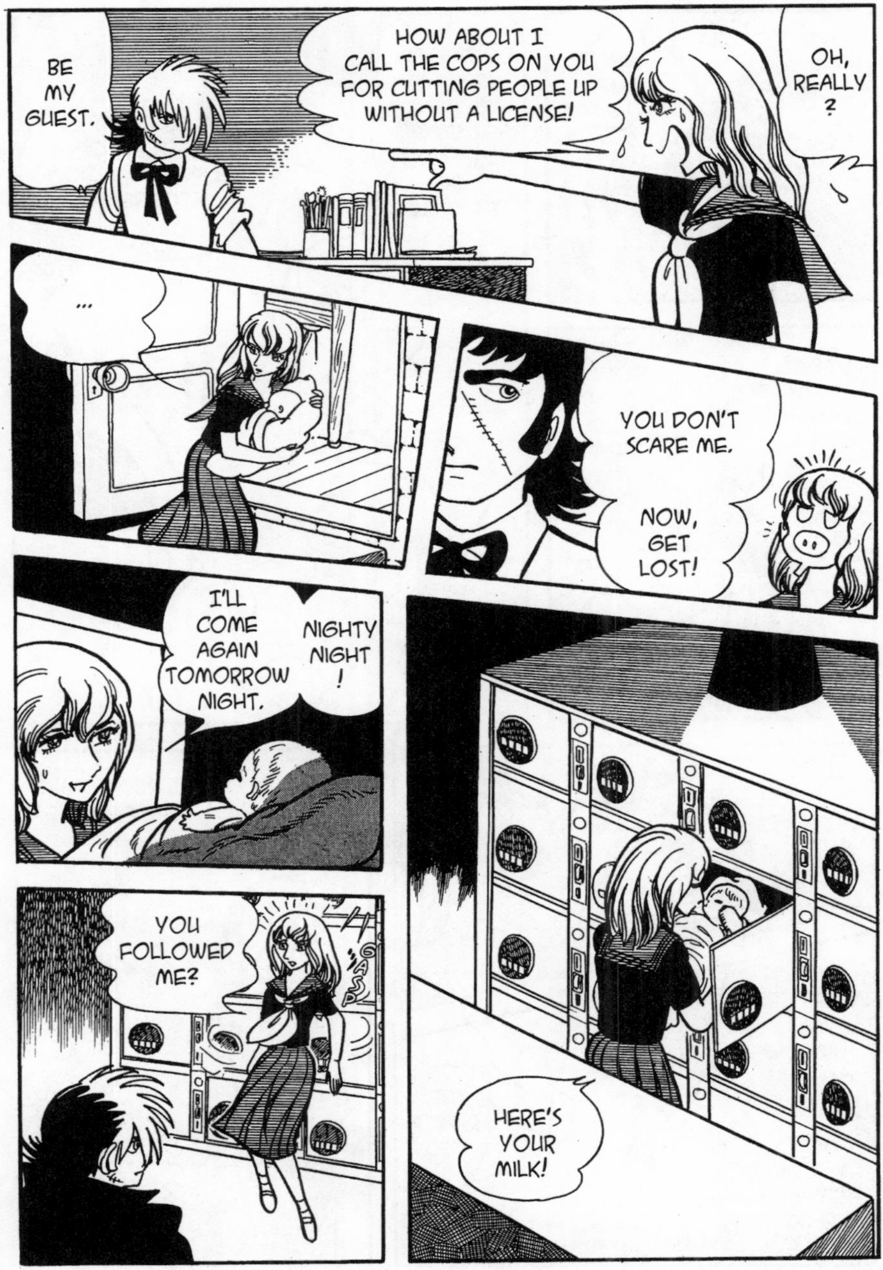
OH, REALLY?
HOW ABOUT I CALL THE COPS ON YOU FOR CUTTING PEOPLE UP WITHOUT A LICENSE!
BE MY GUEST.
YOU DON'T SCARE ME.
NOW, GET LOST!
...
HERE'S YOUR MILK!
NIGHTY NIGHT!
I'LL COME AGAIN TOMORROW NIGHT.
GASP
YOU FOLLOWED ME?

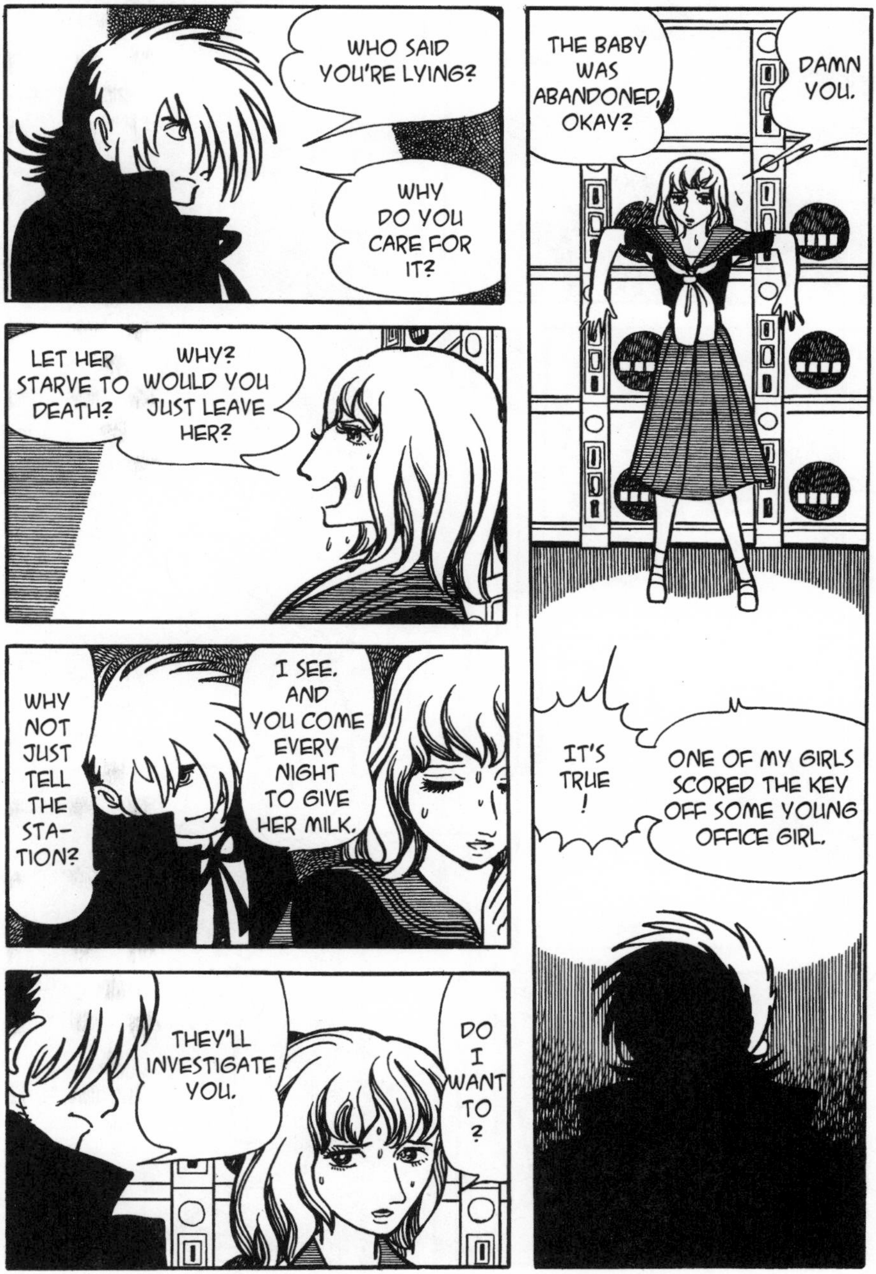
DAMN YOU.
THE BABY WAS ABANDONED, OKAY?
ONE OF MY GIRLS SCORED THE KEY OFF SOME YOUNG OFFICE GIRL.
IT'S TRUE!
WHO SAID YOU'RE LYING?
WHY DO YOU CARE FOR IT?
WHY? WOULD YOU JUST LEAVE HER?
LET HER STARVE TO DEATH?
I SEE. AND YOU COME EVERY NIGHT TO GIVE HER MILK.
WHY NOT JUST TELL THE STA- TION?
DO I WANT TO?
THEY'LL INVESTIGATE YOU.

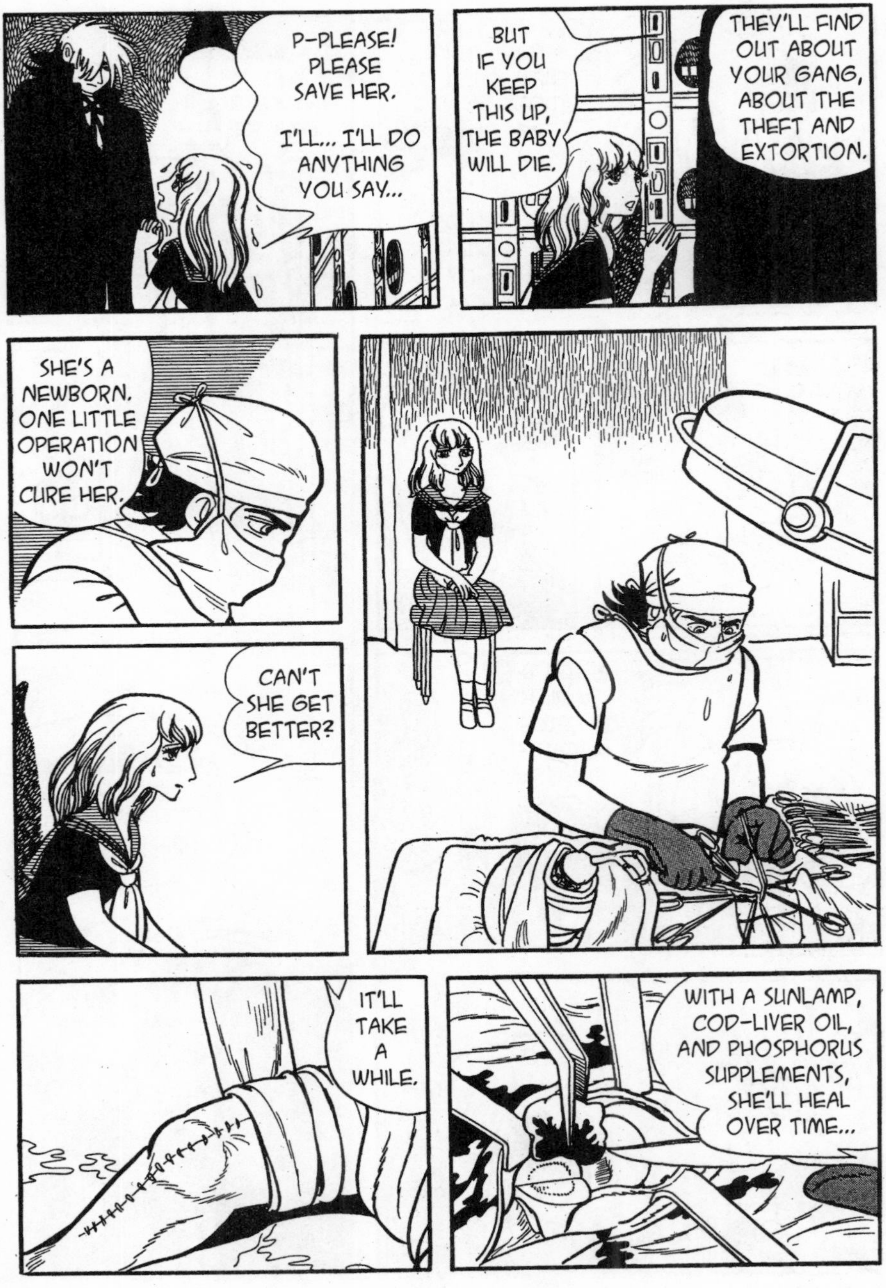
THEY'LL FIND OUT ABOUT YOUR GANG, ABOUT THE THEFT AND EXTORTION.
BUT IF YOU KEEP THIS UP, THE BABY WILL DIE.
P-PLEASE! PLEASE SAVE HER.
I'LL... I'LL DO ANYTHING YOU SAY...
SHE'S A NEWBORN. ONE LITTLE OPERATION WON'T CURE HER.
CAN'T SHE GET BETTER?
WITH A SUNLAMP, COD-LIVER OIL, AND PHOSPHORUS SUPPLEMENTS, SHE'LL HEAL OVER TIME...
IT'LL TAKE A WHILE.

YOU'RE AN ODD ONE, AREN'T YOU?
A MEAN GIRL LIKE YOU, CARING FOR A BABY?
THERE YOU GO, ASKING STUPID STUFF.
AHA!
YOU'RE GOING TO GET BETTER!
GOOD GIRL! NIGHTY NIGHT.
A WHOLE MONTH SINCE YOUR OPERATION! IT'S GONE BY QUICKLY!
YOU FETCH THAT BABY EVERY NIGHT LIKE YOU'RE FETCHING A SUITCASE?
YEAH ...
GIVE UP AND REPORT HER TO THE STATION.
NO WAY !
ORATOTOMANIM

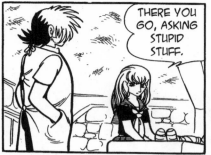

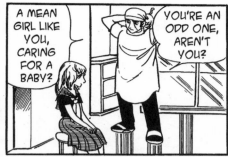

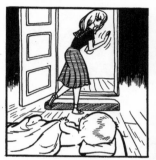

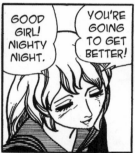

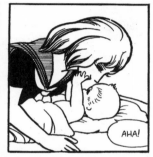

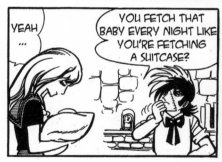

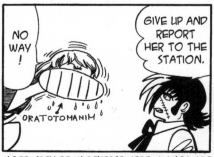

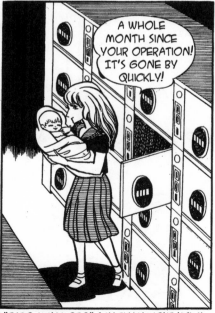

NOTE: SPELLED IN REVERSE HERE, MANGA ARTIST "TARO MINAMOTO" SKILLFULLY WOVE VISUAL GAGS INTO HIS OFTEN SERIOUS WORK.

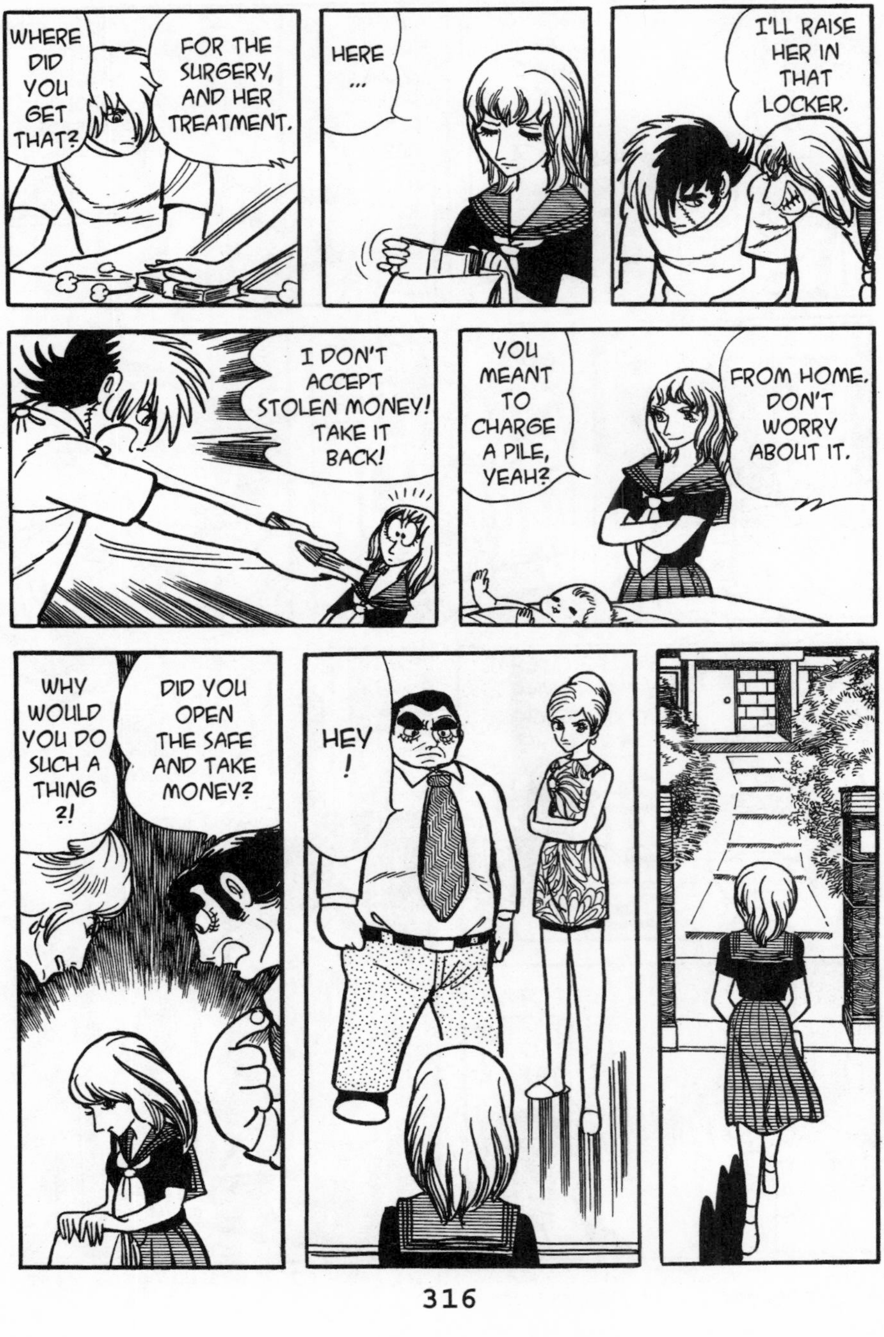
I'LL RAISE HER IN THAT LOCKER.
HERE ...
FOR THE SURGERY, AND HER TREATMENT.
WHERE DID YOU GET THAT?
FROM HOME. DON'T WORRY ABOUT IT.
YOU MEANT TO CHARGE A PILE, YEAH?
I DON'T ACCEPT STOLEN MONEY! TAKE IT BACK!
HEY!
DID YOU OPEN THE SAFE AND TAKE MONEY?
WHY WOULD YOU DO SUCH A THING?!

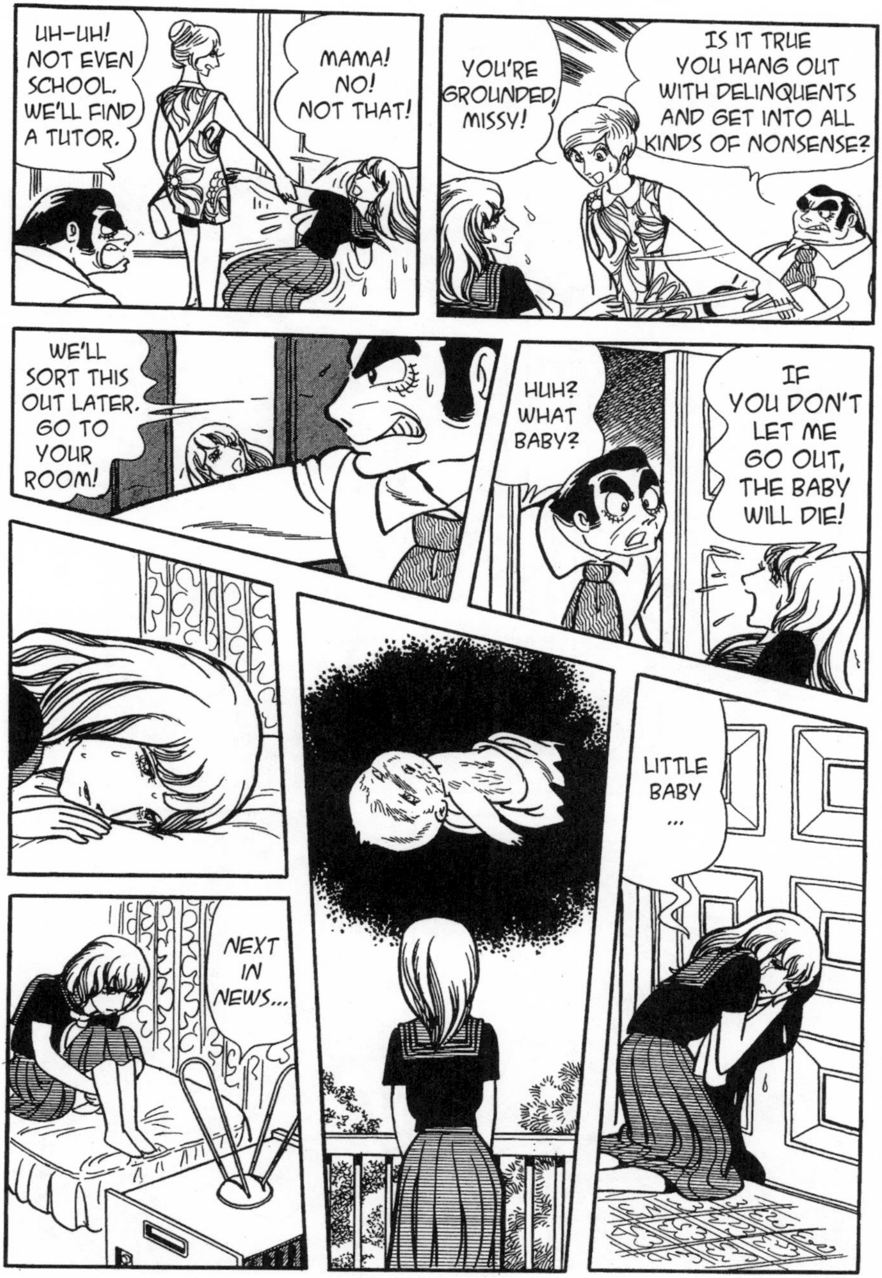
IS IT TRUE YOU HANG OUT WITH DELINQUENTS AND GET INTO ALL KINDS OF NONSENSE?
YOU'RE GROUNDED, MISSY!
MAMA! NO! NOT THAT!
UH-UH! NOT EVEN SCHOOL. WE'LL FIND A TUTOR.
IF YOU DON'T LET ME GO OUT, THE BABY WILL DIE!
HUH? WHAT BABY?
WE'LL SORT THIS OUT LATER. GO TO YOUR ROOM!
LITTLE BABY ...
NEXT IN NEWS...

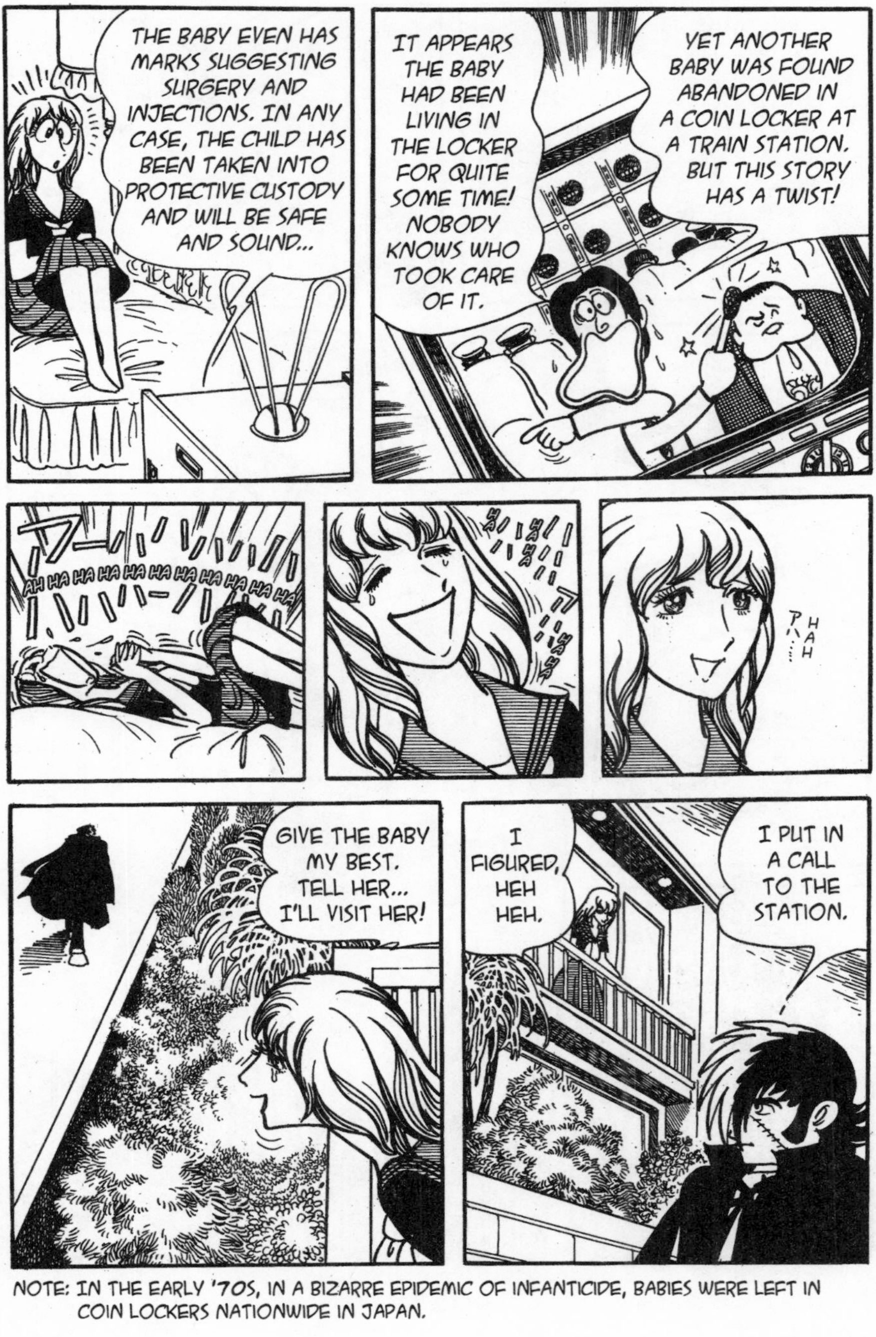
YET ANOTHER BABY WAS FOUND ABANDONED IN A COIN LOCKER AT A TRAIN STATION. BUT THIS STORY HAS A TWIST!
IT APPEARS THE BABY HAD BEEN LIVING IN THE LOCKER FOR QUITE SOME TIME! NOBODY KNOWS WHO TOOK CARE OF IT.
THE BABY EVEN HAS MARKS SUGGESTING SURGERY AND INJECTIONS. IN ANY CASE, THE CHILD HAS BEEN TAKEN INTO PROTECTIVE CUSTODY AND WILL BE SAFE AND SOUND...
HAH HAH
AH HA HA HA HA HA HA HA HA HA HA HA
I PUT IN A CALL TO THE STATION.
I FIGURED, HEH HEH.
GIVE THE BABY MY BEST. TELL HER... I'LL VISIT HER!

NOTE: IN THE EARLY '70S, IN A BIZARRE EPIDEMIC OF INFANTICIDE, BABIES WERE LEFT IN COIN LOCKERS NATIONWIDE IN JAPAN.

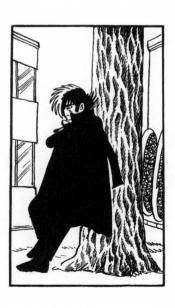